OBSTETRIC VASCULOPATHIES

OBSTETRIC VASCULOPATHIES

Pankaj Desai MD FICOG FICMCH
Consultant and Specialist of Obstetrics and Gynecology
Janani Maternity Hospital, Baroda, Gujarat, India
Formerly
Dean of Students
Medical College, Baroda, Gujarat, India
Associate Professor and Unit Chief
Department of Obstetrics and Gynecology
Medical College and SSG Hospital, Baroda, Gujarat, India
President, Federation of Obstetric and Gynecological
Societies of India (FOGSI), 2007

JAYPEE BROTHERS MEDICAL PUBLISHERS (P) LTD
New Delhi • Panama City • London • Philadelphia

Jaypee Brothers Medical Publishers (P) Ltd

Headquarters
Jaypee Brothers Medical Publishers (P) Ltd
4838/24, Ansari Road, Daryaganj
New Delhi 110 002, India
Phone: +91-11-43574357
Fax: +91-11-43574314
Email: jaypee@jaypeebrothers.com

Overseas Offices
J.P. Medical Ltd
83 Victoria Street, London
SW1H 0HW (UK)
Phone: +44-2031708910
Fax: +02-03-0086180
Email: info@jpmedpub.com

Jaypee-Highlights Medical Publishers Inc
City of Knowledge, Bld. 237, Clayton
Panama City, Panama
Phone: + 507-301-0496
Fax: + 507-301-0499
Email: cservice@jphmedical.com

Jaypee Brothers Medical Publishers (P) Ltd
17/1-B Babar Road, Block-B, Shaymali
Mohammadpur, Dhaka-1207
Bangladesh
Mobile: +08801912003485
Email: jaypeedhaka@gmail.com

Jaypee Brothers Medical Publishers (P) Ltd
Shorakhute, Kathmandu
Nepal
Phone: +00977-9841528578
Email: jaypee.nepal@gmail.com

Jaypee Brothers Medical Publishers Ltd
The Bourse
111 South Independence Mall East
Suite 835, Philadelphia, PA 19106, USA
Phone: + 267-519-9789
Email: joe.rusko@jaypeebrothers.com

Website: www.jaypeebrothers.com
Website: www.jaypeedigital.com

Inquiries for bulk sales may be solicited at: jaypee@jaypeebrothers.com

Obstetric Vasculopathies

First Edition: **2013**

ISBN: 978-93-5090-451-0

Printed at Sanat Printers, Kundli

Preface

It has taken more than two decades to write this book. It was very enticing to write it earlier but I knew that if I would fall in that trap, I would come out with a work of a novice. It would have been a book, just adding to the number of books, written in my curriculum vitae rather than giving quality work in your hands. Every step of gaining the knowledge shared in the pages to follow has been evolving for me. It all started with collection of data for a research paper that I presented in XXXII All India Obstetric and Gynecology Congress at Mysore, Karnataka in December 1988, and then there was no looking back. I went on working in the field. People came, joined the team, and left. I remained constant. I am still continuing to learn more and more about this challenging aspect of obstetrics every day. Such is its vastness and are its intrigues that I wonder if it will ever get fully revealed.

More than two decades of focused work in this field, publication of original research papers in different journals, and discussing it on many scientific fora have gone into this book *Obstetric Vasculopathies*. Recurrent miscarriages, preeclampsia, intrauterine growth retardation (IUGR), recurrent stillbirths, and accidental hemorrhage have long been thought to be diverse conditions diffusely related to one another, if at all. Over a period of time, with the advances in understanding of their intricacies, it has now been conclusively proved that these are different manifestations of one common cause—obstetric vasculopathies. With the mention of the word vasculopathies, an obstetrician may perceive these to be diseases of maternal vasculature. However, it gets involved only secondarily with the epicenter of the mischief being at the fetomaternal interface. Initially, only preeclampsia remote from the term was thought to be a result of obstetric vasculopathy. Nevertheless, current thinking has shown that all forms of preeclampsia have their explanation in here. Therefore, the grouping of preeclampsia as remote from the term and preeclampsia of late onset has blurred. Intrauterine growth retardation (IUGR) was considered as a result of preeclampsia. But with the understanding of the etiopathology involved in obstetric vasculopathies, it has been found that there is no cause-effect relation between the two. They are manifestations of the same etiopathology, namely obstetric vasculopathies.

The basic pathology involved in these conditions is vasospasm followed by reperfusion. More than the vasospasm, it is the reperfusion damage that has been found to be more devastating for the clinical manifestations and complications of obstetric vasculopathies to occur. Immunology seems to be at the axis of these changes. Triggered by some largely obscure genetic basis, immunological protective mechanisms, which are supposed to protect the mother from a foreign protein (in this case the fetus) seem to be in a destructive mode in producing obstetric vasculopathies.

An amorphous genetic stimulus appears to have some role in activation of the immunological mechanism that brings about different changes through oxidative changes. What is vaguely called as oxidative stress seems to be the key etiopathological factor, which generates and sustains the processes of vasculopathies. Free radicals of the oxidative process are the main conductors of this orchestra. They bring about different changes of vasculopathies through their agents: the denatured lipids—low-density lipoprotein and very low-density lipoprotein. Syncitiotrophoblasts seem to have the most important critical role in the causation of obstetric vasculopathies.

Understandably, therefore, the entire process is very complex. In this book, current understanding of the processes involved, and on its basis, the management of different obstetric vasculopathies has been covered in great details. The explanations provided in the understanding of these disease processes and the rationale of scientific management have been based on the current literature as well as more than two decades of my work in this field. It is more an exercise of narration and communication between the reader and me.

As I place this book in the hands of the readers I feel very humble. I am sharing facts based on sound scientific data and very carefully drawn conclusions. I seek their blessings in my pursuit of academic excellence at the service of humanity and mankind.

Pankaj Desai

Contents

1. General Aspects of Obstetric Vasculopathies **1**

What are Obstetric Vasculopathies 2

2. Cardiovascular Changes in Normal Pregnancy **4**

Blood Pressure 5
Longitudinal Changes in Cardiac Functions 6
Peripheral Vascular Resistance 9
Changes in Venous System: Any? 9

3. Immunology of Obstetric Vasculopathy **11**

Leads through Recurrent Spontaneous Abortion (RSA) 11
Fetus as an Allograft 11
What Protects the Fetus? 12
Fetus as a Unique Allograft 13
Suppressor Mechanisms in Protection 16
Partner Specificity in Miscarriages 18
Autoimmunity in Recurrent Pregnancy Loss 19
Embryo Decidua Crosstalk in immunology of Obstetrics Vasculopathy 22
Implantation Not a Right of Embryo 23
Results of the Crosstalk 23
Other Contributory Mechanisms 24
What is Spontaneous Resolution? 27
The Miracle of Paradox 28

4. Endothelial Cell Dysfunction and Obstetric Vasculopathy **31**

The Phenomenon of Endothelial Cell Activation 32
Endothelial Activation and Prostaglandins 33
Plasminogen and Allied Procoagulant Activity—A Manifestation of Endothelial Cell Activation 34
Antiphospholipid Antibodies Act through Procoagulant Mechanism 34
Endothelial Cell Adhesion Molecule Disturbances 35
Components of Fibronectin 36
Vascular Endothelial Growth Factor (VEGF) 37
Endothelin 37
Other Molecules Contributing to Endothelial Cell Activation 38

5. Oxidative Stress and Obstetric Vasculopathies **42**

What is Oxidative Stress 42
Our Basic Study 43
What is a Free Radical? 43
Oxidative Stress and Health 44
The Mischief of Free Radicals in Vascular Walls 45
Lipid Peroxides: the Agents of Oxidative Stress 45
Lipid Metabolism in Normal Pregnancy and its Bearings in Abnormal Pregnancy 47

Placental Lipid Peroxidation 54
Clinical Manifestations 57
Reperfusion 57
Innate Maternal Reducing Systems 59
The Family of Free Radicals 61
Vascular Endothelium and Oxidative Stress 62
Inefficient Second Wave of Trophoblastic Invasion 63
Nitric Oxide in Obstetric Vasculopathy 65
Placental Atherosis in Obstetric Vasculopathy 69
Extracellular Reducing Systems 70
Exercise and Prevention of Obstetric Vasculopathies 74
Treatment Bearings 76

6. The Placenta, Trophoblasts and Obstetric Vasculopathies 80
Basic Process of Normal Placenta and Placentation 80
Oxygenation and Trophoblastic Differentiation 83
Faults in Fetomaternal Linkage at Placenta and Obstetric Vasculopathy 84
Maternal Environment Preventing Trophoblastic Invasion 84

7. The Genetics of Obstetrics Vasculopathies 86
Basis for Reviewing the Role of Genetics in Obstetric Vasculopathies 86
Challenges to the Genetic Studies in Obstetric Vasculopathies 87
Mammalian Studies 88
Application of Genetic Models 89
Examining Associations 89
Fetal Contributions: Any? 89
Reverse Associations 91
Immunology and Genetics 91
Inputs from Animal Models 92
Epigenetic Features in Preeclampsia 92

8. Obstetric Vasculopathies and their Effects on Heart 95
Hemodynamics in Normal Pregnancy and During Obstetric Vasculopathies 95
Effect of Preeclampsia on the offspring—Any? 97

9. Obstetric Vasculopathies and their Effects on the Renal System 98
Vulnerability of Renal System 98
Special Features of Renal Failure in Obstetric Vasculopathies 99
Kidney Lesions 101
Renal Function Alterations in Preeclampsia 107

10. Obstetric Vasculopathies and their Effects on the Central Nervous System 111
The Privileged Status of Central Nervous System (CNS) 111
Pathological Lesions in Preeclampsia 112
Psychiatric Complications Following Obstetric Vasculopathies: Any Correlation? 113

11. Obstetric Vasculopathies and their Effects on Hematological System **114**

Alteration in Coagulation Factors (other than Platelets) and Procoagulants 114

Alteration in other Cellular Components of Blood 115

Review of Coagulation Alterations in Obstetric Vasculopathies 116

12. Obstetric Vasculopathies and their Effects on the Liver **120**

Pathological Changes in the Liver 121

Liver in Hemolysis Elevated Liver Enzymes Low Platelets (HELLP) Syndrome 122

13. Ophthalmic Features in Obstetric Vasculopathy **124**

Retinal Edema 125

Central and Peripheral Cause of Visual Alterations 125

14. Vascular Responses in Obstetric Vasculopathy **127**

Blunted Vascular Response 127

Placental Ischemia 128

Animal Experiments 128

Hard Facts Emerging from Animal Experiments 134

15. Clinical Profile of Obstetric Vasculopathies **136**

Hypertension 136

Proteinuria 140

Edema 141

Other Laboratory Parameters 142

16. Differential Diagnosis of Obstetric Vasculopathies **144**

Preeclampsia and Chronic Hypertension 144

Transient Hypertension 146

Renal Diseases 146

Hepato-Hematological Involvements 147

17. Predicting Obstetric Vasculopathies **148**

Overview of Available Predicting Measures 148

Application of Predicting Systems for other Uses 149

The Amorphous Characterizations of Pathogenesis and Clinical Features 149

Overview of the Types of Tests 150

Negative to Positive Predictive Value 151

Conditions Based Tests 151

An Ideal Test 151

Clinical Tests 151

Urinary Tests 153

Hematological Cellular and Non-cellular Indices 154

Epidemiological Indices 158

Color Doppler in Obstetric Vasculopathies: The Game Changer 159

18. Prevention of Preeclampsia and other Obstetric Vasculopathies **164**

What is the Difference between Disease and Derangement? 165

Preventing Obstetric Vasculopathy is a Challenge 167

Which Subjects may Benefit Out of Preventive Measures 167
Measures Prevent Occurrence or Prevent Worsening 169
Preventive Measures of Obstetric Vasculopathies 173
Prevention of Eclampsia 184

19. Color Doppler in Obstetric Vasculopathies **187**
Color Doppler in Early Pregnancy 187
Third Trimester Color Doppler in Obstetric Vasculopathies 192
Color Doppler for Discontinuation of Antithrombotic Agents 199
Fetal Aortic Doppler Studies 201

20. Cardiotocography in Obstetric Vasculopathies **204**
Physiology and Cardiotocography 204
Hypoxia and Fetal Heart Rate 207
Cardiotocographies in Subjects with APA Syndrome 208
Color Doppler and Cardiotocography Correlation 208

21. Treatment of Obstetric Vasculopathy: Recurrent Miscarriages **212**
Corticosteroids: Not Used Any More 212
Folic Acid 213
Low Dose Aspirin 214
Heparin 215
Progesterone is Treatment of Immunological Miscarriages 215
Treatment of a Subject of Miscarriage Always for Prevention 217

22. Treatment of Obstetric Vasculopathy—Preeclampsia **218**
Limitations of Blood Pressures as an Indicator of Severity 218
Early Diagnosis and Alert Surveillance 219
Do Subjects of Preeclampsia Need Admission 220
Management on Hospitalization 220
Antihypertensives 221
Induction of Labor in Pregnancy Induced Hypertension (PIH) 226
Methods of Induction of Labor 229
Cesarean Section in Pregnancy Induced Hypertension (PIH) 232
Post Delivery Care 232

23. Treatment of Obstetric Vasculopathy: Accidental Hemorrhage **235**
The Etiopathology of Accidental Hemorrhage 235
The Clinical Effects of Accidental Hemorrhage 236
Cardiotocography Changes in Accidental Hemorrhage 237
Ultrasonography in Accidental Hemorrhage 238
Obstetric Management of Accidental Hemorrhage 238
Cesarean Section in Accidental Hemorrhage 239
Medical Management 239

Index *241*

CHAPTER

1

General Aspects of Obstetric Vasculopathies

CHAPTER OUTLINE

- What are Obstetric Vasculopathies

INTRODUCTION

Human reproduction is the most challenging, most complex and still the most dangerous of all physiologies in the human body. As if by magic, it takes hardly any time for the process of physiology to get diseased and get pathological. During the course of my journey through the science of obstetrics, adverse outcomes always intrigued me. As its student, my mind always got filled with the most powerful words of science: Why? How? What?

As a junior resident in the labor ward I once received two mothers of Pregnancy-induced Hypertension (PIH) back-to-back. First one was 37 weeks pregnant, had a BP of 150/100, had edema and trace of albuminuria. The second subject had only 22 weeks pregnancy, a BP of 160/110, edema and very high albuminuria. The first subject went on to deliver normally a 2.9 kg child who was healthy and alive. The second subject of the same disease had to be induced as her BP progressively got more dangerous. The baby could not be salvaged and she took a long time to get her BP pulled back to normal. She stayed in the hospital for nearly 3 months. Many such patients came and went and each time I got challenged, "Why she had this outcome? Why not the others"?

As a couple of years rolled by, I started getting these mothers for subsequent obstetric performances. In her next pregnancy, the first mother who had a milder form of the disease came with no PIH or any other high-risk factor. She delivered vaginally uneventfully and left. The second mother (who had a severe form of the disease and that too very early in pregnancy) came in her next pregnancy with a fetal demise at 10 weeks of pregnancy. The third time she had an IUGR with accidental hemorrhage. She incidentally managed to reach 34 weeks. She had to be sectioned out (LSCS) and went home after nearly a month of stay with us. Her BP had shot up nearing delivery and took nearly a month again for it to come back to normal. Concurrently her baby too needed on initial admission in the neonatal intensive care unit (NICU) as we used to call and then a close monitoring. The silver lining was that the mothers did go home with this live baby.

Seemingly diverse obstetric conditions: Severe PIH remote from term, IUGR, accidental hemorrhage and fetal demise all occurred in the same mother in different pregnancies. Are those interlinked conditions? If yes what way they are interlinked? What binds them together? Do they have some long-term effects? Above all, what causes them? How does one treat them?

Those were the early years of the decades of 80s. The institution where, I worked did not have any facilities for ultrasound leave aside a color Doppler then. Aspirin was still scoffed at. We had just begun to use magnesium sulfate to treat eclampsia. There were no computers to manage the data and at best we had calculators to calculate the statistical indices. Our first study on this matter titled preeclampsia remote from term was presented at the All India Conference of Obstetrics and Gynecology at Jaipur. It showed interesting results. This was the harbinger of more than two decades of diligent and dedicated study of these conditions which are now clubbed as obstetric vasculopathy.

WHAT ARE OBSTETRIC VASCULOPATHIES

In simplest terms obstetric vasculopathy means disease of vessels resulting from an obstetric event. Though this is the first step to the understanding of obstetric vasculopathies, it is the simplest and most preliminary step. Immediately from here, the complexity of this science begins. It is indeed this complexity that makes it very beautiful but challenging, intriguing and therefore invitive for its keen students to decode its mysteries.

Obstetric vasculopathy is not the vasculopathy that occurs in the maternal vascular system. It is the vasculopathy that occurs at the fetomaternal interface. Inherited probably by the genetic propensity at the fetomaternal system, there occurs a series of changed at this interface which invites seemingly totally diverse and apparently unrelated conditions.

In early understandings it was perceived that one condition leads to the other. But as advances in understanding increased, it became clear that this is not a cause-effect relationship but are fruits of the same pathology. In the initial years, only a few conditions were attributed to obstetric vasculopathy viz,

- Recurrent spontaneous miscarriages (RSA)
- Intrauterine growth retardations (IUGR)
- Preeclampsia and preeclampsia remote from term
- Accidental hemorrhage
- Chorea gravidarum.

However, with scientific research going in details of these conditions, more specifics and complexities added up. Currently obstetric vasculopathies include:

- Recurrent spontaneous missed abortions of late first trimesters and second trimesters.
- Accidental hemorrhage with association of IUGR or Preeclampsia remote from term

- Fetal demise of non anomalous pregnancies with association of any one of the above conditions.

With the etiopathology becoming clearer over a period of time, it became apparent that the differentiation of preeclampsia remote from term from preeclampsia was unnecessary and was therefore subsequently dropped.

Newer additions also continued which included hyperhemocystenemia. SLE associated pregnancies are a special class. They have a magnified manifestation of vasculopathy thereby enabling a closer look at this miraculous but mysterious phenomenon. While still on lupus, I am reminded of a very thought provoking incidence that took place with me in 1980. It was during my internship in internal medicine that we were allowed to attend a PG case presentation. Incidentally in one of these presentations, one guest from abroad who was visiting my institution was also present. The case being presented was that of SLE. This subject was not pregnant. A professor in internal medicine remarked that this was a rare case. The visiting guest did not agree. He said that he wanted to visit the clinical wards. To the surprise of many of us, he pointed out so many admissions that could be having lupus in association. I do not know if this was followed up with any further investigations or was just scoffed at. I, too, had completely forgotten this incidence. It was nearly a decade later that I suddenly recollected the event when more and more diverse obstetric conditions started associating with obstetric vasculopathy. Lest I may be misunderstood, I wish to clarify that all obstetric vasculopathies are not SLE but SLE does produce obstetric vasculopathy. I would however like to highlight that immunology of and its disturbances have indeed a big role to play in obstetric vasculopathy.

CHAPTER

2

Cardiovascular Changes in Normal Pregnancy

CHAPTER OUTLINE

- Blood Pressure
- Longitudinal Changes in Cardiac Functions
- Peripheral Vascular Resistance
- Changes in Venous System: Any?

INTRODUCTION

Obstetric vasculopathy is the derangement in the vascular system of the pregnant woman. To understand a derangement well, one has to first know what is normal and physiological. After this to understand the abnormality becomes easier.

Maternal system undergoes massive changes due to the conceptus. These are due to:

- Progressively increasing demands of the conceptus
- Need for the maternal system to supply increase amount of blood with least resistance
- Certain physiological changes, both in the mother as well as the conceptus which can put a load on the maternal systems.

In simplest words the maternal cardiovascular system brings about these changes by:

- Increase in the total blood volume during pregnancy
- Reduction in peripheral resistance and decrease in resistance to the blood flow to critical organs and systems
- Changes in the rate, rhythm, contractility and efficiency of her cardiac pump musculature.

The pregnant mother is able to achieve all this through a complex interaction and coordinated interplay between the heart, blood vessels and vascular pools like the placenta. There is an alteration in neurological control, circulating humoral substances and certain structural and functional changes in the maternal systems. It is of interest to note that the early gestation modulations of physiological mechanisms are through conceptus-based mechanisms rather than maternal.[1]

Incessant growth of the fetus coupled with continual placental pool increase brings about changes in cardiovascular functions ceaselessly. Most of these changes are as a direct result of increase in requirements of the fetus and maternal adaptation to the same.

BLOOD PRESSURE

Due to a large low resistance pool of blood flow that develops in the uterus, maternal blood pressure declines late in II trimester and midtrimester. Before the advent of color Doppler, this midtrimester fall in BP was used for screening individuals at a high-risk for developing obstetric vasculopathies especially preeclampsia.

The spiral arterial moulding that follows the second wave of trophoblastic invasion leads to the formation of low resistance pool at the placental bed. Absence or incompetent second wave of this trophoblastic invasion leads to development of increased vascular resistance. Before the maternal system actually starts registering a rise in her BP there occurs a failure of BP to fall in midtrimester. This fall in B.P in midtrimester precedes the rise in BP in subjects who are to develop PIH. Midtrimester fall in BP was used by clinicians to predict the possibility of PIH. It is customarily believed in clinical practice that there is a significant drop in BP as early as late first trimester in women with a normal pregnancy outcome when compared to those who subsequently developed preeclampsia.

Animal Studies

In animal experiments interesting changes have been documented. Maternal cardiovascular adaptations occur in normal pregnancy, systemically, and within the uterus. Transient structural remodeling of endometrial spiral arteries normally occurs in human and mouse pregnancies. In mice, this depends on uterine natural killer cell function. Using normal and immune deficient mice, it was investigated if spiral artery remodeling critically regulates gestational mean arterial pressure and/ or placental growth. Radiotelemetric transmitters were implanted in female mice. Hemodynamic profiles to a dietary salt challenge and to pregnancy were assessed. Implantation sites from noninstrumented females were used for histological morphometry.

Both normal and immune deficient mice had normal sensitivity to salt and showed similar 5-phase gestational patterns of mean arterial pressure correlating with stages of placental development, regardless of spiral artery modification. After implantation, mean arterial pressure declined during the preplacental phase to reach a midgestation nadir. With gestation day 9, opening of placental circulation occurred. This led to rise in pressure, reaching baseline before parturition, whereas heart rate dropped.

Heart rate stabilized before parturition. Placental sizes deviated during late gestation when growth stopped in normal mice but continued in immune deficient mice. As an indication of the potential for abnormal hemodynamics, 2 pregnant females delivering dead offspring developed late gestational hypertension. This study characterizes a dynamic pattern of blood pressure over mouse pregnancy that parallels human gestation.[2]

Recent studies have shown that several changes noted in cardiovascular and uteroplacental systems occurring during normal murine pregnancy have striking similarities to humans and can be accurately measured using newer ultrasonographic techniques. Further studies are needed to evaluate changes in these vascular beds in mouse models of diseases such as preeclampsia and intrauterine growth restriction.[3]

Diurnal Variations in BP

One more feature that has a clinical bearing as regards blood pressure change is the pattern of diurnal variation. As is found in all blood pressure recordings in all healthy human beings, BP tends to fall during sleep. This does not occur in preeclamptic pregnancies. In some subjects this entire pattern of diurnal variation may be reversed in preeclampsia.

It has an indirect clinical bearing. Subjects in whom there is a possibility or are already showing an early rise in BP, diurnal variation is abolished. These subjects consistently report to the clinicians with complaints of inability to have a good quality, peaceful and sound sleep. They usually report with difficulty in sleep maintenance though sleep induction is usually not a problem.

LONGITUDINAL CHANGES IN CARDIAC FUNCTIONS

It is of interest to know that changes in cardiac function occur very early in pregnancy. This may be as early as the luteal phase of the menstrual cycle.[4] Savu O et al assess the performance of the left ventricle (LV) in normal, uncomplicated pregnancies while considering the actual LV load and shape. Cardiac output increased during pregnancy because of a higher stroke volume in early pregnancy and a late increase in heart rate, whereas total vascular resistance decreased. Progressive development of eccentric hypertrophy was observed, which subsequently recovered postpartum. Sphericity index decreased from the first to the third trimester and returned postpartum to values comparable to the control. Although higher LV stroke work was noted toward the third trimester.[5]

This seems to be guided by principles of preparation for the advancing pregnancy and labor. Development of a state of hypercoagulability is one such classic example of preparedness shown by the maternal system to the challenges that the mother's coagulation system may face with advancing pregnancy and during labor.

Stroke Volume and Heart Rate

Cardiac output is the multiplication product of cardiac rate and stroke volume. A rise in cardiac output could be due to increase in either one or both. The rise in cardiac output is a function of increase in heart rate till about 32 weeks of pregnancy. Increase in heart rate is not very significant clinically. But it serves the function of increasing the cardiac output well. Similarly the volume of blood emitted at every heart beat, expressed as stroke volume increases in early pregnancy. It steadies by 15 weeks of pregnancy. Both these rises get reflected in the rise in cardiac output during pregnancy.

How Does the Heart Increase the Cardiac Output?

It is not very difficult to understand this apparently complex phenomenon. The cardiac muscle acts as a pump. Increase in cardiac output means the pump needs:

- More fluid to push
- It has to increase its pumping capacity and
- There should be an unhindered out flow system.

All the three in combination will increase the output and therefore the amount of blood that reaches the target organs and tissues.

Increase in fluid supplied to the heart is ensured by the increase in preload. In states of health this preload is efficiently pumped out through a robust cardiac musculature. The efficiency of cardiac musculature also increases in healthy and uncomplicated pregnancy. The final step of smooth and unhindered outflow is ensured by the reduced peripheral resistance in normal pregnancy.

As regards the pumping efficiency, all three components that can contribute to better pumping are increased. The cardiac musculature increases in thickness, the size of the cardiac chambers is also increased and the contractile power of the cardiac muscle mass and size leads to increased amount of blood being efficiently pushed out. A small but significant contribution to this comes from the increase in heart rate. All of these together combine with each other as a team effort to bring about an increase in cardiac output.

While it is true that there are so many changes in the cardiac structure and function, it need not be forgotten that none of these alterations reach the level of abnormality of pathological proportions. To illustrate this with an example: increase in size of the cardiac chambers never goes to the levels of what can be called as a cardiomegaly. Cardiomegaly is a pathological state while increase in cardiac dimensions is physiological.

Vascular Response to Increase Cardiac Output

One very important aspect that should complement is the change in the vascular bed to accommodate increased cardiac output. The amount of blood in circulation and the amount of push out being done by the heart are both increased in normal pregnancy. To accommodate this significant increase in the volume of blood forced out more powerfully by the heart the vascular channels through which the blood circulates also gets more accommodative. The mechanism by which the body does this, is the vascular channel modeling done by the second wave of trophoblastic invasion. This converts the vascular channels especially at the voluminous fetomaternal interface to be a low resistance pool. Consequently the blood volume meets less resistance and can flow easily.

Expansion of the plasma volume and an increase in red blood cell mass begin as early as the fourth week of pregnancy, peak at 28 to 34 weeks of gestation, and then plateau until parturition. Plasma volume expansion is accompanied by a lesser increase in red cell volume. As a result, there is a modest reduction in hematocrit, with peak hemodilution occurring at 24 to 26 weeks. The blood volume in pregnant women at term is about 100 mL/kg.[6]

However, changes of vascular modeling occurs relatively late in pregnancy. On the other hand, the changes in blood volume, etc take place much earlier. As a result, body has to make certain changes early in pregnancy too. This change is the change in oscillatory pressure along the vessels lining. This is a very interesting phenomenon.

Oscillatory Pressure and Propulsive Pressure (Fig. 2.1)

The vessel wall has two types of pressures to bear when the blood mass strikes it on getting pumped out from the heart. One pressure is generated along the vessel wall which does not have any propulsive function. It gets distributed along the vascular lining. It is like the force that lashing waves generate on the rocks along the seashore. This is the oscillatory pressure that is generated by the blood pushed out from the heart along the vessel wall.

The other pressure is the *propulsive pressure*. It is that component of the total pressure on the vessel wall other than oscillatory pressure. It is the pressure that actually propels the blood through. This pressure is functionally important as it propels the blood forward. It is influenced by the pulsatility of the vessel wall therefore plays a very important role in facilitating the increase blood volume and power of flow.

Due to increased pulsatility, the oscillatory pressure is effectively combated. The vessels walls are able to withstand the force of the lashing of blood being pumped out of the heart. That component of increased pulsatility which is not used in resisting the onslaught of oscillatory pressure is used to propel the blood forwards. Increased pulsatility of the vessel wall, therefore, accommodates the increased blood volume being pushed out of the heart of the pregnant subject, efficiently. This occurs early in pregnancy.

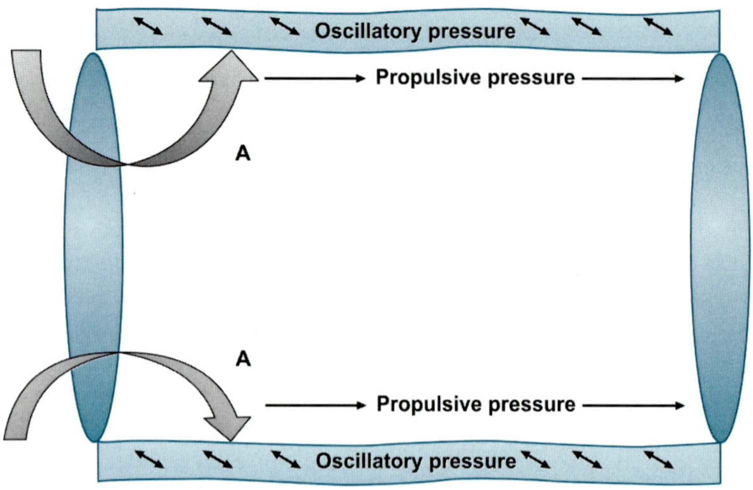

Fig 2.1: Oscillatory and propulsive pressures

Blood enters that vessel well and strikes the well with great force (A). This force generates vibrations along the vessel well and is called the oscillatory pressure. The remaining component of the pressure with which blood component enters the vessel, propagates the blood further as propulsive pressure

In obstetric vasculopathy, there is an interesting breakdown of this accommodative mechanism. In preeclampsia, the spasmodic vessels initially accommodate the oscillatory pressure. Rise in BP that occurs, causes the blood to flow with a much greater pressure. The vessels especially the arteries respond by further increasing their pulsatility. As a result they are able to first let the nonpropulsive force efficiently distributed along the vessel wall without breaking. Also, the propulsive component of these vessels is increased whereby the blood can flow through narrowed vessel lumen without much problem. However, it should be borne in mind that the power of accommodation of the vessels is not limitless. At some unpredictable stage, the vessel wall gives way. This is seen in accidental hemorrhage, intracranial hemorrhage in severe eclampsia and subcapsular hemorrhage in liver.

PERIPHERAL VASCULAR RESISTANCE

The body of the gravida makes all possible arrangements to ensure a smooth and unobstructed blood flow to the critical organs of her body including the uterus. Reduction in peripheral resistance is one more mechanism by which this is ensured. Peripheral resistance seems to be most vulnerable to pathological onslaught of obstetric vasculopathies. Rise in peripheral resistance due to different complimentary processes makes the maternal system sense the challenge faced by circulating blood stream. The mother therefore raises her blood pressure and the clinician diagnoses it as preeclampsia. In a study published in 2012 it has been found that during normal pregnancy there is an increase in cardiac output, and decrease in blood pressure and peripheral arterial resistance whereas central aortic properties are less altered. The increased ventriculo-arterial coupling index during normal pregnancy indicates a decrease in left ventricular function not fully compensated for by vascular adaptation.[7]

CHANGES IN VENOUS SYSTEM: ANY?

It goes without saying that while massive accommodation changes are taking place in the heart, blood volume and cardiac output, the arterial changes are also correspondingly accommodate the outflow from the heart. Concurrently the venous musculature and tone also adjust to some extent to these changes. Not much is known on this aspect of the cardiovascular system changes. The venous walls seem to be passively accommodative. This is due to a very weak muscular wall in their structure. In absence of a muscular resistance, the venous vessels are able to dilate passively without a need for large adjustments. Thus the passive accommodations by venous system assisted by strong skeletal muscle activity that surround these venous lining (e.g. gastrocnemius muscles) propel the increased venous circulation towards the heart in pregnancy. Venous system, therefore, does not undergo much change.

REFERENCES

1. Barrette V, Adams M, Croy B. Endometrial decidualization does not trigger the blood pressure decline of normal early pregnancy in mice. *Biol Reprod.* 2012;86(3):66.
2. Burke S, Barrette V, Bianco J, Thorne J, Yamada A, Pang S, et al. Spiral arterial remodeling is not essential for normal blood pressure regulation in pregnant mice. *Hypertension.* 2010;55(3):729-37.
3. Khankin E, Hacker M, Zelop C, Karumanchi S, Rana S. Intravital high-frequency ultrasonography to evaluate cardiovascular and uteroplacental blood flow in mouse pregnancy. *Pregnancy Hypertens.* 2012;2(2):84-92.
4. Spaanderman M, Van Beek E, Ekhart T, Van Eyck J, Cheriex E, De Leeuw P, et al. Changes in hemodynamic parameters and volume homeostasis with the menstrual cycle among women with a history of preeclampsia. *Am J Obstet Gynecol.* 2000;182(5):1127-34.
5. Savu O, Jurcuţ R, Giuşcă S, van Mieghem T, Gussi I, Popescu B. Morphological and functional adaptation of the maternal heart during pregnancy. *Circ Cardiovascular Imaging.* 2012;5(3):289-97.
6. Foley M. http://www.uptodate.com/contents/maternal-cardiovascular-and-hemodynamic-adaptations-to-pregnancy. April 2012
7. Estensen M, Grindheim G, Remme E, Swillens A, Smiseth O, Segers P, et al. Systemic arterial response and ventriculo-arterial interaction during normal pregnancy. *Am J Hypertens.* 2012;25(6):672-7.

CHAPTER

3

Immunology of Obstetric Vasculopathy

CHAPTER OUTLINE

- Leads through Recurrent Spontaneous Abortion (RSA)
- Fetus as an Allograft
- What Protects the Fetus?
- Fetus as a Unique Allograft
- Suppressor Mechanisms in Protection
- Partner Specificity in Miscarriages
- Autoimmunity in Recurrent Pregnancy Loss
- Embryo Decidua Crosstalk in Immunology of Obstetrics Vasculopathy
- Implantation not a Right of Embryo
- Results of the Crosstalk
- Other Contributory Mechanisms
- What is Spontaneous Resolution?
- The Miracle of Paradox

INTRODUCTION

Having firmly established that vasculopathy occurs at the fetomaternal interface which produces a series of obstetric adverse outcomes, it is imperative to know as to what is responsible for this phenomenon.

LEADS THROUGH RECURRENT SPONTANEOUS ABORTION (RSA)

There are explainable and unexplainable causes of RSA. The classic example of explainable causes includes the anatomical defects of the genital tract, both congenital and acquired. However the most intriguing and therefore the most challenging amongst all causes still remain immunological causes. They are very complex to understand and a challenge to treat. Nevertheless they prove very vital leads to the understanding of obstetric vasculopathy.

FETUS AS AN ALLOGRAFT

It is well understandable that the fetus is immunologically a very dynamic structure. It bears an expression of maternal as well as paternal antigens on itself. Any foreign protein that enters a human body generates a series of immunological reactions in the host. These are the responses that ultimately destroy the entrant to protect the host. On these very lines the fetus is also a graft, albeit an allograft that is transplanted in the mother's body. It has on itself an expression of maternal and paternal alloantigens. The fetus, therefore, behaves as a transplanted graft. It has been a big challenge for all transplant scientists to understand how does the fetus quiescence the host reaction and generates a peaceful acceptance. This is the key to any graft acceptance.

There is no reason why the fetus also should not be treated as a graft. Attempts are bound to be made by the maternal immune system to reject it. The paternal alloantigens are foreign to the maternal immune system. They generate the graft-host reaction. The maternal antigens are not foreign to the mother. They are her own. Therefore, the mother accepts those antigens. But the paternal antigens have no business to expect such a warm welcome and tolerance by the mother's system.

Now that it has been understood that the fetus is an allograft which too has an expression of antigens, the question that arises is why does the fetus escape from the rejection phenomenon? Not only does the fetus not get rejected but it is also made to thrive and is nourished. On one side are the protective mechanisms in the mother that readily reject any foreign graft and on the other are the maternal system that tolerates, accepts, nourishes and ensures that the fetal allograft thrives. What provides this privileged status to the fetus? How does this miracle occur? The antigens that have been found to have a big bearing on this entire phenomenon are the antigens of the major histocompatability complex (MHC). These antibodies have been documented to bind the cells of the fetus and the trophoblast.

WHAT PROTECTS THE FETUS?

Due to ethical constraints most of the understanding of human pregnancy and immunological response comes from studies in mice. Mice, too, have a hemochorial pregnancy and are therefore providing valuable insight into the understanding of human pregnancy tolerance.

Small Size

The small size of the embryo does help in protecting it. The effectors cells from the maternal system that may have strayed into the fallopian tube or the peritoneal pelvic fluid fail to detect this small embryo. Also, due to this small size there is no interaction between the maternal lymphatic systems and the embryo. This also prevents the detection of the embryo while it transits from the fallopian tube to the uterus. Hill (1987) demonstrated that if, for whatever reason, the macrophage effector cell system does get activated, it effectively releases destructive cytokines like tumor necrotizing factor alpha (TNF-α) and granulocyte macrophage colony stimulating factor (GM-CST) Interleukin-1, Interleukin-6 and others.[1] This can lead to implantation failure following embryo damage. The fact that these inflammatory substances do play a very important role in protection – destruction interplay of the fetal allograft has been demonstrated in another study. It was found that for the first time that Allograft Inflammatory Factor-1 (AIF-1) was expressed in uterus. The expression level was associated with the population size of macrophage and varied during the estrous cycle and the pregnancy period. The augmented expression of AIF-1 with concomitant expressions of TNF-α and nitric oxide synthase 2 (NOS_2) mRNA in poly (I:C) injected mice suggests a correlation between AIF-1 production and fetal resorption.[2]

Zona Pellucida

The shield provided by the zona pellucida plays a very valuable role in the failure of maternal protective system while the embryo is in its phase of transit migration. It is not exactly understood as to whether the zona provides a physical barrier to the detection by the maternal protective systems only or also makes the embryo hypoantigenic. The role of zona in protecting the conceptus is confined to the transit. This is proved by it getting shed off just before implantation. It is not required once the embryo reaches the uterus. One study has shown that the zona pellucida thickness has an important influence on in vivo fertilization and implantation processes, but not on birth.[3]

Paralysis of Maternal Protector Systems and Pregnancy

In the days when hysterosalpingography and Rubin's tubal insufflation tests were still popular for tubal patency testing, clinicians know that there used to be successful pregnancies just after performing these tests. This was more consistently observed after hysterosalpingography and is attributed to the transient paralysis or ablation of maternal macrophage effectors systems. This is the explanation to how the fetal embryo gets protected in transit. However the bigger challenge lies in protecting, implanting and bringing about a thriving growth of the conceptus.

Hypoimmunogenic Embryo

The mechanisms of protection of embryo from getting destroyed by the maternal protective systems also include its hypoimmunogenicity. The embryo is always low in creating immune reaction. As has been stated in previous pages, there are different types of antigens expressing on its surface. These include products of the MHC or Major Histocompatability Complex (H) such as HLA and non-MHC or minor histocompatability (h) gene complexes. It is interesting to note that expression of (H) is shut off before implantation. This is an important change in the embryo to render it hypoantigenic.[4]

It seems the hormone leptin, which is primarily produced by adipose tissue, is a critical permissive factor for multiple reproductive events (in the mouse), including implantation. Throughout development leptin patterning suggests that it is a component of the subcortical maternal complex with as yet unknown significance in preimplantation development.[5]

FETUS AS A UNIQUE ALLOGRAFT

A question arises in the investigators' mind as to why does the fetus not get rejected. This is extremely complicated but very interesting phenomenon. The conceptus has two mechanisms of immunologically active strata. One is the fetus itself and the other is the trophoblast. The fetal tissue is immunologically susceptible to recognition and rejection by the mother. This would occur if there is a direct interaction between the fetal surface and the maternal lyhmphomyeloid cells. In animal experiments it has been found that if the fetal tissue is directly injected into the thigh of mice, there is an immediate rejection of this tissue.[6] Direct contact between the maternal lymphocytes and fetal cells can also occur if there is an intrauterine transfusion accidentally or spontaneously. This leads to fetal rejection.

Entry of maternal cells in fetal circulation and entry of fetal cells into maternal system is rare. But the maternal system has a big advantage. It has a very competent effector system and the intruding fetal cells are quickly and efficiently eliminated from the maternal system. If at any instance there is a failure of any of these systems graft-versus host (GVH) diseases get manifested.

On the flip side, the phenomenon of fetal microchimerism has been found to have interesting bearings in this aspect. The fetal cells can persist in a wide range of woman's tissues following a pregnancy or an abortion and she becomes a chimera. Fetal cells have been found in the maternal circulation and they were shown to persist for the entire life in humans, thus demonstrating long-term engraftment and survival capabilities. Microchimerism is a subject of much interest for a number of reasons. Studies of fetal microchimerism during pregnancy may offer explanations for complications of pregnancy, such as preeclampsia, as well as insights into the pathogenesis of autoimmune diseases which usually ameliorate during pregnancy. The impact of the persistence of allogenic cells of fetal origin and of the maternal immunological response to them on the mother's health is still not clear. On the beneficial side, it has been proposed that genetically dissimilar fetal microchimerism provides protection against some cancers, that fetal microchimerism can afford the mother new mechanisms of protection to some diseases, that fetal microchimerism can enlarge the immunological range of the mother improving her defense against aggressor. Fetal cells are often present at sites of maternal injury and may have an active role in the repair of maternal tissues.[7]

Now let us see a very intriguing phenomenon: The estimated instance of passage of maternal lymphocytes is believed to be rare but at 1 in 50 to 1 in 100 embryos. We have seen that any instance if such an exchange occurs, the fetus gets rejected. Thus the estimated spontaneous resorption rate (in mice) and abortion rate in humans should be around 1 to 2% (1 in 50 to 1 in 100). But in actual clinical practice, this rate is much higher. Thus there is some more to explain then mere lymphocytes of mother playing havoc.

This is where the second strata of immunological activity beyond the conceptus steps in and this stratum is the stratum of trophoblast. It is well-established since the mid 1980s that the trophoblasts are very specialized forms of tissues as regards genetic expression is concerned. There are two groups: One that is found primarily at the fetomaternal interface between the fetoplacental capillaries and maternal blood (fetal interface) second is at the maternal interface in contact with the decidua.

Fetal trophoblasts are essentially dependant on paternal genetic material for their survival and development. However, if there is only paternal genetic material pathological pregnancies like gestational trophoblastic diseases develop. This means the maternal genetic expression on the trophoblast helps in creating a balance. It is well known that there is an uncontrolled growth of trophoblastic tissue in hydatidiform mole. This uncontrolled growth is checked by the expression of maternal genetic material on trophoblast which brings about the normal fetal growth and development.

It is very interesting to note that in absence of maternal genetic expression, the trophoblasts have a field day. This paradox is worth understanding. The maternal immune system is derived from the mother and therefore should not give any resistance to growth or survival of its own material. However, the paternal contribution is alien to the maternal effector system. The latter is supposed to react and protect the maternal system by eliminating any foreign genetic material. Nevertheless at the fetomaternal interface a complete reversal of this phenomenon occurs. Instead of eliminating the tissue with paternal genetic expression (foreign to the mother), it actually brings about a growth of these trophoblasts.

A complete foreign or alien genetic maternal seems to promote trophoblastic growth. Only paternal genetic expression however brings about uncontrolled growth as is seen in hydatidiform mole. It seems such an uncontrolled growth is effectively prevented by the maternal genetic material. Thus at the level of the trophoblast a totally paradoxical situation develops. Foreign genetic material promotes growth and genetic material from the host check this growth or may even hamper this growth. It seems the trophoblast have a privileged status. This privileged status is given to the syncitiotrophoblasts.

An important characteristic of most trophoblasts is their capacity to resist rejection by the host antigen specific effectors mechanism. This privileged status of the trophoblast is the key to the survival and growth of a partly foreign genetic material on the conceptus in an alien environment (the maternal environment).

The early invasion of the trophoblast into the maternal spiral arterioles and their resistance to maternal elimination systems is the key to healthy pregnancy outcome. As a corollary to this, any impendence or failure to this invasion can lead to complete rejection of fetal tissue. This is seen in miscarriages. In subjects in whom the trophoblasts partially resist maternal rejection, manifestations of other obstetric vasculopathies result. Thus PIH and IUGR are a result of partial rejection by the host.

Hence it gets well established that paternal genetic expression is the key to the survival of fetal tissue. It is the paternal genetic material which is the growth driver in the trophoblast and subsequently in the fetus. The trophoblasts are extremely resistant to maternal rejection due to paternal genetic expression which is a privileged status. This resistance is intrinsic.

The entire spectrum of normal fetal growth and development along with resistance to rejection gets explained. At one end of the spectrum is a total failure of trophoblast to resist the maternal rejection systems. This results in a miscarriage. At the middle of the spectrum is an array of obstetric vasculopathies where there is a partial rejection or partial activation of maternal effectors systems not killing the conceptus but producing diseased states. On the other extreme of the spectrum is a hydatidiform mole. In this there is only paternal genetic expression and no maternal expression. This gives a field day to the trophoblasts leading to their uncontrolled growth. Therefore there is a strong genetic platform for the immunological basis for obstetric vasculopathies. These will be revisited in the pages to follow.

SUPPRESSOR MECHANISMS IN PROTECTION

In this section we shall be seeing one more unique and amazing phenomenon that takes place at the level of the decidua which plays an important role in the successful nidation and then a proper growth of the fetus. At this stage it will be worthwhile noting that all these protective mechanisms act partly in tandem with each other and partly independent to achieve the ultimate goal of a successful pregnancy outcome. Scrupulous understanding of these mechanisms will play a pivotal role in our understanding of the processes involved in causation and management of obstetric vasculopathies.

Just before implantation, workers like Brierley and Clark and Daya et al have shown that unique populations of cells develop in the uterine lining. These are the suppressor cells. They are unique in ways more than one. They are developed under the hormonal influence and not under the influence of antigens. They are locally generated confining themselves to the uterine lining and not all across the mothers' body. They are relatively large cells resembling the structure and function of T cells. [8,9] So as to understand the function of these suppressor T cells, there is a need to introduce the readers to the concept of DTH or Delayed Type of Hypersensitivity reaction. This DTH has important role. If DTH is generated before time it can prove lethal to the process of successful implantation. However the same process of DTH is important later to maintain proper growth of the conceptus postimplantation.

Now let us see why these suppressor T cells get generated in the uterine lining. Firstly they have a capacity to keep the maternal macrophages at bay. Secondly, they delay the generation of DTH preventing its occurrence in first 4 days. If DTH occurs as early as first day of implantation it will sense an allergen like antigen in the implanting conceptus and thereby bring about changes to cause its rejection. This also includes activating macrophages. Whether the suppressor T cells can keep the macrophages at bay individually or through the delay in generation of DTH is not known.

By the fifth postimplantation day these large T cell suppressors get replaced by smaller suppressor cell population. This replacement is necessary as the new population of cells have a different role to play besides protecting the conceptus. They also have a function to generate potent immunological molecule RGF-B which promotes new blood vessel formation and growth. These are early steps being taken to generate growth of the conceptus.

Before we go further into depth of understanding the role of these new suppressor cells, we need to quickly revise some basic facts. The conceptus is half alien to the mother. Therefore the tendency of the maternal protecting systems to reject and eliminate it is understandable. Through a series of complex but amazing mechanisms the conceptus protects itself from getting eliminated. At the same time, the maternal protective systems help the conceptus to successfully implant and then nidate and grow.

So as to understand this complex phenomenon a little more easily, one can draw a parallel in something that is occurring in the world, so obviously. Every large and thriving country has a problem of illegal migrants. India too has such a problem. To put it simplistically, the conceptus is such an illegal migrant. Illegal immigrants devise different mechanisms by which sneak in through the Indian borders. So as to avoid detection it may sneak in at night or through porous areas on the Indian borders. Once within the territory of India, politicians who may have been bribed or may have same political ulterior motives generate mechanisms by which this migrant gets some foothold either at some shanty dwelling or as a guest of some host without getting detected. Soon the politician becomes his protector and generates illegal housing, ration benefits and subsequently even gets him a voting right. The migrant under the patronage of his protector soon starts getting accepted in his new country. He starts growing in acceptance, starts his own business or gets some other employment. As time passes, he grows so much in stature that even becomes on accepted leader thereby influencing the entire host mechanism in its favor.

This is exactly what the fetus does. As pregnancy advances it grows in size and maturity and influences the entire maternal physiology in such a way that it may even endanger the mother's life to ensure its own survival. This newly generated smaller suppressor cell crop has the capacity to suppress destruction of the embryo by releasing a potent immune suppressive molecule like transforming growth factor β (TGF-β). This molecule seems to be inhibitive to natural killer cells (NK cells) and suppresses the plethora of destructive cytokines like Interleukin 3 (IL-3). Thus this TGF-β seems to have a potent capacity to block nearly all maternal effectors systems.[10,11]

As has also been mentioned before a couple of pages, this TGF-β also generates new vessels. Therefore, it seems that this potent molecule not only protects the conceptus that is implanting but also lays the foundation for its subsequent sustenance and growth. TGF-β also promotes generation of extracellular matrix and may alter hemostatic mechanisms (uq).

It seems TGF-β and TNF-α has a point to point antagonizing mechanism as regards to their effects on immune mechanisms.[12] While one protects and prepares for the growth and development of the conceptus, the other is a potent protector of the mother. TNF-α is all out to destroy any immunologically alien molecule, in this case the conceptus. It gets neutralized by TGF-β.

From a bird's eye view it seems the general opinion is that the fundamental protective mechanism must be located locally at the contact plate, between the maternal and fetal tissues. Immunologic investigations proved the presence of specific systems which block the function of antipaternal maternal antibodies, as well as formation of cytotoxic maternal T-cells to paternal antigens. The system preventing rejection of graft during pregnancy is functioning at the level of maternal and fetal tissues. The protective mechanisms are coded by genes of MCH region, locus HLA-G.

Protective mechanisms in the placenta: The placenta protects itself against antibody mediated damage. A high level of complement regulatory proteins (CD46, CD55 and CD59), being the response to the synthesis of complement fixing maternal antibodies to paternal antigens and regulation of the placental HLA expression as a preventive reaction of the fetoplacental unit to the influence of maternal CTL, are the most important protective mechanisms of placenta.

Protective mechanisms shared by the placenta and uterus: Protective mechanisms common both for placenta and uterus are as follows: expressions of Fas ligand prevention of infiltration of activated immune cells, regulation of immunosuppression which prevents proliferation of immune cells and high natural immunity (Na cells and macrophages) of the decidua.[13]

PARTNER SPECIFICITY IN MISCARRIAGES

In early 90s there was a trend to classify women who abort as *primary aborters* and *secondary aborters*. Primary aborters were those mothers who aborted all her pregnancies and never had a successful outcome. On the other hand secondary aborters were those who at some time or the other have had at least one successful outcome. By successful outcome, it was meant as a live birth. Interestingly primary abortions seemed to be partner specific and secondary aborters, aborted irrespective of the partner. Though this classification did not become clinically popular, it raised some interesting questions.

It is possible that partner specific abortions could have a genetic basis but non-partner specific abortions have an explanation beyond the faulty genetic material. This is where the immunological explanation started becoming popular. Currently it is accepted that majority of abortions result from immunological problems. This problem can be simply worded as failure to prevent rejection. It is very interesting to note that 25% of mothers threaten a miscarriage but only 10% actually abort. This means that while the maternal system is all out to reject it (threatened abortion), the fetal system protects itself from the rejection onslaught and a successful outcome results. If fetal heart activity can be detected in the first trimester, more than 90% conceptus gestate successfully. Thus the onus of initial survival of the fetus against the maternal onslaught is not on the shoulders of the mother but on the fetus itself.

Also the clinical phenomenon of threatened miscarriage is merely a clinical expression of the ongoing conflict between the fetal system to survive and the maternal system to destroy. As has been hinted in some of the preceding pages cytokines have a very important role to play in this process. It is well known that there are a set of protective cytokines and destructive cytokines. This activity occurs throughout the maternal vascular channels. As a result of this, there is an injury and rupture of vascular system resulting in threatened miscarriage clinically.

However, it is not necessary that the destructive cytokines should win or lose. The war may go on any side. If the destructive cytokines win, the mother aborts. If protective cytokines win, it results in a favorable outcome. But this entire process mediates through the vascular bed irrespective of the result. As a result threatened miscarriage is far more prevalent than actual miscarriage. This complex interplay of cytokines is tackled separately in sections to follow.

While the trophoblasts have an intrinsic capacity to resist maternal immunologic destruction, it should be noted that a certain **IA** antigens have an important role to play in this. This immune response associated antigens (**IA** antigens) associate with a variety of foreign molecules and allow their recognition by T helper /DTH cells. Animals deficient in **IA** antigens cannot mount an immune response to defined epitopes.

The gene coding of **IA** genes have been called immune response genes. A difference in **IA** expression causes maximum proliferation of responding T cells.[14] Interestingly these **IA** antigens are absent on the trophoblast. This could be one of the mechanisms by which the trophoblasts resist maternal destruction responses.

Of late, the roles of HLA and MCHs in human pregnancy have been found to be limited. The other responses though similar are equally interesting and intriguing. It has been suggested by proponents of HLA sharing hypothesis that recurrent abortion represents a heterogeneous group of subjects and this sharing is relevant only to a subgroup.[14] In that case the two major subgroups proposed are:

- Primary aborters: They abort with one partner and have a significant HLA sharing. They have no live births.
- Secondary aborters: They have one or more live births, no HLA sharing, may abort with several partners and may possess antibodies to paternal cells.[11]

All these mechanisms of immune recognition, tolerance and rejection play an important role in recurrent miscarriages due to immune causes.

Primary aborters and non-immunological basis: By and large discussion on primary and secondary aborters hovers around immunological basis for the same. However, there are some who believe that primary aborters may have a predisposition for maternal meiosis errors resulting in digyny. Digyny (also digynia) refers to the process of a diploid ovum becoming fertilized by a monoploid sperm. The result of digyny is a triploid zygote. A case report supporting the concept that some women have a predisposition for maternal meiosis errors resulting in digyny have also been published.[15] Similarly anatomical corrections have also ended in successful pregnancy outcome in primary aborters. There is a report where septoplasty allowed successful delivery in a primary aborter with six previous first trimester miscarriages.[16] It would, therefore, be wise if these rarer occurrences are kept in mind while one evaluates a subject of recurrent miscarriages before attributing all of them to obstetric vasculopathy.

AUTOIMMUNITY IN RECURRENT PREGNANCY LOSS

A smaller but important group associated with obstetric vasculopathy is that of autoantibodies. Amongst a variety of autoantibodies that have been found to have an association with obstetric vasculopathies, antiphospholipid antibodies have been found to have the most consistent and reproducible association.

Antiphospholipid Antibodies

Antiphospholipid antibodies are a diverse group of antibodies that were first described Wassermann as early as in 1906. But it was only in 1952 that Country and Hartman described them in patients with SLE. Soon it became obvious that antiphospholipid antibodies can exist without any connective tissue disorders. These are a diverse family of autoantibodies which share a common reactivity with negatively charged phospholipids.

Many members have been described to constitute the group of antiphospholipid antibodies. Of these only three have been found to have a clinical bearing. These are:

- Biological false seropositive for syphilis (BFSPS)
- Anticardiolipin antibodies (ACA)
- Lupus anticoagulant. (LAC)

A word regarding BFSPS: The reactivity of serum of many patients of recurrent miscarriages to phospholipids falsely testing positive for syphilis was intriguing. Many subjects tested positive for syphilis did not have any other stigma of syphilis. This brought two facts to light: 1) These subjects never had syphilis, and 2) They had a consistent adverse obstetric outcome.

Lupus anticoagulant or LAC antibodies are autoantibodies which prolong phospholipids dependant coagulation assays by reacting with negatively charged phospholipids. Interestingly while LAC has been associated with SLE they are more often than not found in subjects without SLE. Most of these subjects only have manifestations of obstetric vasculopathies without any association with SLE. Anticardiolipin antibodies or ACA as they are popularly known are so named because these groups of antibodies were originally extracted from bovine heart tissue.

The Role of a Cofactor

In early 1990s workers like Matsuura had evinced interest in the role and need of a cofactor in the activity of anticardiolipin antibodies in obstetric vasculopathies.[17] It seems the ACL (anticardiolipin) antibodies when released from a result of infection like syphilis behave differently than those released out of an autoimmune process. Whereas the ACL antibodies of autoimmune origin need a cofactor for its activity, ACL antibodies released from other sources do not need a cofactor. This cofactor has been identified as β2-glycoprotein1 (β2GP1).[18] It was postulated that the cofactor β2GP1 may:

1. Inhibit intrinsic phase of coagulation
2. May inhibit platelet activation and
3. Is an antiphospholipid binding protein

These three processes are critical in causation of obstetric vasculopathies.

Prevalence of APL

This is an interesting aspect of the autoantibodies. In general population also APL antibodies have been demonstrated. But in all of these obstetric vasculopathy did not occur (£). Around this time association between APA and preeclampsia remote form term was investigated by us and we found that 53.3% of subjects tested positive. Of these, low positive were 17.9%, moderate positive were 50.0% and strong positive were 32.1%.[19] It is understood that low levels of APL antibodies are important to cause obstetric vasculopathies. Therefore, when the cutout values are higher, a significant association with obstetric vasculopathies can occur. This means a mere presence of APL antibodies at low levels do not have much clinical bearing. Therefore mere presence of APL antibodies is not an indication for starting any treatment. Case controlled studies have also demonstrated that APL antibodies have a direct bearing in causation of obstetric vasculopathies.[20]

However the study by Infante-Rivard needs a special mention. This study which did not show such an association suffered from a handicap. These workers had included single miscarriage also in their study. It proved two points: 1. Single miscarriages are not associated with APL, and 2. The study got diluted by this inclusion of single miscarriages and therefore became less reliable.[21]

Pathogenesis

The basic problematic nucleus for obstetric vasculopathy is at the fetomaternal interface. As in its alloimmune counterpart, in autoimmune causes of obstetric vasculopathies also the basic mischief occurs at the level of the placenta. In a normal physiological change of pregnancy the trophoblasts invade the maternal spiral arterioles. They destroy the arteriolar intima and replace the endothelial cell lining. Thus there is a conversion of the fetomaternal interface to a low resistance pool of blood which is critical to development of a healthy pregnancy.

Under the effect of APL antibodies these changes do not occur. Instead of destruction of the muscular and elastic tissue by the invading trophoblasts, the vessels get loaded by the immune complex deposits after decidual necrosis. The vascular bed in that case fails to form the low resistance pool of blood. In actuality it becomes a high resistance point Impoverished of effective blood supply. The conceptus fails to get nourished resulting into a series of adverse obstetric outcomes. All these are grouped as obstetric vasculopathies. In early phases of pregnancy there is a miscarriage, in late pregnancy there is IUGR. Besides these the obstetric vasculopathies also include PIH, accidental hemorrhage and fetal death.

Platelets

Having understood the effect of APL antibodies on the vessel walls at fetomaternal interface, it would now be worthwhile examining the role of APL antibodies on other cells and tissues. These effects may not be principally acting to cause obstetric vasculopathies but contribute in some way to same. Amongst these, effect on platelets has been studied in details. It has been found that APL antibodies have no effect on inactivated platelets. But they bind with activated platelets. Phospholipids are found to have been distributed at the platelet cell membranes when activated. This causes a local dysfunction of hemostatic mechanism which is critical for proper placentation and maintenance of normal pregnancy.

Disruption of Thromboxane Prostacyclin Mechanism

For normal caliber and proper perfusion of maternal vascular system a balance between prostacyclin thromboxane activities is critical. During normal pregnancy there is a bias of the balance to tilt towards vasodilatory system prostacyclin. Though some disruption seems to be occurring in the prostacyclin thromboxane balance system in presence of APL antibodies to what extent it produces the consequences of obstetric vasculopathies is a matter of conjecture.

Protein C Activation

One more mechanism by which APL antibodies may be acting is by activation of protein C. This is achieved through a protein present on the vascular endothelium called thrombomodulin. This protein has to be bound to phospholipids for activation of protein C. In some subjects, APL antibodies inhibit this mechanism.

Also for its activity protein C needs a cofactor known as protein S. It has been found that once bound to platelet membranes, the protein C-protein S complex inhibit coagulation factors Va and Xa. This activity is inhibited by APL antibodies. However, this effect has not been consistently found suggesting that it is prevalent only in some subjects with obstetric vasculopathy.

Thus the primary mechanism of APL activity is the action on the vascular bed directly as has been stated in preceding pages. Through this the APL antibodies prevent the destruction of vascular intima and elastin so critical for vascular modulation. At the same time other mechanisms simply act as adjuvants to this main mechanism.

Is there a Crossover between Different APL Antibodies?

It is interesting to note how advances in science refine the understanding of various disease processes. In early and mid 1990s, it was thought that there is a considerable crossover between three main types of APL antibodies of clinical importance viz,

1. ACL antibodies
2. LAC and
3. BFPS antibodies.

However, in early 2000, it was found that such crossover does not exist. Therefore, if a clinician or a scientist wants to investigate a subject of obstetric vasculopathy for autoimmune association, it will be necessary for them to assess both—ACL antibodies as well as LAC in any particular subject. Initially it was thought that only ACL antibody assessment would suffice. But in 2005, it was found that both need to be assessed. In absence of any clinical leads to suspect syphilis assessment of BFPS is not of use in subjects with obstetric vasculopathies.

Interestingly, there is one study that studied midluteal phase uterine artery blood flow through Doppler assessment in nonpregnant women having a history of recurrent spontaneous abortions. It was found that uterine arteries PI values in RSA patients were significantly higher with respect to those found in the control group. When patients were grouped according to the different RSA causes, the highest PI values were found among patients with uterine abnormalities, antiphospholipid antibodies syndrome and unexplained RSA in that order. The authors suggested that increased resistance to uterine blood flow may be an important contributing factor to some causes of RSA and may represent an independent indication of the risk of pregnancy loss.[22]

EMBRYO DECIDUA CROSSTALK IN IMMUNOLOGY OF OBSTETRICS VASCULOPATHY

In the initial years when this concept of crosstalk got afloat in science, it was thought that it is confined only to lower animals and may not be in humans. Over a period of time, it has been found to be universal and therefore very much in human beings also.

IMPLANTATION NOT A RIGHT OF EMBRYO

Just because the fertilization is successful, it is not the right or privilege of the embryo to get implanted. It has to generate a series of changes in the decidua (mother) and in its own self to make it nidable. This is conceptually similar to the phenomenon of sperm capacitation. Capacitation is the one before the last step in the maturation of mammalian spermatozoa and is required to render them competent to fertilize an oocyte. This step is a biochemical event; the sperm move normally and look mature prior to capacitation. In vivo this step typically occurs after ejaculation, in the female reproductive tract. In vitro, capacitation can occur in sperm that have either undergone ejaculation or have been extracted from the epididymis. The uterus aids in the steps of capacitation by secreting sterol binding albumin, lipoproteins, proteolytic and glycosidase enzymes such as heparin. Non-mammalian spermatozoa do not require this capacitation step and are ready to fertilize an oocyte immediately after release from the male. After this capacitation the sperm must undergo activation involving the acrosome reaction. Just because the sperms are deposited in the vagina they do not have a right or a capacity to fertilize the ovum. The sperm has to develop a capacity through the process of capacitation to render its fertilizing potential unmasked. This capacitation takes place predominantly while the sperm travels through a long journey in the cervix through the cervical crypts. This distance is of nearly 2 miles if not more. Even while attempting intrauterine insemination (IUI) the sperms have to be processed in the laboratory. Only after this processing, can the sperm be left in the uterine cavity deep. In absence of this process, it is well known that the success rates of fertilization are negligible. Thus nothing in nature comes by a matter of right. Every phenomenon or to that matter every tissue, organ or cell have to work hard to achieve its fall function.

Coming back to the blastocyst endometrium crosstalk this interesting phenomenon seems to have far reaching bearings on favorable obstetric outcome.

RESULTS OF THE CROSSTALK

As soon as the blastocyst comes into existence, it begins negotiating with different cell linings in the maternal reproductive system to achieve an implantation. The decidua responds to the signals emanating from the blastocyst to bring about a series of changes upon its own self to allow implantation. One of the most significant changes is the activation of progesterone receptors in the luteal phase of the menstrual cycle. This activation is most in the decidua though it seems there may be some amount of activation in other cell linings of the female reproduction system also.

When activated, these receptors have a capacity to bind with DNA and promote transcription.[23] Another change that occurs concurrently as a result of the series of changes at the decidua is the increase in expression of genes of prolactin (PRL) and insulin growth factor binding protein (IGFBP-1). Mak et al investigated the importance of this genetic expression in comparison with autoantibodies. They used monoclonal cardiolipin antibody ID2. It was found that the genetic expression of PRL and IGFBP-1 was markedly reduced in presence of ID2. They used an irrelevant antibody to serve as control. The genetic expression of PRL and IGFBP-1 was markedly reduced only in presence of ID2 and not in presence of the irrelevant antibody. This shows the specific nature of these antibodies to produce the critical changes.[24]

Another interesting phenomenon that occurs in presence of an immunological challenge is defective syncitialization of the decidua. This results in increasing placental apoptosis and impairment of trophoblastic invasion. For a complete and competent placentation, this phenomenon of syncitialization is very important. The trophoblasts invade into the extravascular interstitial segment as well as the endovascular segment of the deciduas. It seems that it is the endovascular infiltration which becomes absent or defective in presence of an autoantibody challenge. The extravascular interstitial segment however remains unaffected. While this is so well demonstrated in the presence of an autoantibody challenge, there is no reason not to apply this even in presence of an alloimmune challenge. One of the manifestations of this was reduction in substances like adrenomedullin. In one study, it was shown that adrenomedullin is decreased in preeclampsia because of failed response to epidermal growth factor and impaired syncitialization.[25] Thus, in presence of an immunological challenge a foundation stone for defective placentation is laid resulting in series of obstetric vasculopathies.

There are three possible mechanisms by which APL antibodies seem to be inhibiting an efficient trophoblastic invasion and syncitialization.

1. By binding to the trophoblastic cell surface or damaging the trophoblasts directly.
2. Binding to the maternal vessels and destroying the generation of a healthy milieu for trophoblast endothelium interaction.
3. Formation of endovascular plugs.

These mechanisms may be acting singly or in combination. Basically to cut the long story short, the trophoblastic invasion and activity becomes defective.

OTHER CONTRIBUTORY MECHANISMS

APL antibodies seem to generate some other changes in vivo to produce hostile environment for the fetus. One of them is failure to block complement activation. Complements like C3 and C4 have been found to play an important role in protecting the host by destroying the foreign graft. In a successful pregnancy implantation and growth, maternal protecting mechanisms need to be blunted. APL antibodies generate such environments that the complement C3 and C4 activation is blunted. Once C3 and C4 get activated the intrauterine environment becomes hostile to the trophoblasts and a destruction of effective trophoblastic invasion occurs. This leads to destruction of the fetal graft. This clinically manifests as missed abortion.

Defective Generation of Syncitiotrophoblasts

Syncitiotrophoblasts are the key trophoblasts that protect the fetus graft from getting rejected. These syncitiotrophoblasts are privileged cell linings that have a series of defense mechanisms that prevent the fetus from getting rejected. One of the ways by which the alloimmune or autoimmune mechanism of obstetric vasculopathies occurs is failure to generate competent syncitiotrophoblasts. As is well known cytotrophoblasts fuse with one another to generate this specialized syncitiotrophoblast lining.

Trophoblast molecules like Integrin and Cadherin have an important role to play in this generation of defective syncitiotrophoblasts. There are two types of Integrins—one that inhibit trophoblastic invasion like In-1 and others that promote trophoblastic invasion like In-5.

Cadherins (named for "calcium dependent adhesion") are a class of Type 1 transmembrane proteins. They play important roles in cell adhesion, ensuring that cells within tissues are bound together. They are dependent on calcium (Ca++) ions to function, hence their name. The cadherin superfamily includes cadherins, protocadherins, desmogleins, and desmocollins, and more. In structure, they share cadherin repeats, which are the extracellular Ca++-binding domains. There are multiple classes of cadherin molecule, each designated with a prefix (in general, noting the type of tissue with which it is associated). It has been observed that cells containing a specific cadherin subtype tend to cluster together to the exclusion of other types, both in cell culture and during development.

Cadherin VE and Cadherin E are two subtypes of the large family of Cadherins that cause an effective fusion of cytotrophoblasts leading to a genesis of competent and effective syncitiotrophoblast. These two cadherin subtypes are believed to have an important role in aggregation, differentiation and subsequent fusion of cytotrophoblasts. These three phenomena subsequently result in generation of effective syncitiotrophoblasts.

It seems that APL antibodies IgG cause a down regulation of VE Cadherin and upregulation of E cadherin. These regulations cause refractoriness to effective Cadherin activity. This ultimately leads to failure of one or all three mechanisms needed for genesis of competent syncitiotrophoblasts.

Incompetent GnRH Activity

Besides the complex link between the immunology and genetics in successful pregnancy outcome, endocrinal components are also having a key role to play in this process of trophoblastic activity. GnRH is the step where immunological failures may be occurring. APL antibodies blunt the GnRH activity thereby disturbing the healthy hormonal milieu that is required for promoting a healthy pregnancy foundation.

Privileged Status of Syncitiotrophoblasts

One of the most intriguing phenomenon that occurs in human body in particular and in the entire living kingdom in general is the phenomenon of reproduction. Further more in this reproduction the array of changes that take place to allow the fetus allograft to be tolerated, kept alive and nourished is still more intriguing and even sometimes a scary phenomenon. Not a single step in this is simple. Offering simplistic explanations to these would amount to bordering inexactitudes.

In the society mothers are supposed to be most loving and most protective about her children. But in the process of reproduction, she consistently and continuously tries to destroy the fetus allograft. This should not come as a surprise because the fetus has immunologically two components—the component from the mother and the component from the father. The immunological fetal component that has been received from the mother is her own. This is innate to her. As a result, she has no problems in tolerating this component. However the paternal component is immunologically alien to her. It is a foreign protein. Universally, foreign proteins invite stormy reactions from the protective systems of the host. This is well-understandable. If foreign proteins enter the body systems and are not quickly eliminated, they can destroy the host. Therefore the host defense system has to generate a series of responses to eliminate it. The paternal immunological component of the fetus is such a foreign protein. It is not treated any differently by the maternal immune systems. The latter tries all its might to eliminate and destroy the alien. However miraculously it may seem the fetus allograft survives.

One of the big roles that are played by a series of actors in this phenomenon is the one that is played by the syncitiotrophoblasts. As is well known these syncitiotrophoblasts are very specialized cells. The cells of cytotrophoblasts merge or fuse with each other to form the syncitiotrophoblasts. Syncitiotrophoblasts have the capacity to shield the fetus from the maternal onslaught. Syncitiotrophoblasts are immunologically very efficient. They can physically resist destruction by the maternal immune responses. Not only this, the syncitiotrophoblasts have an amazing capacity to protects the fetal system and make it grow. This can serve as important lessons for transplant scientists.

The biggest bugbear of transplant science is rejection. Preventing this rejection is a big challenge for them. It is therefore proposed that if the transplant scientists can create artificial syncitiotrophoblast system, the entire rejection phenomenon can be relegated to history. An efficient artificial syncitiotrophoblast system will protect the graft (in transplant sciences a non-allograft). Just as in the reproductive system, the fetal allograft is allowed to survive and even protected by the host (mother) due to syncitiotrophoblasts, on the same lines as the host system will at the least ignore and not eliminate the graft.

Immune diversity between the mother and fetus is very important. The fetus is expected to be immunologically diverse from the mother because of the component it receives from the father. If the fetus is immunologically similar to the mother, the mother will eliminate it. It seems the syncitiotrophoblasts are programmed to protect only immunologically diverse grafts. If the fetus is immunologically distinct from the mother, it will be protected nurtured and made to grow. If it is similar to the mother it will be eliminated.

Syncitiotrophoblasts sense the immunologically different entity of the fetus and mount a protective response. Understandably this immune differentiation of the fetus has its roots in the father. If one step is traced behind one can understand that if the father is immunologically different from the mother, the fetus will also be different. If the father and therefore the fetus are immunologically different, the syncitiotrophoblasts will mount a successful protective response. As a corollary if the mother and the father are immunologically similar the syncitiotrophoblasts will be rendered hypoefficient. They will then fail to mount a protective response and thereby create an elimination of the fetus. This explains the immune rejection in reproduction leading to the clinical entity of fetal demise.

WHAT IS SPONTANEOUS RESOLUTION?

In clinical practice one sees the reality of spontaneous resolutions in subjects with recurrent missed abortions. This is most pronounced in whom once the fetal heart activity is demonstrated and then lost. These are usually immunological losses. There is a need to explain spontaneous resolution at this stage. This is the happening in which the mother who was repeatedly rejecting the fetal allograft just starts tolerating it after a series of immunological losses. Spontaneous resolution is also attributable to the maternal immune system learning to tolerate the fetus. Vaccination science can help understanding this phenomenon of immune tolerance better.

In vaccination science, it is a well-known fact that the first dose generates an attenuated response and needs a booster dose for a complete protective response. In the same way it is possible that the maternal system too learns to tolerate the fetal allograft efficiently in subsequent pregnancies. This results in a favorable outcome after failures due to obstetric vasculopathies. This vaccination model as it can be called may be working in some subjects showing a spontaneous resolution.

Nevertheless in clinical practice it also happens that a subject may have a spontaneous and total resolution in third or fourth pregnancy but again some manifestation of an adverse obstetric outcome in fifth or sixth pregnancy. In one of our studies related to preeclampsia remote from term (an allied vasculopathy to recurrent miscarriages) we found that long-term follow up of these cases showed interesting results—59.8% developed PE in next pregnancy, 24.4% developed PE of severe type, Fetal outcome was consistently poor. There was a high-risk for missed abortions and IUGR. These subjects had very high chances of chronic hypertension.[26]

So why is it that some subjects show adverse obstetric outcomes inspite of a successful pregnancy (spontaneous resolution)? The only possible explanation is that in some subjects, the requirement of booster is repeated. Thus after a successful pregnancy outcome due to the maternal system completely tolerating that pregnancy again the system slips back to a non-protection mode and needs one or more pregnancies to evince one more protective response. In vaccination, declining levels of immune responsiveness is time based. But in human pregnancies with immunological failures, it is not-time based. It means that time between the occurrence of a successful pregnancy outcome and the next pregnancy which fails is not important. In vaccination it is important. It is only on this time factor that booster doses and timings are decided. It, therefore, seems that the vaccination model seems good to understand how maternal systems may learn to tolerate a fetal allograft. Accepted that it is not completely applicable in reproductive immunology, this model however helps to understand the process better and easily.

At the same time, the event of spontaneous resolution is attributed to the generation of efficient syncitiotrophoblast system. In subjects who show an obstetric vasculopathy after a spontaneous resolution, it seems that the key lies in the generation of proficient syncitiotrophoblasts. With every pregnancy there is a generation of new syncitiotrophoblasts. Drawing from the vaccination model, the maternal system may influence in generating an efficient syncitiotrophoblast system once the threshold has been crossed. In such subjects there is no recurrence of obstetric vasculopathies. But in those subjects in whom there is a recurrence, the maternal system has a limited influence or no influence to cause generation of efficient syncitiotrophoblasts. In them obstetric vasculopathies recur even after one successful live birth. In which subject this would occur is not predictable. To what extent does the paternal component of the fetus influences this is also not known.

However, one fact gets solidly crystallized. The syncitiotrophoblasts have a very important role in protecting the conceptus from rejection. Also they have a privileged status enabling them to generate a miracle of paradox.

THE MIRACLE OF PARADOX

Leads to Transplant Scientists

Any miracle if at all it occurs is intriguing and magnificent. Such a paradox is occurring continuously in this process of host-graft interaction. A mother readily tolerates, nourishes and makes the fetus grow. However the mother rejects an implant if the donor of the implant is the father of her child. The fetus (child) has two immunological contributions. One is from the mother which is innate to the maternal system. The other component is received from the father. This is alien to the maternal system. Why then does the mother reject the kidney donated by the father and tolerate the fetus allograft provided by him. Interestingly the physical size of the kidney may be just 1% of the full grown mature fetus still the hundredth time smaller kidney gets rejected coming from the incompatible father but the fetus coming from him is nourished and nurtured. This is the paradox. It becomes further intriguing and amazing as one examines this phenomenon in still further depth.

When the MHC antigens on the mother and the father were studied it was found that more sharing of these antigens better the possibility of the mother accepting the father's kidney. On the other hand more the sharing of the antigens, poorer the chances of the fetus being tolerated. In other words, if the father is immunologically similar to the mother his kidney (or to that matter most other organs) get accepted in the maternal milieu. He is called a compatible donor. However the fetus bearing the immunological contribution from the same compatible father has a much larger chance to get rejected. If there is a HLA-sharing (MHC similarity), the fetus fails to protect itself and the mother fails to nurture the pregnancy. If there is an MHC sharing between the mother and the father the fetus gets rejected but not the father's organs. On the flip side if they are immunologically diverse their organs get rejected but not their fetus.

Concept of Artificial Syncitiotrophoblasts and Organ Transplants

On this basis an exciting proposal can be forwarded. If transplant scientists can create an artificial syncitiotrophoblasts it will solve their problem of immune rejection. Under the protection of artificial syncitiotrophoblasts, the transplanted organ will be transferred into the host. The rejection response mounted by the host will outright be blunted by the artificial syncitiotrophoblast system. Queerly in the human body, diverse the immune systems of the mother and the father lesser are the chances of immune rejection. This means if the parents have less HLA sharing, their chances of having an obstetric vasculopathy are low. On the same lines, if the transplant scientists find the donor and the recipient to be immunologically diverse, they would under the protection of the artificial syncitiotrophoblasts be able to exchange organs better. If two individuals are immunologically similar or compatible, currently they can donate organs to each other but can't tolerate pregnancies from each other. These pregnancies suffer from obstetric vasculopathies. Under the protection of syncitiotrophoblasts they too can sire each other's pregnancies without facing the challenge of immune rejection and clinical manifestations of obstetric vasculopathies.

So for the organ transplant world these artificial syncitiotrophoblasts will protect donated organs from getting rejected. For obstetricians they will prevent pregnancies getting rejected and develop clinical manifestations of obstetric vasculopathies.

REFERENCES

1. Kayaaltı Z, Tekin D, Aliyev V, Yalçın S, Kurtay G, Söylemezoğlu T. Effects of the interleukin-6 (IL-6) polymorphism on toxic metal and trace element levels in placental tissues. *Sci Total Environ.* 2011;409(23): 4929-33.
2. Shimada S, Iwabuchi K, Watano K, Shimizu H, Yamada H, Minakami H, et al. Expression of allograft inflammatory factor-1 in mouse uterus and poly(I:C)-induced fetal resorption. *Am J Reprod Immunol.* 2003;50(1):104-12.
3. Marco-Jiménez F, Naturil-Alfonso C, Jiménez-Trigos E, Lavara R, Vicente J. Influence of zona pellucida thickness on fertilization, embryo implantation and birth. *Anim Reprod Sci.* 2012;132(1-2):96-100.
4. Bell S, Billington W. Anti-fetal allo-antibody in the pregnant female, *Immunol Rev.* 1983;75: 5-30.
   Bell S, Billington W. Humoral immune responses in murine pregnancy. III. Relationship between anti-paternal alloantibody levels in maternal serum, placenta and fetus. *J Reprod Immunol.* 1983;5(5):299-310.
5. Schulz L, Roberts R. Dynamic changes in leptin distribution in the progression from ovum to blastocyst of the pre-implantation mouse embryo. *Reproduction.* 2011; 141(6):767-77.
6. Woodruff M, Anderson N. The effect of lymphocyte depletion by thoracic duct fistula and administration of antilymphocytic serum on the survival of skin homografts in rats. *Ann N Y Acad Sci.* 1964;120: 119-28.
7. Boyon C, Collinet P, Boulanger L, Rubod C, Lucot JP, Vinatier D. Fetal microchimerism. benevolence or malevolence for the mother? *Eur J Obstet Gynecol Reprod Biol.* 2011; 158(2):148-52.
8. Brierley J, Clark D. Characterization of hormone-dependent suppressor cells in the uterus of mated and pseudopregnant mice. *J Reprod Immunol.* 1987;10(3):201-17.

9. Daya S, Clark D, Devlin C, Jarrell J. Preliminary characterization of two types of suppressor cells in the human uterus, *Fertil Steril.* 1985;44(6):778-85.
10. Clark D, Falbo M, Rowley R, Banwatt D, Stedronska-Clark J. Active suppression of host-vs. Graft reaction in pregnant mice. IX. Soluble suppressor activity obtained from allopregnant mouse decidua that blocks the cytolytic effector response to IL-2 is related to transforming growth factor-beta. *J Immunol.* 1988;141(11):3833-40.
11. Tsunawaki S, Sporn M, Ding A, Nathan C. Deactivation of macrophages by transforming growth factor-beta. *Nature.* 1988;334(6179):260-2.
12. McIntyre J, McConnachie P, Taylor C, Faulk WP. Clinical, immunologic, and genetic definitions of primary and secondary recurrent spontaneous abortions. *Fertil Steril.* 1984;42(6):849-55.
13. Milasinović L, Bulatović S, Ilić D, Ivanović L, Zupanski M. Adaptation of the immune system as a response to pregnancy. *Med Pregl.* 2002;55(7-8):305-8.
14. Clark D. The immunology of recurrent abortion. In. John Bonnar, (Ed) *Recent Advances in Obst and Gynecology*. Churchill Livingstone, New York. 1990;16:25-42.
15. Check J, Katsoff B, Summers-Chase D, Breitbart J. A case report supporting the concept that some women have a predisposition for maternal meiosis errors resulting in digyny. *Clin Exp Obstet Gyneco.* 2009;36(2):133-4.
16. Choe J, Check J, Chern R. Septoplasty allows successful delivery in a primary aborter with six previous first trimester miscarriages. *Clin Exp Obstet Gynecol.* 2009;36(1):15-6.
17. Matsuura E, Igarashi Y, Fujimoto M, Ichikawa K, Koike T. Anticardiolipin cofactor(s) and differential diagnosis of autoimmune disease. *Lancet.* 1990;336(8708):177-8.
18. McNeil H, Simpson R, Chesterman C, Krilis S. Antiphospholipid antibodies are directed against a complex antigen that includes a lipid-binding inhibitor of coagulation: beta 2-glycoprotein 1 (apolipoprotein H). *Proc Natl Acad Sci USA.* 1990;87(11):4120-4.
19. Desai P. RSA: Current Concepts. *Indian Jr. Clinical Practice.* 1992;3 (6):13-15.
20. Do Prado A, Piovesan D, Staub H, Horta B. Association of anticardiolipin antibodies with preeclampsia: a systematic review and meta-analysis. *Obstet Gynecol.* 2010; 116(6):1433-43.
21. Infante-Rivard C, David M, Gauthier R, Rivard GE. Lupus anticoagulants, anticardiolipin antibodies, and fetal loss: A case-control study. *N Engl J Med.* 1991;325(15):1063-6.
22. Lazzarin N, Vaquero E, Exacoustos C, Romanini E, Amadio A, Arduini D. Midluteal phase Doppler assessment of uterine artery blood flow in non-pregnant women having a history of recurrent spontaneous abortions: correlation to different etiologies, *Fertil Steril.* 2007;87(6):1383-7.
23. Rai R, Tuddenham E, Backos M, Jivraj S, El'Gaddal S, Choy S, et al. Thromboelastography, whole-blood hemostasis and recurrent miscarriage, *Hum Reprod.* 2003;18(12):2540-3.
24. Mak I, Brosens J, Christian M, Hills F, Chamley L, Regan L, et al. Regulated expression of signal transducer and activator of transcription, Stat5, and its enhancement of PRL expression in human endometrial stromal cells in vitro, *J Clin Endocrinol Metab.* 2002;87(6):2581-8.
25. Hongshi L, Jamal D, Kaufman S, Guilbert J. Adrenomedullin is decreased in preeclampsia because of failed response to epidermal growth factor and impaired syncitialization. *Hypertension.* 2003;42: 895-900.
26. Desai P, Chandrasekhar G, Udvani H H, Hazra M. Preeclampsia of early onset. *Jr of O and G of India.* 1988;38 (5):548.

CHAPTER

4

Endothelial Cell Dysfunction and Obstetric Vasculopathy

CHAPTER OUTLINE

- The Phenomenon of Endothelial Cell Activation
- Endothelial Activation and Prostaglandins
- Plasminogen and Allied Procoagulant Activity—A Manifestation of Endothelial Cell Activation
- Antiphospholipid Antibodies Act through Procoagulant Mechanism
- Endothelial Cell Adhesion Molecule Disturbances
- Components of Fibronectin
- Vascular Endothelial Growth Factor (VEGF)
- Endothelin
- Other Molecules Contributing to Endothelial Cell Activation

INTRODUCTION

One constant feature mentioned in works of all those who have tried to explain the etiopathology of obstetric vasculopathy is endothelial cell dysfunction. Endothelial cells are lining the vascular walls. They are in other words located between the vascular smooth muscles in the vessel wall and the flowing blood column. All secretions and releases from these cells consequently have a direct access to the entire body. In turn they also have vulnerability. Therefore, for all cellular and soluble plasma constituents in circulation, this can include the cytokines, the lipoproteins, platelets and prostaglandins, peroxidized and unperoxidized lipid molecules and all other particles and secretions in circulation. It is estimated that they occupy a surface area of about 1000 m.[1,2]

Due to this strategic location and resultant access to diverse circulating substances, endothelial cells can directly modulate the tone of the vessels. Along with, they also modulate the processes of coagulation and vascular permeability. The vascular tone is maintained by the endothelial cells by striking a balance between the circulating vasodilatory and vasoconstrictive substances. The body needs a potent, well-balanced and well-toned vascular system. This is achieved by modulating the tone of the vessel musculature. As has been previously mentioned blood does not come in direct contact of the vessel wall and therefore is relatively remote from the smooth muscles lining them. Endothelial cells are interceding between the vessel walls and circulating blood column. Therefore, the body has to mediate its actions through endothelial cells.

Amongst the obstetric vasculopathies preeclampsia is one where vascular tone has a very important cause. Vascular tone is maintained in the human body by striking a balance between vasoconstrictive and vasodilatory substances. The most well-known vasoconstrictive substances active in pregnancy and known to science are endothelin and thromboxane A2 (TXA2). Contralatterally, the most potent vasodilatory substances are nitric oxide (NO) and prostacyclin (PGI2).

In the same way as maintaining balance between dilatory and constrictive substances leads to maintaining of vascular tone, the flow of blood without coagulating is maintained by procoagulants and anticoagulants in circulation. The vascular permeability is controlled by endothelial cells by maintaining the tightness of endothelial cell junctions. Excessively weak cell junctions lead to tissue edema as permeability of vessel wall increases. This is seen in obstetric vasculopathies especially in preeclampsia.

THE PHENOMENON OF ENDOTHELIAL CELL ACTIVATION

Endothelial cell activation is a unique phenomenon. It occurs in the endothelial cells when they are subjected to sublethal injury. This activation process is characteristically found in the generation of atherosclerosis in the body. It seems that the phenomenon of endothelial cell activation is different in non-pregnant states than in pregnancy than that in other pathological conditions involving endothelial damage. Pregnancy related endothelial cell activation is typically characterized by higher levels of both coagulation endothelial markers and endothelial activation markers like matrix metalloproteinases (MMPs). In pregnancy, changes in extracellular matrix composition and matrix metalloproteinase activity also occur and promote vascular remodeling but, only in the uterus.[2]

Endothelial cell activation provoked many workers to suggest simplistically that preeclampsia in particular and obstetric vasculopathies in general are a result of transient atherosclerotic process. This was similar to the suggestion that obstetric vasculopathies result from a process of inflammation. However, the two have been found to have only a small but significant contributory role in the entire complex plethora of etiopathology of obstetric vasculopathies. Endothelial cell dysfunction and resultant activation in obstetric vasculopathies results from variety of factors. These include physical shearing forces, hypoxia, or reactive oxygen species or their metabolites and other circulating constituents.[3]

The intense vasospasm generated in preeclampsia can cause the tearing or shearing force on the endothelial cells leading to their activation. The vasospasm understandably generates a hypoxic microenvironment explaining its contribution in the endothelial cell activation. Reactive oxygen species (ROS) as well as their denatured products are abundant in circulation in obstetric vasculopathies. These denatured products include peroxidized LDL and peroxidized VLDL moieties of lipids. All three in summation, the shearing force, hypoxia and circulating oxidized products lead to endothelial cell activation.

The process of endothelial cell activation may occur only at the fetomaternal interface or can occur in the entire maternal vasculature. This depends on the manifestation of obstetric vasculopathy that may be involved in. This could be well-understood in two clinical entities encompassed in obstetric vasculopathies: preeclampsia and IUGR. In preeclampsia this activation of endothelial cells occurs all throughout the body systems and in IUGR it is confined to the fetomaternal interface.

Renal glomerular capillary endotheliosis is one entity where endothelial cell activation takes place in preeclampsia in renal system. This is histologically characterized by swelling of endothelial cytoplasm and obliteration of endothelial fenestre.[1] These are thought to be the best characterized examples of such a lesion.[4-5] Similarly, lesions attributable to endothelial cell activation have been described in other organs of the body of the preeclamptic subject. This includes lesions in the liver, uterus and extrauterine organ systems and tissues.

Circulating Markers of Endothelial Activation

Many markers have been identified in experimental and clinical investigations which are supposed to indicate the endothelial activation process. They have been reported in preeclampsia thus:

- Increased circulating concentration of endothelin-1
- Increased levels of fibronectin in circulation.[6]
- Decreased levels of circulating vasodilator prostacyclin.[7]
- Increased levels of circulating thrombomodulin.[8]

ENDOTHELIAL ACTIVATION AND PROSTAGLANDINS

Prostaglandins are acknowledged as markers of endothelial cell activation. During normal pregnancy, there is a very important balance between vasodilatory prostaglandins like thromboxane with vasodilatory prostaglandins like prostacyclin. All throughout pregnancy the bias of the female pregnant body is towards the prostacyclin. However, during obstetric vasculopathies, this bias is lost. Prostacyclin production is tilted against prostacyclin. It has been found that the plasma urinary secretion of prostacyclin is reduced in preeclampsia.[7]

This altered prostaglandin production is due to the circulating peroxidized lipid molecules in preeclampsia. Denatured lipids directly affect the cyclooxygenase pathway that is so critical in generating prostaglandins from arachidonic acid. Placentas from subjects with obstetric vasculopathies are known to produce more thromboxane and peroxidized lipids when compared with normal placenta. The entire pathophysiology of production and circulation of lipid peroxides is discussed in great details in chapter 5. It seems that endothelial cell activation is one of the resultant insults of this etiopathology.

On the other hand, endothelial cell activation is not the only change contributing to the etiopathology of preeclampsia. The cellular and chemical manifestation of this process provides many useful markers in the prediction of obstetric vasculopathies and its allied adverse obstetric outcomes. It seems that endothelial cell activation following a series of sublethal injuries provide the ROS needed for the process of lipid peroxidation that is taking place in the intercellular matrix. If this entire etiopathology is to be summarized at this stage it could be done.

Functional slowing of maternal blood pool at fetomaternal interface and endothelial cell activation occurs concurrently. The VLDL and dense small lipid particles of LDL have a tendency to walk in and out of the intercellular matrix. In the eventuality of the process of endothelial cell activation, when the lipids walk into the intercellular matrix they come in close contact of the ROS released by the activated endothelial cells. These ROS then peroxidize or in simpler terms denature the lipid particles. The lipid particles that are so denatured when go back to the circulation serve as agents of free radicals. Wherever the denatured lipids go they activate the endothelial cells and at the same time and initiate the cyclooxygenase pathway alterations in such a way that the thromboxane release is increased. This leads to vasospasm and resultant clinical manifestations of obstetric vasculopathies.

PLASMINOGEN AND ALLIED PROCOAGULANT ACTIVITY—A MANIFESTATION OF ENDOTHELIAL CELL ACTIVATION

Any cell is a complete structure with a series of life sustaining and protecting mechanisms in place for its survival. Sublethal injuries that lead to endothelial cell activation therefore expectedly produce a plethora of other changes and releases. One of these is a release of plasminogen proteins and plasminogen activation. It is well-known from basic human physiology that plasminogen is one of the final critical steps that subsequently leads to formation of plasmin. This plasmin is necessary for the ultimate formation of a coagulum or a thrombus.

Endothelial cell activation leads to plasminogen activator inhibitor type 1 (PAI-1) to increase. In normal pregnancies uncomplicated by obstetric vasculopathies, PAI-1 is actually reduced at the fetomaternal interface. Thus, the bias towards reduced local thrombosis and good quality of blood circulation is established. Increase in PAI-1 has been well documented in obstetric vasculopathies.[9] Circulating levels of PAI-1 were found to be directly correlated with the severity of obstetric vasculopathies.[10]

ANTIPHOSPHOLIPID ANTIBODIES ACT THROUGH PROCOAGULANT MECHANISM

In a wide spectrum of immunological causes of adverse obstetric vasculopathies, antiphospholipid antibodies were identified very early to be one of the causes. Antiphospholipid antibodies are acting through their procoagulant action. There are other procoagulant molecules that have also been subsequently identified to be acting through this mechanism. In a series of obstetric vasculopathy leading to preeclampsia remote from term, 25% women had functional protein S deficiency, 18% demonstrated hyperhemocystenemia and 29% had detectable levels of antiphospholipid antibodies.[11] Increased expressions of other procoagulant proteins have been reported. These include the likes of von Willebrand's factor, platelet activating factor, ß-thromboglobulin, cellular fibronectin and thrombomodulin. These are used to differentiate preeclampsia of obstetric vasculopathy origin from preeclampsia of other causes.[12,6]

Factors that produce hypercoagubility are hyperhemocystenemia, anticardiolipin antibodies, and increased levels of procoagulant proteins like tissue proteins, von Willebrand's factor and the like. Of the several relevant endothelial cell associated anticoagulant proteins like antithrombin III, protein C, and protein S are reduced. These substances are anticoagulants. Reduction in their expression reduces an anticoagulant environment. This by default produces hypercoagulant state.

In summary, therefore, these agents get functionally affected or lead to endothelial cell activation. These in turn produce an imbalance of pro and anticoagulation milieu in a pregnant subject in favor of procoagulants. This subsequently leads to the activation of the entire cycle of etiopathology of obstetric vasculopathy. The molecules like antiphospholipid antibodies can directly activate the endothelial cells at the fetomaternal interface very early in pregnancy. They generate their clinical effects therefore very early leading to fetal demise and subsequent miscarriage.

ENDOTHELIAL CELL ADHESION MOLECULE DISTURBANCES

The process of endothelial cell activation following sublethal injury leads to a series of changes at the fetomaternal interface as well as in the entire maternal vasculature. Procoagulation to anticoagulation balance getting disturbed in favor of procoagulation has been examined in the preceding section (P***). One more change that occurs due to endothelial cellular activation is the release or activation of some specific cell adhesion molecules. Two principle cell molecules that have been identified are fibronectin and van Willebrand's factor.

Fibronectin molecule ultrastructure alteration gives a valuable insight resulting from endothelial cell activation. Fibronectin molecules remain in extracellular matrix very close to the endothelial cells. Their ultrastructure study reveals that they have a fibrillar structure. Under the process of endothelial cell activation this fibrillar structure gets disturbed or distorted. Due to this distortion there is a loss of a chemotryptic protease-sensitive isotope. It precipitates a loss of fibronectin fibrillar structure.

The loss of fibronectin fibrillar structure leads to activation of neutrophils which in turn leads to amplified destruction of fibronectin fibrillar structure. Thus an amplified and amplifying vicious circle is generated. Endothelial cell activation, besides leading to fibronectin ultrastructure disturbance also leads to proactive secretion of fibronectin and molecules like von Willebrand's factor from the activated endothelial cells.

The process of active secretion of these molecules provides the supply chain of fibronectin to the fire of endothelial cell activation by Interleukin-1. This sets the stage of further generation of the same vicious cycle causing stepwise cascading effect snowballing into a full blown reaction. The constant supply of fibronectin that is required to sustain this cycle is provided by the activated endothelial cells. This is how the process is activated, maintained and amplified. In reality, the activated endothelial cells are not releasing fresh fibronectin for maintaining this vicious cycle. Infact fibronectin is getting secreted for restoring. However, on ground zero this has a totally reverse result. On ground zero it adds fuel to fire.

The fresh supply of fibronectin inadvertently starts providing raw material to sustain the vicious cycle.

Besides these pathophysiological consequences, alteration in fibronectin levels serves as a useful marker for endothelial injury. Elevated fibronectin means active vicious circle. Active vicious circle means there is endothelial injury and resultant cell activation.[13]

There are some allied observations on fibronectin. The majority of fibronectin in circulation is a result of hepatocytes.[14] The correlation of stasis in circulation of blood with increased fibronectin is of important pathophysiological consequence. Vascular flow impediment and stasis is critical for the generation of denatured lipid molecules. Helping actively in this is the vasospasm found so consistently and globally in obstetric vasculopathies.

One more phenomenon which has been found to increase fibronectin is hypoxia. Hypoxia is also a very important feature of obstetric vasculopathy. It, therefore, seems apparent that all significant events that produce obstetric vasculopathies and sustain them lead to increase fibronectin levels.

COMPONENTS OF FIBRONECTIN

With multiple sources of fibronectin becoming obvious it is quite possible that the total mass of fibronectin may reflect these molecules from heterogeneous sources. These heterogeneous sources could be shedding off from hepatocytes, vascular stasis as well as hypoxia. The total mass is also having a contribution from the active secretion by activated endothelial cells. Luckily these heterogeneous contributors to fibronectin have different isomers of fibronectin. The cellular fibronectin (cFN) expresses two extra domains of fibronectin – ED-A and ED-B. This ED-A fibronectin is non-hepatic in origin.

Therefore, when one assesses ED-A, it shows fibronectin that has been released by the process of endothelial cell activation. Thus assessment of ED-A fibronectin is more sensitive marker for the endothelial cell activation process. Increase levels of ED-A fibronectin means endothelial cell activation. Lockwood and Peters demonstrated that ED-A cellular fibronectin increase precedes development of preeclampsia. Therefore, the potential of using this component for predicting obstetric vasculopathies is very high. Robert Taylor and James Roberts (1) have further qualified the utility of cellular fibronectin in differentiating hypertensive disorders of pregnancy. They have demonstrated that increase in cellular fibronectin especially the ED-A is increased in preeclampsia as a component of obstetric vasculopathy.

Contrastingly, cellular fibronectin is not increased in other forms of hypertension found in pregnancy. This includes hypertension without proteinuria and/or edema as well as hypertension where there was no maternal or fetal morbidity. Not only these observations prove the sensitivity of cellular fibronectin in predicting preeclampsia but also help in differentiation of the types of hypertensive disorders of pregnancy. It also has the potential to predict maternal and fetal outcome by differentiating the subtypes of hypertensive disorders of pregnancy.

VASCULAR ENDOTHELIAL GROWTH FACTOR (VEGF)

While we are on predicting preeclampsia and differentiating the types of hypertensive disorders of pregnancy, it was perceived that VEGF levels should alter in preeclampsia is edema and proteinuria. Both of these are a result of increased vascular permeability. Increased vascular permeability is dependent on VEGF also known as vascular permeability factor. It is VEGF that plays an important role in increasing the vascular permeability in preeclampsia. Understandably therefore VEGF levels are expected to be elevated in preeclampsia. Considerably higher levels of VEGF have indeed been demonstrated by Cooper JC et al.[15]

Further detailing of this increase in VEGF was done to identify the source. Cooper JC et al[16] have studied the placental VEGF-mRNA levels. These were found to be decreased in preeclampsia. This proves that VEGF in preeclampsia is not of placental origin and is of maternal vascular in origin. VEGF levels rapidly increased when retinal epithelial cells were exposed to molecules of oxidative stress like superoxide or hydrogen peroxides.[17] This goes on to prove that VEGF is maternal vasculature in origin and is sensitive to oxidative stress.

Clinical Bearing

There is a very important clinical bearing of the finding that VEGF is essentially non-placental in origin. Obstetric vasculopathies wherein the etiopathology is confined to the placenta there is no clinical edema is found in IUGR and abruptio placenta the latter when not associated with preeclampsia. In both of these, there is clinically no edema. VEGF also known as vascular permeability factor gets essentially released by the activated endothelial cells of maternal vasculature. Therefore, in conditions where the maternal vasculature endothelial cells are not involved, there is no increase in vascular permeability as a result there are no clinical feature of edema. In clinical practice there is a belief that if preeclampsia is not accompanied by edema and only with proteinuria, it is a grave combination. This also seems to be a clinical myth from the behavior of VEGF. The circulating levels of VEGF are not increased by worsening preeclampsia. Also, no correlation is found between the levels of VEGF and obstetric outcome in preeclampsia. This proves that VEGF cannot be used to prognosticate preeclampsia.

ENDOTHELIN

One more circulating protein in preeclampsia is endothelin. Endothelin has different subtypes. The subtype Endothelin-1 (ET-1) is the most potent vasoconstrictor in human pregnant subject ET-1 like all forms of endothelin is released by the activated endothelial cells. However, it is of interest to know that ET-1 is not found in circulation before preeclampsia becomes clinically evident. Therefore, ET-1 has no predictive value. This is in contrast to protein like fibronectin which are able to predict preeclampsia.

Also, ET-1 is not found to have a placental origin. This characteristic of ET-1 is similar to VEGF. In one study, ET-1 levels were studied in blood from uterine vein and antecubital vein. The former indicates blood from placental origin and the latter from general vascular bed. It was found that ET-1 levels were distinctly higher in the antecubital blood. However, they were negligible in blood from uterine vein.[18] This proves that the source of ET-1 is non-placental. Maternal endothelial cells when sublethally injured and activated, release ET-1. Placenta has no role to play in this. It is consequently possible that thromboxane that is released due to endothelial activation and resultant lipid peroxidation initiates the vasospasm in obstetric vasculopathy. The origin of increase in thromboxane is both placental and non-placental. Therefore, the vasospasm generated at fetomaternal interface is attributable to thromboxane-prostacyclin balance getting tipped in favor of thromboxane. However for subsequent maintenance and even amplification of the process of vasospasm ET-1 steps in. It generates vasospasm in the entire maternal vessel bed and produces its clinical complications and manifestations of preeclampsia.

Two interesting studies need to be interpreted with caution as regards ET-1 is concerned. Kubota et al[19] showed that expression of ET-1 mRNA is increased in villous placenta from women with preeclampsia. Also, Genbacev et al[20] demonstrated that villi cultured in hypoxic conditions in-vitro mimic the cellular changes noted in preeclampsia. However in subjects of preeclampsia the expression of ET-1 mRNA in placenta remains dormant. It does not engineer the synthesis of ET-1. Also, the in vitro studies of hypoxically cultured villi elaborating ET-1 seems not to be occurring in pregnant subjects in any significant or notable amount. In clinical practice, ET-1 remains essentially non-placental in origin and probably has an amplification role in vasospasm in preeclampsia in the maternal vasculature.

OTHER MOLECULES CONTRIBUTING TO ENDOTHELIAL CELL ACTIVATION

While the discussion is focused on endothelial cell activation it will be relevant to examine other contributors to the orchestra that also directly or indirectly cause endothelial cell activation. It is being described as an orchestra because it is not a chain of events that produce endothelial cell activation. It activity of these activators in quick succession that lead to endothelial cell activation. While many such molecules have been identified, it is possible that these may not be the only ones. There may be still some unknown molecules to medical science which also may be contributing to the process of decidual cell activation. Admittedly, the biggest player in this game is the oxidized lipid molecules, LDL. Even amongst the LDL the dense low molecular weight LDL molecules have been found to be the principle game player in this entire process.
The others are described as under:

Immunological Antibodies

Immunological basis of obstetric vasculopathies have been discussed at length in chapter 3. Amongst these immunologically active molecules the antiphospholipid antibodies are causing direct endothelial cell activation. Elevated levels of IgG and IgM antibodies have been consistently reported in women with preeclampsia remote from term. It is worthwhile nothing that a separate evaluation of IgG and IgM antibodies does not have any clinical significance especially in regards to antiphospholipid antibodies. The two only indicate the avidity of these antibodies but have no clinical bearing different from each other.

Cytokines

Cytokines have caught the attention of investigators in this aspect of science of obstetric vasculopathies since a very long time. A series of such "destructive" cytokines have been identified which are also causing endothelial cell activation. The principle player in this family is TNF-α (Tumor Necrosis Factor-α).

Formed Elements in Blood

A series of cellular components of blood have also been found to play important role in the process of decidual cell activation. These include:

- Platelets
- Neutrophils
- Placenta membrane micro vesicles.

Toxins

Historically preeclampsia was called pre-eclamptic toxemia or even plain and simple toxemia. This was with a presumption that by whatever mechanism some toxins are released by the placenta leading to development of preeclampsia. It was subsequently disproved as no such toxin was identified into circulation of pre-eclamptic women. This led to change in name from preeclamptic toxemia to plain and simple preeclampsia. However, inspired by those early presumptions some groups of workers do indulge in the activity of identifying or at least searching for the ever elusive toxin. Such efforts have also been made in the possible agents ("toxins") that might be causing decidual or maternal vascular endothelial cell activation.

Metallothionein has been proposed as a toxic factor which may be causing endothelial cell activation.[1] However, there are more questions than answers to this metallothionein and its action on the endothelium. It is believed that this agent metallothionein binds with circulating cadmium to produce a complex. It is stated that manifestations of cadmium toxicity leads to a syndrome similar to preeclampsia.[21] It is being flaunted as the possible but hitherto elusive toxin that produced "pre-eclamptic toxemia". By and large results on this are inconclusive.

Besides these heavy metals, another contributor to endothelial cell activation process is calcium. Clinical research has shown that calcium supplementation reduced the incidence of preeclampsia.[22] However, these were not proved consistently.[23] It was however found that supplementing calcium does not reduce preeclampsia universally. It reduces preeclampsia only in communities where dietary intake of calcium is low. But this inconsistency in results vis-à-vis occurrence of preeclampsia in relation to calcium drives a conclusion that the role of calcium deficiency in endothelial activation is at best inconsistent.

However, there is no denial of the fact that endothelial cell activation has a big role to play in obstetric vasculopathies. It is caused and influenced by many factors. Understanding the complexity of the factor and the intricacies of the process of endothelial activation can hold the key to the treatment of obstetric vasculopathies.

Angiogenic Factors

One review addresses translational aspects of preeclampsia by synthesizing information on preeclampsia pathogenesis, describing diagnostic biomarkers that predict disease, and suggesting strategies to lessen adverse outcomes. The review feels that key to this understanding is the role of cardiotonic bufodienolides, with marinobufagenin (MBG) as the prototype, and angiogenic factors in preeclampsia pathogenesis. Data from a rat model believed to mimic human preeclampsia show that urinary excretion of MBG increases before the onset of hypertension and proteinuria and that affected animals have an increased vascular leakage and blood brain barrier permeability. Angiogenic imbalance occurs with the onset of the syndrome in this model. Also, this review reports that MBG levels in preeclampsia patients exceed those in normal pregnancy and that angiogenic factors are altered in patients showing signs and symptoms of overt disease. In vitro administration of MBG inhibits cytotrophoblast function and triggers hyperpermeability in endothelial cell monolayers. This review advances the hypotheses that MBG precedes preeclampsia; MBG causes disruption of tight junction proteins leading to vascular leak via activation of MAPK which triggers apoptotic mechanisms resulting in further endothelial dysfunction leading to edema with the release of angiogenic factors. This review provides new evidence about the role of MBG and vasoactive intermediates in preeclampsia pathogenesis including the neurologic sequelae and may reveal new therapeutic targets for the prevention of preeclampsia complications.[24] This requires further investigations.

REFERENCES

1. Taylor R, Roberts J. Endothelial Cell Dysfunction. In: *Chesley's Hypertensive Disorders of Pregnancy,* Lindheimer M, Roberts J, Cunningham F (eds). Ct. 2nd Edn. Stamford, Appleton and Lange: Pg 395-430.
2. Slavik L, Prochazkova J, Prochazka M, Simetka O, Hlusi A, Ulehlova J. The pathophysiology of endothelial function in pregnancy and the usefulness of endothelial markers. *Biomed Pap Med Fac Univ Palacky Olomouc Czech Repub.* 2011;155(4):333-7.
3. de Groot C, Taylor R. New insights into the etiology of preeclampsia, *Ann Med.* 1993; 25(3):243-9.
4. Bell ET. Renal Lesions in the toxemias of pregnancy. *Am J Pathol.* 1932;8(1):1-42.
5. Schneider C. The active principle of placental toxin; thromboplastin; its inactivator in blood; antithromboplastin. *Am J Physio.* 1947;149(1):123-9.
6. Taylor R, Crombleholme W, Friedman S. High plasma cellular levels correlate with biochemical and clinical features of preeclampsia but cannot be attributed to hypertension alone. *Am J Obstet Gynecol.* 1991;165: 895-901.
7. Remuzzi G, Marchesi D, Zoja C, Muratore D, Mecca G, Misiani R, et al. Reduced umbilical and placental vascular prostacyclin in severe preeclampsia. *Prostaglandins.* 1980;20(1):105-10.

8. Hsu C, Iriye B, Johnson T, Witter F, Hong S, Chan D. Elevated circulating thrombomodulin in severe preeclampsia eclampsia. *Am J Obstet Gynecol.* 1993; 169(1):148-9.
9. Paidas M, Haut M, Lockwood C. Platelet disorders in pregnancy: implications for mother and fetus. *Mt Sinai J Med.* 1994;61(5):389-403.
10. Shaarawy M, Didy H. Thrombomodulin, plasminogen activator inhibitor type 1 (PAI-1) and fibronectin as biomarkers of endothelial damage in preeclampsia and eclampsia. *Int J Gynecol Obstet.* 1996;55(2):135-9.
11. Dekker G, de Vries J, Doelitzsch P, Huijgens P, von Blomberg B, Jakobs C. Underlying disorders associated with severe early-onset preeclampsia. *Am J Obstet Gynecol.* 1995; 173(4):1042-8.
12. Hsu C, Copel A, Hong S, Chan D. Thrombomodulin levels in preeclampsia, gestational hypertension and chronic hypertension. *Obstet Gynecol.* 1995;86(6):897-9.
13. Forsyth K, Levinsky R. Fibronectin degradation; an in vitro model of neutrophil mediated endothelial cell damage. *J Pathol.* 1990;161(4):313-9.
14. Hynes RO. The role of fibronectin in cellular behavior. *Results Probl Cell Differ.* 1980; 11:112-23.
15 Cooper J, Sharkey A, McLaren J, Charnock-Jones D, Smith S. Localization of vascular endothelial growth factor and its receptor, FLt, in human placenta and decidua by immunohistochemistry. *J Reprod Fertil.* 1995;105(2):205-13.
16. Cooper J, Sharkey A, Charnock-Jones D, Palmer C, Smith S. VEGF mRNA levels in placentae from pregnancies complicated by preeclampsia. *Br J Obstet Gynecol.* 1996; 103(12):1191-6.
17. Kuroki M, Voest E, Amano S, Beerepoot L, Takashima S, Tolentino M. Reactive oxygen intermediates increase vascular endothelial growth factor expression in vitro and in vivo. *J Clin Invest.* 1996;98(7):1667-75.
18. Rust O, Bofill J, Zappe D, Hall J, Burnett J Jr, Martin J Jr. The origin of endothelin-1 in patients with severe preeclampsia. *Obstet Gynecol.* 1997;89(5 Pt 1):754-7.
19. Kubota T, Kamada S, Hirata Y, Eguchi S, Imai T, Marumo F et al. Synthesis and release of endothelin-1 by human decidual cells. *J Clin Endocrinol Metab.* 1992;75(5):1230-4.
20. Genbacev O, Joslin R, Damsky C, Polliotti B Fisher SJ. Hypoxia alters early gestation human cytotrophoblast differentiation/invasion in vitro and models the placental defects that occur in preeclampsia. *J Clin Invest.* 1996;97(2):540-50.
21. Chisolm J, Handorf C. Further observations on the etiology of preeclampsia: mobilization of toxic cadmium-metallothionein into the serum during pregnancy. *Med Hypotheses.* 1996;47(2):123-8.
22. Purwar M, Kulkarni H, Motghare V, Dhole S. Calcium supplementation and prevention of pregnancy induced hypertension. *J Obstet Gynaecol Res.* 1996;22(5):425-30.
23. Levine R, Hauth J, Curet L, Sibai B, Catalano P, Morris C J. Trial of calcium to prevent preeclampsia. *N Engl J Med.* 1997;337(2):69-76.
24. Uddin M, Allen S, Jones R, Zawieja D, Kuehl T. Pathogenesis of preeclampsia: marinobufagenin and angiogenic imbalance as biomarkers of the syndrome. *Transl Res.* 2012;160(2):99-113.

CHAPTER

5

Oxidative Stress and Obstetric Vasculopathies

CHAPTER OUTLINE

- What is Oxidative Stress
- Our Basic Study
- What is a Free Radical
- Oxidative Stress and Health
- The Mischief of Free Radicals in Vascular Walls
- Lipid Peroxides: The Agents of Oxidative Stress
- Lipid Metabolism in Normal Pregnancy and its Bearings in Abnormal Pregnancy
- Placental Lipid Peroxidation
- Clinical Manifestations
- Reperfusion
- Innate Maternal Reducing Systems
- The Family of Free Radicals
- Vascular Endothelium and Oxidative Stress
- Inefficient Second Wave of Trophoblastic Invasion
- Nitric Oxide in Obstetric Vasculopathy
- Placental Atherosis in Obstetric Vasculopathy
- Extracellular Reducing Systems
- Exercise and Prevention of Obstetric Vasculopathies
- Treatment Bearings

INTRODUCTION

Over a period of years obstetric vasculopathies have slowly but surely started showing evidences of a strong association with oxidative stress. The entire gamut of immunological challenge in obstetric vasculopathies gets transferred from etiology to etiopathogenesis. By this it is meant that while immunological challenge lays the basis of obstetric vasculopathies, their clinical manifestations occur due to oxidative stress.

WHAT IS OXIDATIVE STRESS?

Oxidative stress is a phenomenon in which the free radical seeks its balancing partner. This balancing partner—the reducing systems help to stabilize and promote health. In absence of getting effectively neutralized by the reducing systems, free oxygen radicals remain un-neutralized and cause widespread changes leading the different clinical manifestations of obstetric vasculopathies.

OUR BASIC STUDY[1]

- We carried out a systematic evaluation of pro-oxidants and antioxidants in preeclampsia to serve as a basis for our understanding of this disease process
- It confirmed oxidative stress in normal pregnancy and in preeclampsia.
- Natural endogenous antioxidant enzymes activity is enhanced significantly against this oxidative stress, to maintain the state of equilibrium in favor of antioxidant defense
- However in preeclampsia, the antihypertensive therapy showed little change in oxidative stress and like normal pregnancy, body still maintained increased antioxidant enzyme activity
- This indicates that though the antihypertensives may reduce the effect of oxidative stress, they cannot stop the cause of it
- This study proved as the basic first step for us in understanding of this disease process.

WHAT IS A FREE RADICAL?

Each atom has in itself a set numbers of protons effectively balanced by an equal number of electrons. Positively charged subatomic particles, the protons get balanced against the negatively charged electrons (Fig 5.1). However free radicals also known as reactive oxygen species (ROS) are atoms that have an un-neutralized electron (Fig 5.2). They have an extra electron or one proton less. On the other hand, the reducing systems are atoms that have an unbalanced electron. It is, therefore, understandable that a free radical can be like an un-neutralized powerful force. The reducing systems that have an extra or un-neutralized proton provide that electron to the free radical thereby neutralizing it (Fig 5.3). If not effectively and timely neutralized free radicals can produce extensive changes

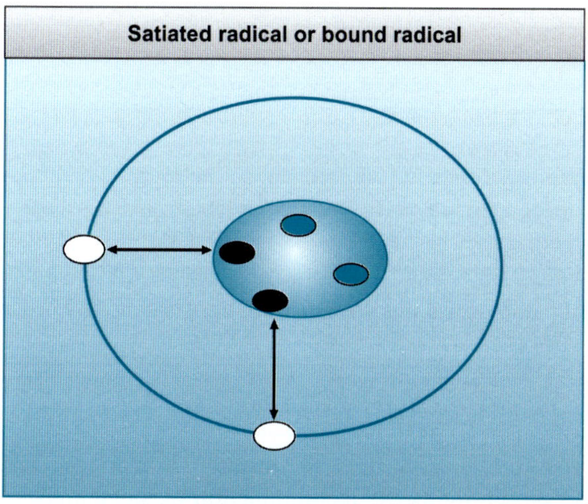

Fig 5.1: Subatomic structure of a bound or balanced atom. Each proton and electron are balanced against each other

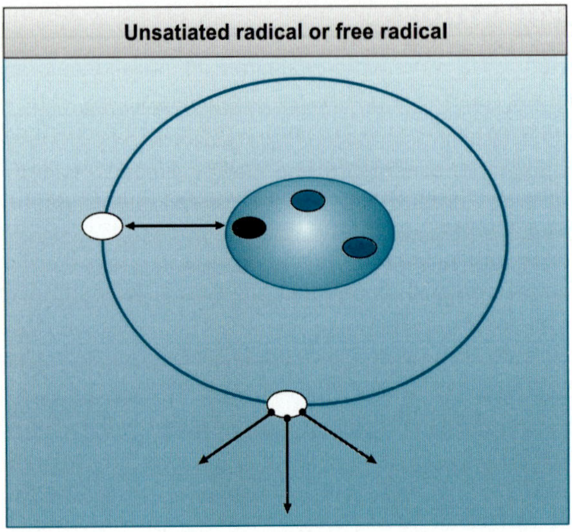

Fig. 5.2: Subatomic structure of a free radical. The electron is unpaired

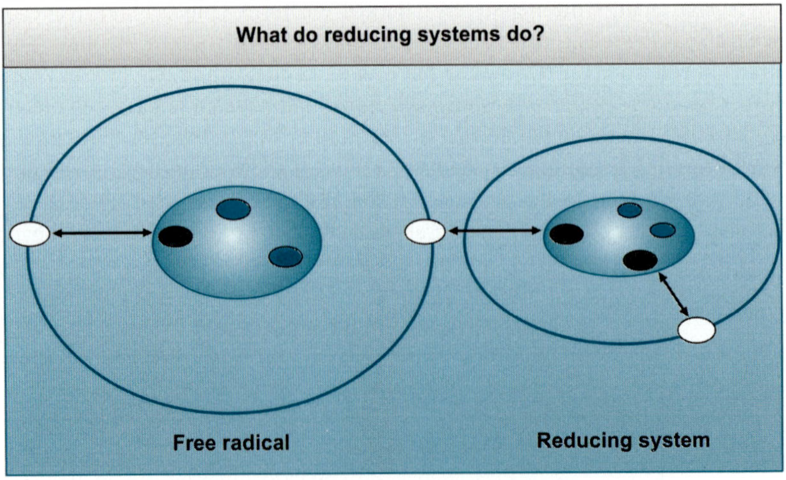

Fig 5.3: The reducing radical which has an extra proton balances it against the unpaired electron of a free radical

and a series of pathological manifestations. These are disease processes as a result of oxidative stress.

OXIDATIVE STRESS AND HEALTH

Not all processes of oxidative stress are resulting in a disease. Infact some of the complex processes in the body like elimination of metabolites of digestion and removal of dead cells like RBCs and gastric mucosal cells occurs by oxidative free radicals. Very important detoxicating and so called "cleansing" mechanisms of the liver are dependent on free radicals for their successful occurrence. Whilst the body uses the free radical systems to remove the dead tissues and toxic wastes from the body, the effect of this is maintenance of health. By eliminating results of catabolic processes in the body reducing systems maintain many health mechanisms in the body.

This becomes a challenge for therapeutic reducing systems. Therapeutic reducing systems should therefore act in such a way that they counteract only the diseases process which are resulting from oxidative stress. They should not counteract the health promoting oxidative processes. If a reducing system is going to affect both the disease creating mechanisms as well as the health promoting ones, the body would blunt their action. As a result an ideal reducing system would be one that is having no effect on health promoting mechanisms and selectively act only on disease processes. But like any ideal this remains an elusive dream as of now. This explains the lack of consistent treatment response to reducing systems in clinical practice for management of obstetric vasculopathies.

THE MISCHIEF OF FREE RADICALS IN VASCULAR WALLS

As expected, obstetric vasculopathies have their principal nodal activity at the fetomaternal vascular bed. In this interface the basic oxidative stress is generated. The harbinger of this stress is the complex immune interaction between the mother trying to reject the fetus and the fetal systems principally the trophoblast resisting the rejection. This rejection takes place through oxidative stress. A successful rejection leads to full blown fetal demise. In the eventuality of maternal rejection if completely and successfully neutralized by the fetus it leads to a healthy live baby at the other end of the spectrum. Intermediates are other manifestations of obstetric vasculopathies like IUGR, preeclampsia, accidental hemorrhage and probably even some of the preterm births.

The intercellular matrix in the fetomaternal vascular interface is the hot bed of generation of free radicals or ROS. This is the point of maximum activity. It can be compared to the training camps for terrorists. This is the point where free radicals bring about a series of changes which subsequently lead to obstetric vasculopathies.

LIPID PEROXIDES: THE AGENTS OF OXIDATIVE STRESS

Free radicals or ROS themselves do not have the numbers or the capacity to go through the entire maternal vasculature to cause maternal manifestations of obstetric vasculopathies. They need agents which are more universally distributed, readily available and have the capacity to get denatured to produce the changes that ROS want from them. The best agents which are available in the human body are lipid lipoproteins. It is very well-known that lipoproteins are of different densities:

A. The HDL: High density lipoproteins
B. The LDL: Low density lipoproteins and
C. The VLDL: Very low density lipoproteins

The LDL and VLDL are so configured that they have a tendency to go near and sink into the vascular cell linings. In early pregnancy there is a preponderance of HDLs in the circulation. As a result the lipid goblets are not able to sink within the intercellular matrix. With advancing normal pregnancy and in abnormal (vasculopathic) early pregnancy, the lipid distribution changes in favor of LDLs and VLDLs who sink closer to the intercellular matrix (Figs 5.4 and 5.5). Once

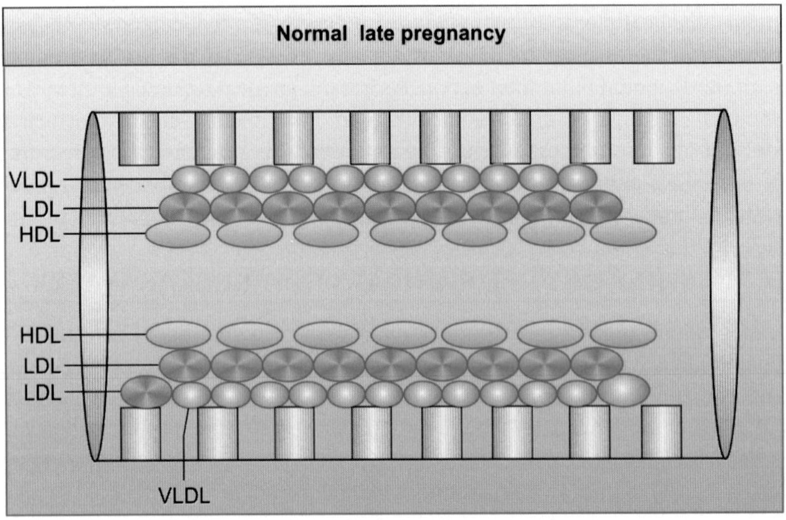

Fig 5.4: Disposition of fat globules during normal late pregnancy. The LDL and VLDL are closer to the cell wall

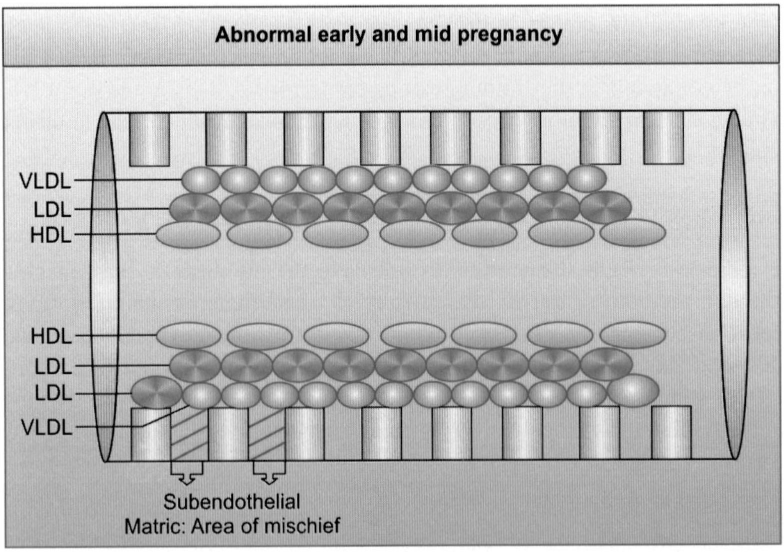

Fig. 5.5: Disposition of fat globules during abnormal early and mid pregnancy when vasculopathic process is on. The LDL and VLDL are closer to the cell wall

they are here the free radicals pounce on them to denature them (Fig 5.6). However for this to occur there is some need for the blood stream to slow down. This is brought about by the innate tendency of genetically susceptible women to have a minimal vasospasm. These are transient occurrences and occur intermittently. On their own, these vascular impendence tendencies do not have the capacity to produce significant clinical manifestations.

Nonetheless they effectively impede the vascular flow to give the time and opportunity to the VLDL and LDL molecules to sink to the intercellular matrix. Once they are in the matrix the ROS are readily available and waiting to denature them producing lipid peroxidation. As soon as the vascular impedance of transient nature is relieved the denatured lipid peroxides are flushed into the system during reperfusion (Fig 5.7). Wherever they go they bring about a tilt in prostacyclin-thromboxane balance. The balance is tipped towards thromboxane producing a vasospasm. It is universally known that the principal and most consistent change universally seen in obstetric vasculopathies is vasospasm and the genesis of vasospasm is a result of the ROS-lipid peroxidation.

LIPID METABOLISM IN NORMAL PREGNANCY AND ITS BEARINGS IN ABNORMAL PREGNANCY

The dyslipidemia of obstetric vasculopathy is best understood by understanding the normal lipid changes in physiology of pregnancy. Lipids are carried into circulation primarily as lipoproteins which are composed primarily of free and esterified lipid proteins also known as apolipoprotein and phospholipids.[2] The two

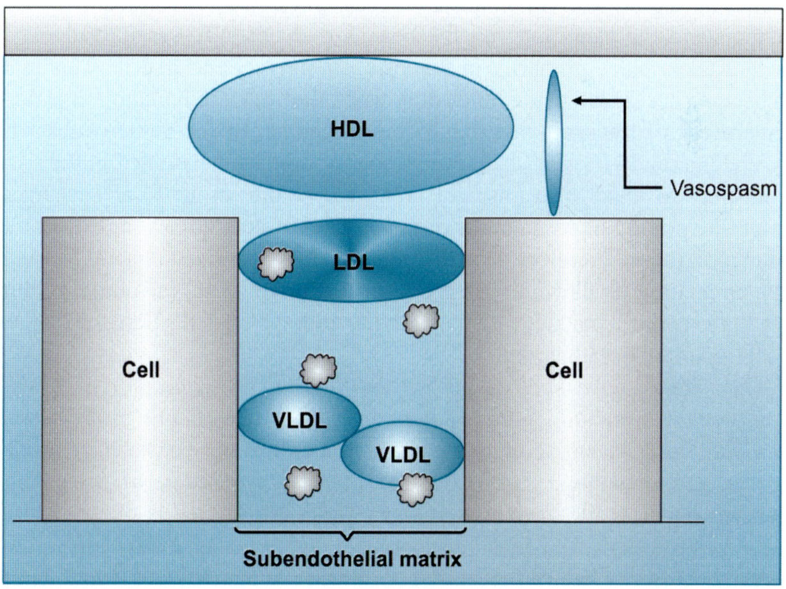

Fig. 5.6: Changes in the intercellular matrix during vasospasm. VLDL and LDL molecules sink between the cells in the intercellular matrix and undergo denaturation by free radicals that have been generated there

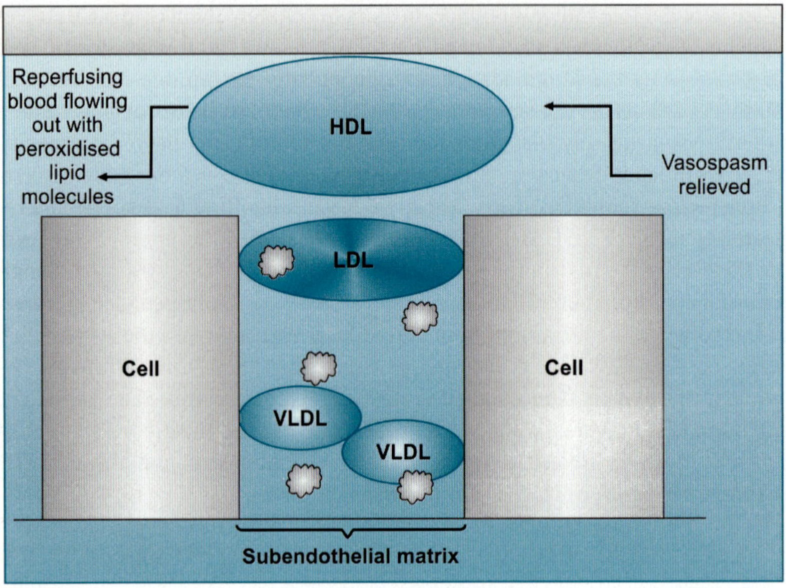

Fig. 5.7: The denatured fats are flushed into circulation during reperfusion causing a damage wherever they go

main triglyceride carrying lipoproteins are chylomicrons and very low density lipoproteins (LVDL). The two main cholesterol containing lipoproteins are low density lipoproteins (LDL) and high density lipoproteins (HDL).

The entire process of lipid transport needs to be closely examined if one wants to understand the causation and the behavior of obstetric vasculopathies. The mischief takes place primarily in the vascular intercellular matrix. This matrix will become accessible to the lipids only when they are in circulation. It is during their process of transport that they come in contact of the vessel walls where they undergo and series of changes. Stationary lipids are stationed in the tissues do not play so much of a mischief. They are neither prone to any changes at storage site nor are likely to undergo the process of pathological destruction and dysfunction there. Therefore, stored lipids are of very limited clinical bearing. It is the circulating lipids which are most susceptible to changes. While in transit, these lipids come in contact with the vascular endothelial wall. Here they undergo the all important desaturation.

When lipids have such an important bearing in causation of obstetric vasculopathies why do obese women not suffer consistently from obstetric vasculopathies? All obese or overweight women are not consistently prone to obstetric vasculopathies. This is because obesity or the state of "overweight" is labeled on basis of stored or stationary lipid stores. One is obese if his/her lipid stores are high. But in clinical practice these young overweight mothers may not necessarily have an increased or altered circulating lipid levels. Till that time as the circulating lipid levels are not altered obstetric vasculopathies would not manifest. This is the explanation to why all overweight/obese women do not develop obstetric vasculopathies. Further interestingly the security of obstetric vasculopathy that a subject faces is not dependant on the degree of overweight or obesity. Thus in clinical practice an obese woman may just register a mild preeclampsia while an overweight woman may have a fulminant form of obstetric vasculopathy. While on the stationary and circulating lipids, one more clinical manifestation gets explained. This is the finding in clinical practice that even lean pregnant subjects develop obstetric vasculopathy. This is again because a subject is labeled as lean on basis of her weight (dependant on stationary and stored adipose tissue). On the other hand, her obstetric vasculopathy develops on basis of circulating lipids.

In the early weeks and months of pregnancy the HDL levels are high in circulation. As pregnancy advances circulating levels of LDL and VLDL start increasing. The serum lipid levels are significantly higher in all the trimesters of the pregnant women than in the controls. There was a steady increase in the serum lipid levels with increasing gestational age. A significant positive correlation is observed between the lipid fractions and the different trimesters of pregnancy. Total Cholesterol: HDL ratio is decreased significantly in pregnant women, with increasing gestational age. This goes on progressively till term.[3] Relative insulin resistant states of late pregnancy have a vital role to play in these happenings. It is very well-known that pregnancy is a diabetogenic state though all pregnancies may not manifest clinical diabetes. This relative insulin resistance progressively increases as pregnancy advances. As soon as delivery occurs the relatively altered insulin sensitivity is restored to normal and the potential diabetogenic state is reversed. Insulin resistance does not clinically manifest as loss of euglycemic states in all pregnant subjects. In most blood sugar levels do not cross their thresholds to be labeled as overt diabetes. However, the relative insulin resistance is reflected in circulating insulin levels which are consistently increased. Placental growth hormone seems to have a very important role in this. Placental growth hormone induces maternal insulin resistance and thereby facilitates the mobilization of maternal nutrients for fetal growth.[4]

Placental growth hormone is produced by trophoblast. This hormone becomes detectable in maternal serum during the first trimester of pregnancy. Its concentration increases as term approaches and becomes undetectable within one hour of delivery. Placental growth hormone has important biological properties, including lipolytic activity.[5] This presumably boosts the release of free fatty acids and glycerol releasing them into circulation thereby increasing the substrate for VLDL production.

It is also off interest to know that under the effect of estrogen, VLDL gets readily released from the liver stores into circulation. Also the lipolytic activity gets so influenced that with advancing pregnancy VLDL and LDL remain in circulation for a longer period of time. Basically these changes are taking place to maximize the transfer of maternal essential fatty acids to the fetus. Before the clinical picture of preeclampsia becomes obvious dyslipidemia has been documented to occur. Disturbed lipid metabolism has been noted as a feature of preeclampsia as early as in 1924. However its importance was not well-understood.

With the insights into the etiopathology of obstetric vasculopathies becoming obvious, the reasons for these changes in lipids were not amazing. The process of lipid peroxidation at intercellular matrix in the vascular bed leads to denaturation of circulating VLDL and LDL. Their denaturation mobilizes more and more of lipid peroxides to maintain the supply of "unadulterated" VLDL and LDL. Thus the laboratory change would be a significant increase in circulating VLDL and LDL levels in subjects with obstetric vasculopathy as pregnancy advances. As soon as the parturient delivers these circulating increased levels get precipitously reduced. This may not match with a reversal of manifestations of obstetric vasculopathies.

This is understandable. The maternal attempt to increase levels of circulating VLDL and LDL was to maximize the supply of essential fatty acids to the fetus. However with the parturient delivering the baby, this need gets annulled. The maternal systems which in presence of lipid peroxidation was compensating for this loss only with an aim to provide critical levels of circulating essential fatty acids to the fetus has no need now to continue the overdrive. As a result of this, the circulating raised levels of LDL and VLDL reverse very fast in obstetric vasculopathies once delivery occurs.

The changes of obstetric vasculopathies too start undergoing the change for reverse. But these changes do not match with changes in maternal circulating VLDL and LDL levels. This is because the process of denaturation of lipid moieties continues even on smaller number of these lipids. Changes of preeclampsia including hypertension may take weeks to reverse. Sometimes the BP may strike the base apparently giving the signal that the process is over. However, soon after a week or so the BP registers a high again. Sometimes, the BP may follow a disciplined and graded reversal. On some other times and in some other subjects the BP may not show any change for a couple of days or a week and then start declining. Again, this decline may not necessarily follow a charted pattern. Similar behavior can be seen in other manifestations of obstetric vasculopathies including edema or proteinuria as well. Even the potentially devastating changes of renal compromise may not follow any predecided pattern.

This is indeed intriguing but explainable: For the changes of obstetric vasculopathies to occur an entire cacophonic orchestra comes into action. Though termed as cacophonic as it leads to devastating clinical manifestations, it is never dysrrhythmic. It follows a rhythm so as to say there is a well geared method even in this madness. While dyslipidemia is just one segment or section of the entire orchestra in obstetric vasculopathies there are a series of other processes also involved. Thus even if dyslipidemia reverses the other processes may not reverse. Also, the lipids, essential fatty acids are needed to maintain their supply to fetus. Therefore, hyperlipidemia is maintained when the fetus is still in the uterus. The concurrent process of lipid denaturation including lipid peroxidation destroys or threatens to destroy this all important supply chain of essential fatty acids to the fetus. So as to compensate for this, the mother mobilizes more and more essential fatty acids. This explains why the fury and complications of obstetric vasculopathies is at a maximum just before delivery of the fetus. However, after delivery the fodder needed for maintaining the dyslipidemia is quickly reversed. Therefore, the changes do not progress.

But even at lower levels of circulating lipids the process can still maintain itself. Thus, the reversal process takes time. Also, the reversal process does not follow any set pattern. How much time does vasospasm and reperfusion damage need before the body senses that the trigger process is over is entirely dependent on the innate capacity of the maternal system to reverse or close the process. Even at normal levels of circulating lipids (that means in absence of hyperlipidemias) the processes continue. They are totally dependent on maternal circulating LDL and VLDL and need no extra lipid supply. As has been stated the extra supply of lipids was only for the fetus.

The fact that the fury of obstetric vasculopathy is at its maximum just before the end of pregnancy is found all obstetric vasculopathies consistently: BP in preeclampsia is highest coupled with edema and proteinuria just before the delivery. Accidental hemorrhage and its complications are at its peak of activity just before delivery. The process of IUGR occurs unabated and leads to a precipitous decline in fetal fortunes till the time that it delivers. This is explained by the supply of "fodder" for this process being at its maximum till that time that the pregnancy gets terminated.

Serum triglyceride, cholesterol, and free fatty acid concentrations decrease sharply in pre-eclamptic and pregnant controls by 24 to 48 hours postpartum.[6,7] However, the triglycerides and cholesterols then after continue to decrease gradually and this may continue for upto 6 weeks postpartum. These decreasing levels of triglycerides and cholesterol provide the feeder for keeping the lowered intensity of changes of obstetric vasculopathies alive. How fast and by what time the levels of triglycerides and cholesterol hit the base of normalcy will depend on the innate maternal systemic responses. They are different and variable for each mother and the same mother in different pregnancies. Accordingly, the changes of obstetric vasculopathies vary from mother to mother and even in the same mother from pregnancy to pregnancy.

Hypertriglyceridemia and Obstetric Vasculopathies

Fatty acids notoriously contribute to endothelial dysfunction in preeclampsia by several ways: FFA mediated endothelial dysfunction facilitate ROS generation.[8] Generation of ROS is one of the most important steps in obstetric vasculopathies. ROS incite the entire plethora of obstetric vasculopathies. However, one big question that always remains in the mind of the scientific investigator is what generates these ROS. This work is done by the free fatty acids.

There is now an established relation between hyper triglyceridemia and coronary artery disease as well as atherosclerosis. In the realms of oxidative stress monocytes isolated from individuals with hypertriglyceridemia show increased production of superoxides and enhanced binding to endothelial cells. Thus hypertriglyceridemia generate ROS by first increasing the binding of circulating monocytes to endothelial cells. Followed in quick succession these monocytes start generating superoxide. For this, however, the hypertriglyceridemia is the consistent precursor and critical event.

The superoxides critically associated with ROS quickly make the latter alive and available in the intercellular matrix. It is then in this intercellular endothelial matrix that the VLDL and LDL that are walking in and out get ensnared by the ROS to undergo the process of lipid peroxidation. Another important event in this series is the conversion of large LDL particles to small dense LDL particles for the maintenance of the pathology of obstetric vasculopathies which need to be closely understood.

Small Dense LDL Phenotype in Obstetric Vasculopathy

The entire LDL family consists of phenotypically different particles. Its difference is based on their density, size and even chemical structure. It is this phenotype that decides the buoyancy and nature of the LDL particles. In adult healthy females the large LDL particles are predominant. They remain buoyant and away from the vessel wall in circulation. They have a definite estrogenic influence. With menopause appearing these large LDL particles start getting phenotypically metamorphosed to small dense LDL particles.

There is also an intermediate subclass of LDL particles not as small and dense as those found in menopausal women not as large as the LDL particles in other healthy adult non-menopausal females. These are not as buoyant as the large LDL particles. They are found predominantly in the adult males. This variation in LDL particle size and density is under both, genetic as well as non-genetic influence. Amongst non-genetic influence dietary intake and factors like smoking also have an influence on them.

In obstetric vasculopathies there are distinct metabolic changes that produce hypertriglyceridemia. These generally shift the spectrum of LDL subfractions towards a proportional increase of smaller and denser LDL particles [2] Small dense LDL particles are relatively depleted of cholestryl esters, and enriched in protein.[9,10] These small dense LDL particles by the innate size and buoyancy as well as their electronic propensity have an increased proteoglycan binding. This proteoglycan binding makes them susceptible to getting closer to the vessel wall and therefore the vascular endothelium. Once they come in apposition to or in close proximity to the vascular endothelium they move readily in and out of the intercellular matrix of the vascular endothelium. This is where they readily undergo the process of LDL lipid peroxidation. These small dense LDL particles have a major influence and contribution in the occurrence of a series of diseased states. Women with higher levels of circulating small dense LDL develop non insulin-dependent DM more readily. They also had a higher propensity to myocardial infarctions subsequently.

Non-insulin dependent diabetes mellitus and myocardial infarctions are usually the disease of adults and advancing age. This does not hold true for obstetric vasculopathies. Obstetric vasculopathies do not necessarily occur in elderly pregnant women. In clinical practice no definite association is found between obstetric vasculopathies and maternal age. Elderly gravida do seem to have a tendency to develop obstetric vasculopathy especially the superimposed preeclampsia over under running hypertension. Yet all obstetric vasculopathies do not occur only in the elderly gravida. This goes on to show that obstetric vasculopathies create a pathological milieu similar to those in aging. The conversion of large and buyout LDL particles readily to small dense particles is a direct example of the same. It also goes on to explain the findings of atherosclerosis like changes at the fetomaternal interface in subjects with obstetric vasculopathies. This is essentially age independent and by and large reversible in pregnancy.

Interestingly, small dense LDL particles are not only more susceptible to getting drawn towards the vascular endothelium but are also more susceptible to oxidation compared to the large buoyant variety.[11] Proportional increases in small dense LDL with heightened susceptibility to oxidative modification may account for the part of the increased cardiovascular risk in individuals with the small dense LDL phenotype.[12] This may have a genetic basis as genetic copy number variants in myocardial infarction patients with hyperlipidemia.[13]

Interestingly one more characteristic associated with small dense LDL is that these are more susceptible to oxidative degeneration due to decreasing particle size and proportional polyunsaturated fatty acid increase. Concurrently per each small dense LDL particle there is a decrease in reducing systems effectivity It therefore seems obvious that the pitch for occurrence of obstetric vasculopathies is queered very competently and very decisively by the maternal system.

Compared to their more buoyant and larger LDL particles, small dense LDL particles have a greater capacity to stimulate thromboxane synthesis.[2] They also have an increased capacity to increase intracellular calcium in smooth muscle cells. The sum total effect of this is an increased propensity to smooth muscle contraction. Thus the small dense LDL particles lead readily to vasospasm. Interestingly, small dense LDLs have an effect on increasing thromboxane synthesis but they do not concurrently reduce prostacyclin levels. This leads to alteration in thromboxane prostacyclin ratio only by affecting one factor of the ratio and not both. This is unlike many other events in obstetric vasculopathies which affect both the factors of the ratio increasing thromboxane and reducing prostacyclin production.

The correlation between the size of LDL particle and triglycerides is also very interesting. It will have a very important bearing on obstetric vasculopathies. The size of LDL particles reduces from large buoyant variety to intermediate dense variety as pregnancy progresses from 5 to 6 weeks to 36 weeks. This subsequently reverts to prepregnant level nearly completely by 6 weeks postpartum.[2] In a very interesting study which proved this gestational progression of LDL diameter was studied prospectively in ten pregnant nonsmoker subjects. It was found that the LDL particle size was negatively correlated with serum levels of triglyceride.[14] This means as the particles became smaller and denser the triglyceride levels increased

In physiological parlance, the LDL particles were therefore divided into three subtypes. This was based on the size and density of these particles. Particle sizes 1 and 2 were the buoyant variety. Particles of the size 3 were the less buoyant variety. It was found that as pregnancy advanced the size transformed from 1 to 3. In preeclampsia this transformation occurs much faster and much more steeply. It gets reflected in the clinical behavior of preeclampsia. Any pregnant subject becomes more susceptible to preeclampsia as pregnancy advances. Also, in the distinct entity of preeclampsia remote from term this conversion occurs still more briskly.

It is critical for the process of etiopathology of preeclampsia in particular and obstetric vasculopathies in general that this conversion occurs. If and whenever this conversion occurs the LDL III reach the intercellular endothelial matrix. As has been made amply clear LDL particles undergo peroxidation in the matrix to generate and perpetuate the obstetric vasculopathies.

Admittedly, there is at present no direct or indirect demonstration of oxidized lipids in obstetric vasculopathies from vascular channels. This is in complete contrast to unequivocal demonstration of these denatured lipid moieties from vascular spaces in atherosclerosis and their clinical manifestations or associates like diabetes mellitus and myocardial infarction. However the indirect associations are very strong. Till that time that anything contrary to this appears it is safe to conclude that oxidization of LDL is critical and all important for the etiopathogenesis of obstetric vasculopathies.

PLACENTAL LIPID PEROXIDATION

Lipid peroxidation has been found to be a very important event in the etiopathology of obstetric vasculopathies. Lipid peroxidation product malanodialdehyde is increased in placental tissue along with decreased superoxide dismutase (SOD) activity in preeclampsia.[15,16] Interestingly several isoforms of SOD exist. This includes cytosolic copper/zinc and mitochondrial manganese. Superoxide Dismutase (SOD) has a peculiar role in breaking down superoxide. This breaking down leads to protection of the fetomaternal interface from oxidative injury. In preeclampsia there is a reduced SOD activity and a consequent increased oxidative stress. Also, oxidative stress can alter the isoforms of SOD, both cytosolic as well as mitochondrial. This renders the activity of SOD paralyzed or partly hindered. A partly dysfunctional SOD in placenta of subjects with obstetric vasculopathies leads to unchallenged activity of oxidative free radicals resulting in subsequent lipid peroxidation.

Glutathione peroxides have been studied for the peroxidation activity in obstetric vasculopathies including miscarriages.[17] It has been found that glutathione peroxides are relatively decreased in placenta of preeclampsia. This indicates an increased peroxidation activity. Interestingly chemical inhibition of placental glutathione peroxides results in release of hydroperoxides and an increase in the placental thromboxane to prostacyclin output ratio.[18] The relative deficiency of glutathione peroxides in placenta of preeclamptic subjects occurs in conjunction with increase tissue production of lipid hydroperoxides and thromboxane A2.[18] These observations are very important. The process of lipid peroxidation and flushing of the lipid peroxides into circulation has to have an important link with alteration in the prostacyclin to thromboxane ratio in favor of thromboxane. Lipid peroxide molecules have to affect the pathology of vasospasm through this alteration in ratio. Demonstration of decreased prostacyclin production and/or increased thromboxane production in conjunction with increased lipid peroxidation establishes the link between the two.

Once this link is established it becomes easy to understand the plethora of clinical manifestations that occur in obstetric vasculopathies. The basic pathology in all obstetric vasculopathies is vasospasm. Once it is demonstrated that increased lipid peroxidation occurs in conjunction with alteration in thromboxane prostacyclin ratio it is thenafter easy to grasp the clinical manifestations of obstetric vasculopathies.

One can easily understand the fact that even if one of the factors of any ratio is altered the result alters. This means that if prostacyclin production decreases thromboxane supervenes to produce a tilt in balance towards vasospasm. Alternatively if thromboxane production is singularly increased so will be the resultant manifestation. However, in obstetric vasculopathies the alteration that occurs is very thorough. Both the components of the ratio get altered. This makes the pathology more profound and devastating.

Glutathione peroxidase reduction in preeclampsia is in conjunction with increased thromboxane A2 production. Lipid hydroperoxides on the other hand inhibit prostacyclin syntheses activity. While lipid hydroperoxides inhibit the prostacyclin syntheses activity they simultaneously also stimulate the cyclooxygenase component of prostaglandin-H synthase. Cyclooxygenase is a very important molecule to propagate the conversion of arachidonic acid to prostaglandins cycle perpetuation and generation. By stimulation of cyclooxygenase activity, lipid hydroperoxides ensure that the entire prostaglandin production cycle also gets maintained or perpetuated. This is a critical phenomenon. Merely a single or some episodic alteration in thromboxane-prostacyclin ratio would not suffice to bring about a perpetuated series of changes in obstetric vasculopathies. There has to be a system in place which perpetuates the cycle. By influencing the cyclooxygenase production oxidative stress ensures that the pathology gets perpetuated.

Transition Metals in Lipid Peroxidation

Lipid peroxidation is essentially oxidative deterioration of polyunsaturated fatty acids. It is very interesting to find that lipid peroxidation process has a very important role for transition metals including iron for its amplification. As the first step when the free radical also known as ROS comes in contact with the lipid molecules that are susceptible [Poly unsaturated fatty acids (PUFA)] they extract methylene hydrogen from unsaturated fatty acids (LH) forming a lipid radical (L^+). This lipid radical reacts with molecular oxygen to form a lipid peroxyl radical (LOO^+). This LOO* attacks another molecule of LH (unsaturated lipid) to enter a chain. LH gets attacked by LOO* to produce another LOO* which in turn attacks another LH and thereby generating one wheel of the vicious circle (Fig. 5.8)

Concurrently attempts are made to magnify or amplify the LOO* formation. Thus one section of this vicious circle starts interacting with transition metals like Fe* which are dislocated from the intracellular compartments. These transition metals undergo a conversion while amplifying the catalytic conversion of LH to LOO* and LO*. Thus smaller amount of peroxidised lipid radicals is generated by the direct attack of ROS on PUFA, which then enters the same vicious cycle of denaturing LH—unsaturated fatty acids. The same process concurrently gets amplified in its parallel arm when the transition metals like Fe* get involved in the process.

There are some exceptional players also contributing to the process of generating peroxidized lipid radicals. Examples of this are peroxynitrite anion which can initiate the process of lipid peroxidation without requirement of transition metals. They generate LOO* directly in vastly amplified way without

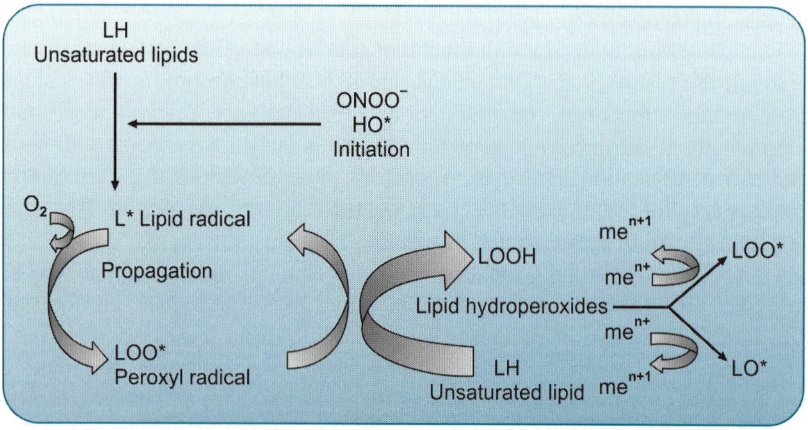

Fig 5.8: Free radical mechanism of lipid peroxidation is initiated when a reactive oxygen species of sufficient power abstracts methylene hydrogen from the unsaturated fatty acid (LH), forming a lipid radical (*). The lipid radical reacts with molecular oxygen to form a lipid peroxyl radical (LOO*). The lipid peroxyl radical attacks another unsaturated lipid forming another lipid radical (that enters the chain) and a lipid hydroperoxides (LOOH) propagation occurs. Once the lipid matrix is seeded with low concentrations of lipid hydroperoxides (LOOH) peroxidation can be amplified by transition metal (me^{n+1}). This catalyzes the conversion of lipid hydroxides to radical species: LOO*and LO*. Bonding of two radical species or reaction with reducing systems such as Vitamin E will slow the peroxidation process

(*Source*: Fig 9.1—Desai P. Reducing systems in preeclampsia: Recent Advances In Obstetrics and Gynecology. Dasgupta S. vol 6, Jaypee Publishers, Delhi, 1st edn. 2003;Pg. 82).

the need to be dependent on the presence of transition metals like Fe*.

While this entire process of lipid peroxidation is on at the intercellular matrix of the vessel wall the circulation of blood has been relatively impeded. In that short period of vasospasm followed by reperfusion, this process gets completed. Also the neutralization of the free radicals by maternal and trophoblastic reducing systems is also taking place concurrently. This means that while the destructive or morbidity causing process of free radical generation and lipid peroxidation is on, so also the activity of healing by reducing systems is also on. These reducing systems not only stop at neutralizing the free radicals but also serve as scavengers eliminating them from the system. In most situations of healthy pregnancy, the process of neutralization and elimination by reducing systems overwhelms the destructive systems. This clinically results in a healthy live birth. If, however, the destructive process gets an upper hand and overwhelms the reducing systems obstetric vasculopathies results.

The process of lipid peroxidation in particular and that of oxidative stress is not always causing a disease process. In fact, there are quite a few processes of health that are dependent on free radicals and lipid peroxidation as has been hinted in previous sections. The classic example of a process which gets propagated thus is the process of activation of the cyclooxygenase component of Prostaglandin-H (PGH) synthase requires the presence of lipid hydroperoxides.[19]

CLINICAL MANIFESTATIONS

Once it is understood why vasospasm in obstetric vasculopathies occur, it will be easy to explain the etiopathogenesis of different clinical manifestations of obstetric vasculopathies. In the eventuality of the process of lipid peroxidation and denaturation occurring uninhibited in early pregnancy, IUGR occurs. There is vascular impendence to healthy oxygen and other vital exchanges at the fetomaternal interface resulting in IUGR.

Vascular impedance from vasospasm throughout the maternal vasculature makes the maternal system sense difficulty in critical blood flow through maternal vascular bed. Once the mother senses that she is unable to maintain effective blood supply to her vital systems due to vasospasm she starts forcing the blood through her vascular channels. This increase in force of blood through the vessels is clinically manifested as hypertension and preeclampsia.

Intermittent vasospasm and reperfusion denudes the vessels of proper protection of its own walls. To what extent is the vasavasorum involved in this is difficult to study. However, the damage to the vessel walls could be a result of both direct injury as well as dysfunctional vasavasorum. The damaged vessel walls can withstand the vasospasm. However, when this spasm is relieved the vessel walls give way. Destroyed integrity of the vessels lead to leakage of blood at the fetomaternal interface, resulting in accidental hemorrhage also known as abruptio placenta.

Initial or early fetal demise occurring at around 8 to 10 weeks may not need the entire ROS-lipid peroxidation process to get activated. A direct annihilation of the embryonic trophoblastic tissue due to immune rejection or defective placentation may be enough for killing the early fetus. This explains the early fetal demise in obstetric vasculopathies.

REPERFUSION

The pathognomonic lesion in obstetric vasculopathies is vasospasm. While this has been the most conspicuous change to the examining eye of the pathologist in actuality it is not the vasospasm that produces the clinical effects. It is infact the reperfusion damage. Reperfusion damage is very intense. Associates of our group carried out an interesting animal experiment.[20] Under strict rules and standards needed for any such experiment, they passed a wire and blocked the circulation through the internal carotid of experimental dogs unilaterally (Figs 5.9 and 5.10). Other side was perfusing the brain of the dogs normally. While this block continued no damage occurred. As soon as the block was removed perfusion was reestablished. Under the effect of this reperfusion profound injuries occurred to the canine brain. Many of them had to be sacrificed. As the next step, they were now perfused wit a strong antioxidant (Kava). However, this antioxidant could at best only partly neutralize the reperfusion damage (Figs 5.11A to C).

The result of this experiment opens up some very interesting insight into the process of reperfusion damage. While it ascertains that it is not the vasospasm but the reperfusion that causes harm it also opens up a bigger challenge. This challenge is related to the limitation of the reducing substances in preventing or reversing the reperfusion damage.

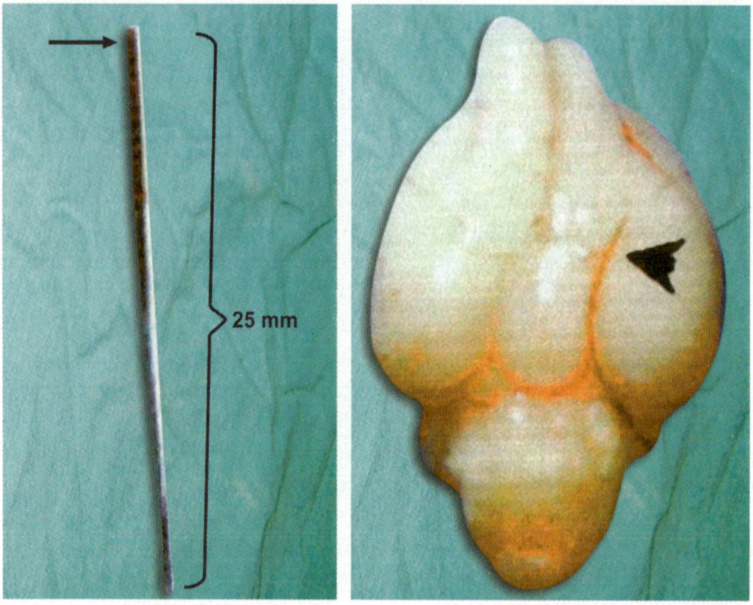

Fig.5.9: The wire used to canulated and block the flow of the carotid artery of the experimental dogs. The brain undergoing ischemic changes

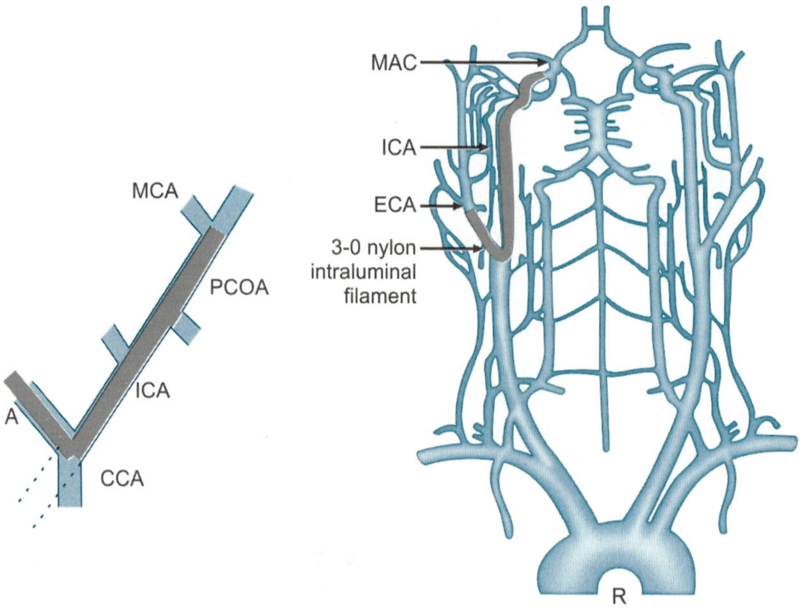

Fig. 5.10: Diagram of the canulated vessel and the anatomy involved

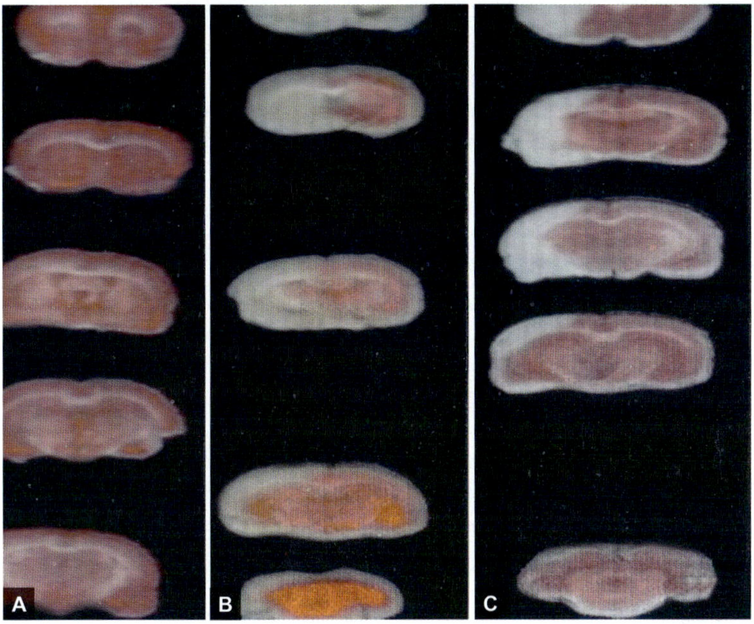

Figs 5.11A to C: Computer generated images of the brains: A. Before canulation, B. After wire canulation, C. After the wire that blocked the circulation is removed and the brains showing profound changes of reperfusion damage

Even in clinical practice it is well-known that reducing substances or antioxidants as they are called are unable to completely ameliorate or prevent obstetric vasculopathies. They can at best limit their damage. However which damage will be limited and to what extent is never predictable. It depends on the maternal systems to undergo the damages of reperfusion and the adequacy of antioxidants for that tissue or body to counteract the oxidative stress resulting in the complications of obstetric vasculopathies.

INNATE MATERNAL REDUCING SYSTEMS

Whereas the mother has to bear the brunt of the fetal graft and undergo a series of changes physiological as well as pathological. The maternal systems also have their protective mechanisms. It is a fact that maternal protective systems are much more power and efficient than any of the pharmacologically active substance administered extraneously. As soon free radicals are generated so are reducing radical also generated. Most of the times, the maternal innate reducing systems are powerful and adequate in amount and strength so as to prevent the injuries by free radicals.

In every pregnancy some amount of sinkage of VLDL and LDL is bound to occur. This is the innate tendency of these molecules to seek the intercellular matrix. Once in the matrix, the free radicals when neutralized by maternal reducing systems, would not be enough to peroxidase the lipid molecules. The lipids that may get peroxidised are in very small amount. While they reach the circulation they do produce a vasospasm. However, at the level of the tissues also the protective guards are present. These are tissue reducing systems. They completely overwhelm the peroxidized lipid molecules rendering them incapable of producing much harm. Once neutralized the peroxidized lipids are not in a position to generate the vasospasm-reperfusion-vasospasm damage chain.

Maternal vasculature during pregnancy has a bias towards maintaining the caliber and thereby effective circulation in the tissues and organs. The thromboxane prostacyclin balance tilts in favor of prostacyclin causing an effective and competent circulation of the organs and tissues. During pregnancy maternal blood tends to be hypercoagulable. It tends to clot easily. This is a protective change that occurs to counteract the blood loss that readily occurs in a pregnant subject most during labor. Inspite of the blood being hypercoagulable, the perfusion of maternal system is excellently maintained. This is a little paradoxical but understandable. This hypercoagulable state, in an intact maternal vascular system is not causing any harm. It also does not clog up the maternal vascular bed.

In the eventuality of failure of maternal reducing systems, devastation follows. It is apparent that obstetric vasculopathies occur not due to one of the following but due to all of these:

- Genetic interplay
- Immune maladaptation
- Imbalance between free oxygen radicals and reducing systems (also known as scavengers in favor of the former)
- Placental ischemia

All four were originally proposed as theories to explain occurrence of PIH. It was believed that one of these produced PIH. However, deeper insights into the entire basket of pathologies of obstetric vasculopathies (including PIH) reveals that all four of them are acting, in combination, to produce obstetric vasculopathies.

Decreased expression of reducing systems thioredoxin and glutoredoxin in placentae from pregnancies with obstetric vasculopathies has been documented.[21] Placental tissues from normal pregnancies were offset against expression of reducing systems from placenta of subjects with obstetric vasculopathies. It was convincingly found that maternal expression of reducing systems was significantly reduced in obstetric vasculopathies. This is interesting. It now becomes apparent that maternal generation of free radicals and resultant perpetuation of spasm-reperfusion-spasm cycle is pronounced in obstetric vasculopathies. Concurrently, there is maternal reduced generation of reducing systems. The free radicals generated in huge and increasing amounts overwhelming the maternal reducing systems. At the same time the maternal reducing system generation is also greatly reduced. Thus increase in generation of ROS is happily perpetuated by reduced production of reducing systems, together combine to produce obstetric vasculopathies.

In non-diseased states, there is a vital role for reducing systems at the level of fetomaternal interface. Distinct and efficient reducing systems have been identified on the trophoblasts. The origin of this could be the trophoblast itself. The trophoblasts have been known to possess an inborn resistance to maternal destructive process. Just as the trophoblastic resilience to maternal rejection is efficient so is their ability to generate protective systems. By generation of these reducing systems on their surface, trophoblasts protect the pregnancy from maternal oxidative stress distribution.

In conditions like PIH, not only are the maternal reducing systems generated in smaller quantities but are also less efficient. In states of maternal health, the maternal reducing systems are in adequate amount and competence to overwhelm and neutralize the oxidative free radicals. But in PIH, reverse occurs. The maternal reducing systems due to smaller amounts and incompetence get overwhelmed. This produces changes of PIH.

Proteins thiol/disulfide oxidoreductases such as thioredoxin, glutaredoxin and protein disulfide isomerase have been found to eliminate ROS. Protein thiol/ disulfide oxidoreductases therefore have an important role in PIH.[21] These results indicated that pre-eclamptic pregnancies were exposed to oxidative stress and the protein thiol/disulfide oxidoreductases were adaptively induced for protection in pre-eclamptic placentae.[2]

A diverse array of cellular and extracellular fluid reducing systems has evolved to control and compartmentalize but not necessarily eliminate the production of ROS.[2] Reducing systems examined in normal and pre-eclamptic pregnancies include the enzymatic reducing systems (Superoxide dismutase catalase and glutathione peroxidase) and transition metal binding proteins (Transferrin, ceruloplasmin and ferritin). These are also low molecular mass which serve as scavengers which directly, primarily and exclusively target free radical and protects in the extracellular compartment.[2] These include water soluble forms of ascorbate, glutathione and protein thiols, and uric acid. They also include lipoprotein and membrane soluble forms including OC-tocopherol (Vitamin-D).[22]

THE FAMILY OF FREE RADICALS

Most free radicals fall in the category of reactive oxygen species (ROS) and superoxide anion radical (O_2^{+}) and also reactive oxygen derivatives that do not contain unpaired electrons, such as hydrogen peroxide (H_2O_2), hypochlorus acid (HOCL) and peroxynitrite anion ($ONOO^-$).[2] Systems altered to generate ROS during postischemic reperfusion include mitochondrial respiration, neutrophil NADPH oxidase, xanthenes oxidase and cyclooxygenase.[2] On similar lines one animal experiment showed exogenous melatonin protects against ischemia/ reperfusion induced oxidative damage to mitochondria in rat placenta emboldening these researchers to suggest that melatonin could be useful in treating obstetric vasculopathies.[23] Interestingly iron delocalized from its normal intracellular compartments during ischemic damage will also promote ROS generation upon reoxygenation and reperfusion.

While examining this very virulent but clinically important family of free radicals it may be relevant to revisit the reperfusion and reoxygenation concept in brief. It is also important to understand that this reperfusion also simultaneously generates free radicals while flushing the peroxidized radicals (Fig. 5.12).

When this process is confined to the fetomaternal interface it results in IUGR. When it gets expanded to the entire maternal vasculature it results in PIH

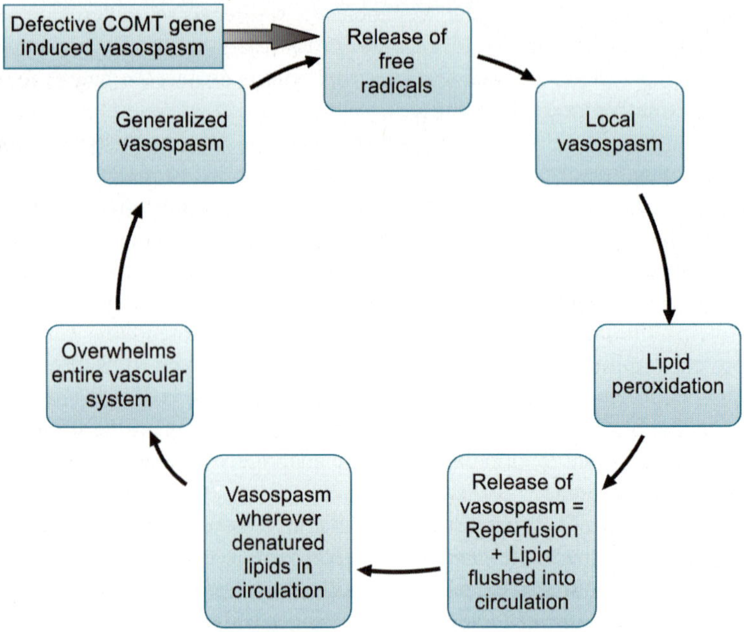

Fig. 5.12: Generation and release of free radicals

clinically. Poverty of quality placentation makes placental sinus walls susceptible to ischemic damage causing it to be rendered asunder resulting in clinical abruptio placenta or accidental hemorrhage.

In initial understanding of obstetric vasculopathy it was thought that maternal vasospasm of PIH extends as vasospasm in the placenta causing IUGR. However, with this complex interplay becoming obvious, it is now clear that PIH and IUGR do not share cause-effect relationship. They are two manifestations of the same pathophysiology. To make it simple – PIH and IUGR do not have a mother (PIH) to daughter (IUGR) relationship. They have a sister to sister relationship both resulting from the same pathophysiology at different locales.

VASCULAR ENDOTHELIUM AND OXIDATIVE STRESS

Vascular endothelium pays the price of its continuous exposure to blood. Besides the many contents of blood that brush past the vessel wall, the active components leave great effects on the vascular endothelial lining. Whereas circulating lipids have a positive effect on the cell wall, the state of dyslipidemia produces a diseased state or endothelial cell dysfunction. VLDL and LDL particles have a capacity to walk in and out of the intercellular matrix due to their cell size and their electronic configuration. This makes them susceptible to denaturation by cell derived oxidative particles. To protect them, the intercellular matrix has reducing systems which protect these lipids.

Two events provided some leads for the scientists in understanding the etiopathology of obstetric vasculopathies. One of them is neutrophil activation suggesting a process of inflammation and the other is the process of lipid peroxidation. Neutrophil activation occurs with the process of obstetric vasculopathy and resolves with delivery irrespective of the obstetric outcome. On the other hand, lipid peroxidation is elevated before and continues even for some time after delivery. In reality lipid peroxidation may go on in the body at a much attenuated level all throughout life indicating the possibility of some role played by the same in the aging process or atherosclerosis.

Yet in obstetric vasculopathies the process of neutrophil activation seems to get much more profound in the presence of uninhibited lipid peroxidation. This prompted some workers to suggest that the entire process of obstetric vasculopathy is an inflammatory response. One study measured Alpha-1 antitrypsin (AAT) an anti-protease, anti-inflammatory and tissue-protective molecule in preeclampsia. It was on the basis of unopposed inflammation might be contributing to preeclampsia, AAT levels were studied to know whether preeclampsia is associated with lower than normal levels. It was found that there was an association between lower AAT levels and severe preeclampsia during pregnancy. But it was wisely concluded that further studies are required to identify the mechanism behind the association, and the possibility of safe AAT augmentation for individuals with insufficient circulating AAT.[24] However, it is clear that anti-inflammatory agents fail to stem obstetric vasculopathies. Thus, inflammatory process may be at the most a side process in obstetric vasculopathies with very minimal modifying role.

INEFFICIENT SECOND WAVE OF TROPHOBLASTIC INVASION

Trophoblasts seem to be very specialized cell lining. At the first step or first wave they have a very big anchoring role. The first wave of trophoblastic invasion anchors the placenta with the maternal surface. This occurs early in pregnancy. It may be as early as one week of pregnancy and may get completed by four weeks of pregnancy. Near simultaneously another amazing phenomenon is occurring: this is the generation of the second wave of trophoblastic invasion.

This second wave of trophoblastic invasion has an extremely specialized function. It is confined to the uterine vasculature maternal spiral arterioles. These trophoblasts mould and modify the spiral arterioles in such a way that the latter get shielded off from maternal circulating substances which may alter the caliber of the vessels readily. They also cause the destruction of the muscular wall of the spiral arterioles to make them a low resistance pool of fetoplacental circulation. It seems that there may be hypoxia-inducible factor (HIF) transcription factors. These direct the cellular responses to low oxygen. This in turn influences the trophoblast lineage commitment thereby promoting development of the invasive trophoblast lineage.[25]

Once shielded from the maternal influence the fetomaternal vascular pool becomes a near autonomous circulation system. It also has a low impedance flow thereby leading to a specialized efficient gushing blood pool. Whereas the second wave of trophoblastic invasion has a critical role in the creation of this autonomous circulation pool, inefficient or failed second wave leads to a wide array of clinical effects including obstetric vasculopathies. Inefficient, incomplete or failed trophoblastic invasion leaves unmodified and unmolded spiral arteriole spaces.

While the hypoxic environment may promote trophoblastic generation and growth, beyond a limit it serves a pathological purpose. It, therefore, has a dual purpose of health when in limits, but once uncontrolled they cause impediment to trophoblastic invasion. This impediment sets the stage and sows the seeds for obstetric vasculopathies. Unmolded spiral arterioles plugged by a partly failed trophoblastic invasion second wave become the hotbed for generation of free radicals. These hypo-oxygenated species lay the foundation for obstetric vasculopathies. Also, as a direct effect of this hypoxia the generation of protective reducing systems is both reduced and whatever reducing systems are generated are also poorly competent.

Amongst a series of paradoxical and at times outright antagonistic phenomenon that are occurring at the fetomaternal interface one more is the generation of reactive oxygen species (ROS) in hypoxic environments. On one side there is hypoxia, on the other side there is a generation of oxygen free radicals. It is necessary to restress here that the hypoxic environment generated by the second wave of trophoblastic invasion is critical for sustaining this wave and subsequent vascular remodeling. But if this hypoxic environment goes beyond its critical limitations, it in itself hampers further trophoblastic invasion. Not only this, the same hypoxic environment becomes the hotbed for generation of ROS.

It is also necessary to acknowledge at this stage that though the entire phenomenon of hypoxia generation of ROS and subsequent lipid peroxidation has a critical role to play in causation of obstetric vasculopathy, this may not be the only etiopathological phenomenon. One more phenomenon that may have some modifying role in obstetric vasculopathies is the generation of VEGF.

Generation of VEGF

Vascular endothelial growth factor (VEGF) is known to be decreased in preeclampsia. VEGF production and behavior seems to have very interesting role in the causation pathology of obstetric vasculopathies. VEGF is a signal protein produced by cells at different locations of the body. Their essential role is to stimulate formation of new vessels and maintain these new vessels functionally and structurally (vasculogenesis and angiogenesis). Vasculogenesis means de novo formation of embryonic circulatory systems and angiogenesis means growth and renovation of already existing vascular system. Indirectly VEGFs restore blood supply to the tissues and organs thereby oxygenate the tissues. They have very big role in supporting embryonic development. VEGF is a subfamily of growth factors derived from platelets or platelets derived growth factors. They have a role in health as well as in disease.

Though there are many known types of VEGF, activity of VEGF-A was identified first. Before other types of VEGF were discovered, VEGF-A was only known and therefore was named simply as VEGF. However, later on other types of VEGFs got identified and got names as VEGF-A, B, etc. Basically, all types of VEGF family members act by binding on cell surfaces to receptors. In cases of VEGF there are tyrosinekinase receptors (VEGFRs) on the cell surface. VEGFs bind to VEGFRs to dimerise them. This leads to activation through the process of transphosphorylation. In pregnancy, there has been a high and positive correlation between VEGF and hormones reflecting placental function like HCG

Table 5.1: VEGF type specific functions	
Type	*Function*
VEGF- A	Angiogenesis Increased migration of endothelial cells Increased mitosis of endothelial cells Increased methane monooxygenase activity Increased Avβ3 activity Creation of blood vessel lumen Creates fenestrations Chemotactic for macrophages and granulocytes Vasodilatation (indirectly by no release)
VEGF-B	Embryonic angiogenesis
VEGF-C	Lymphangiogenesis
VEGF-D	Needed for the development of lymphatic vasculature surrounding lung bronchioles
PIGF	Important for vasculogenesis, also needed for angiogenesis during ischemia, inflammation, wound healing, and cancer

and progesterone. It is possible that VEGF production is increased by these two placental hormones having a positive effect on trophoblast development. The functions of different VEGF have been summarized in the Table 5.1

When VEGF were studied during the menstrual cycle it was found that VEGF activity in the form of expression and action was greatly increased in decidual cells of early pregnancy. During menstrual cycle VEGF activity becomes most pronounced when progesterone is added to the estrogen in the secretory phase of the endometrium. In short VEGF and VEGFRs play an important role in implantation and maintenance of normal pregnancy.

Interesting behavior of VEGF and VEGFRs has been found in obstetric vasculopathies. For this a comparison of their levels was done between placenta of obstetric vasculopathies like PIH and IUGR on one side with placenta from normal pregnancy. Some studies found increased expression of VEGF in obstetric vasculopathies[26,27] whereas others found that free vascular endothelial growth factor is not competent to predict development of preeclampsia.[28] It has also been found that the expression of the new growth factor endocrine gland derived vascular endothelial growth factor (EG-VEGF) is high in early pregnancy but falls after 11 weeks, suggesting an essential role for this factor in early pregnancy.[29]

NITRIC OXIDE IN OBSTETRIC VASCULOPATHY

Nitric oxide is one of the most potent vasodilators in human body. Nitric oxide (NO) was once marveled as the molecule of the century and attempts were made to identify its role in conditions of human health and disease. However, in human pregnancy NO seems to have a compensatory role. Its role is limited to one of the several attempts made by the fetomaternal vascular interface to prevent reperfusion damage. This is in contrast to many other systems, tissues and organs of the body where NO is supposed to promote health of these structures and not merely prevent destruction by disease processes. It is now clear that reperfusion damage occurs by liberation of a series of vasoconstrictive and vasospasmodic elements in the system. NO seems to have a role in reversing this vasospasm. In these ecNOS (Endothelial constitutive nitric oxide synthase) gives vital leads.

ecNOS is an enzyme found in the basic constitution of endothelium. It generates NO by catalytic action. In human placenta NO synthesis and generation is not innate but as a reaction or result to reperfusion. It means that NO would appear at fetomaternal interface only as a response to vasospasm and subsequent reperfusion. This is in contrast to some tissue and organ cell lines where NO is present autonomously on its own. It does not appear as a reaction or in response to some vasospasmodic phenomenon. In tissues and organs where NO is innately present, it is believed that its role is in promoting health of these body constituents. But at the fetomaternal interface NO has a responsive role. Its role is to reverse a harm or injury or at best limit an injury. Therefore, probably it does not have so much significance in human pregnancy. Thus, the molecule of the century NO may not be so consistently exalted for human pregnancy.

It has been found that in obstetric vasculopathies the mRNA expression of ecNOS is significantly increased.[30] This reflects the compensatory and protective responsiveness to vascular reperfusion. mRNA expression of ecNOS occurs only after the process of vasospasm and reperfusion sets in. Therefore, increased generation of NO seems to be on adaptive response of the fetomaternal vasculature to poor perfusion in obstetric vasculopathies.

It is by now apparent that this entire process of obstetric vasculopathy has some modulator bearing on it by the process of inflammation. It has been found that when human placental extract is infiltrated in the thighs of rats, there was a distinct attenuation of inflammatory response.[31] In these experimental locations it was also found that besides other factors, NO synthesis was significantly reduced. This observation requires careful understanding. Placental tissue in itself not only does not need the production of NO in absence of obstetric vasculopathies but they positively reduce its generation. It is, therefore, possible that in absence of reperfusion damage, placenta does not need NO. Not only does it not need NO it ensures a reduction in generation of NO in situations where there is no reperfusion damage. Therefore, if the human fetomaternal interface senses that the milieu is conducive to a healthy pregnancy, NO is dispensed with.

Problems with Assessment of NO

There are a series of problems in assessing the role of NO in human pregnancy. Firstly, it is a very labile molecule.[32] Therefore, scientists have tried to use its stable forms for getting circumstantial or indirect evidence to its activity. Studies that have used these metabolites have shown inconsistent results. In fact the results may even be contradictory to each other.

NO is acknowledged as the strongest vasodilator in the body. It may be an antithesis of endothelin ET-1 in this function. This comparison is more metaphorical. It is not suggested that NO and ET-1 are antagonists of one another. NO being a vasodilator it is expected that in human placenta its levels should be low when there is obstetric vasculopathy in the maternal vascular system as well as at the fetomaternal interface. Some studies report low levels of NO in preeclampsia.[33,34] Contradicting this there are some studies that show no change in NO levels in preeclampsia and some even higher levels.[35] These contradictory results are indeed intriguing.

Pathophysiological changes that occur in obstetric vasculopathies also influence circulating level of NO besides its own lability. Renal systems especially the kidneys are known to excrete NO in blood. Nitric oxide levels may be reduced in obstetric vasculopathies. But the renal function also gets reduced or compromised in preeclampsia. Therefore in the event of blood levels of NO getting reduced in preeclampsia, their excretion out of the kidneys also gets reduced. As a result, the circulating blood levels of NO may not register much change.

One more complexity added in assessing the role of NO in preeclampsia is by the fact that there are many other body organs and tissues that also generate NO. Therefore, even if the endothelial contribution of NO may be reduced in its state of endothelial activation non-endothelial contributions neutralize this reduction. It, therefore, seems that the widespread sources of NO, alteration in physiology of different systems of the body in human pregnancy and technical difficulties in measurement of NO levels all contribute to difficulties in assessing the role of NO in preeclampsia in particular and in obstetric vasculopathies in general.

Nitric Oxide and Endothelial Cells

Leads from some in vivo and in vitro studies have given some interesting insights into the possible role of NO in obstetric vasculopathies. These insights are indirect, circumstantial but nevertheless important. In this context, it is relevant to understand the enzyme NO-synthase. NO-synthase is an enzyme that elaborates NO. Increased activity levels of NO-synthase can give an idea of increased levels of NO in the body. There are a series of processes that tend to increases the levels of NO-synthase. At the same time, there are different physiological processes in the body which upregulates this enzyme. By upregulation, NO levels tend to increase as the enzyme that generates it is precedingly increased.

Using this background one needs to understand the role of NO in obstetric vasculopathies. It has been found that endothelial cells exposed to plasma of pre-eclamptic women in vitro tend to increase the levels of NO. This is intriguing. Endothelial cells are supposed to reduce NO levels in preeclampsia. However in vitro they tend to increase the levels of NO. This is a paradox that needs to be understood carefully. Inspite of their limitations all studies that assessed the levels of NO in preeclamptic women showed one consistent finding: NO levels reduce in preeclampsia. This is in total contrast to the results of in vitro studies wherein endothelial cells showed an increase in NO levels when exposed to plasma of preeclamptic women compared to NO levels released by endothelial cells exposed to plasma of normal pregnant subjects.[36,37]

The explanation for these paradoxical observations is very complex but important. Explanation for this which seems to be most rational is the one based on studies from Davidge et al.[37] This group has demonstrated that the LDL component of plasma is responsible for NO release from the endothelium. Further research in this matter showed that lysophosphotidyl choline, a component of oxidatively denatured LDL upregulated nitric oxide synthase (NOS). NOS the enzyme that releases the NO. This NO is then expected to neutralize the oxidized lipid peroxides.[38,39]

It seems likely that in their innate form in the body, NO which is very labile and active gets quickly used up in neutralizing the oxidized LDL. However, in vitro the endothelium is exposed to much diluted plasma. In the diluted plasma the oxidized LDL too gets diluted. The effect of this is the endothelial cells produce nitric oxide (NO) which remains unutilized and registers a rise in levels in vitro when exposed to plasma of preeclamptic women. In vivo the LDL are in innate form. Though their lysophosphotidyl choline component enhances the levels of NO much more by upregulation, these get effectively neutralized by the undiluted in vivo environment by oxidize LDLs.

This complex but plausible explanation needs to be revisited for better understanding though may appear repetitive. One basic fact remains: the oxidatively denatured LDL play havoc in preeclampsia. Like any other healing system in the body, there is a system in place to neutralize these LDL components of the plasma. NO is the principle neutralizer of these denatured LDL molecules. Therefore, in preeclampsia NO is quickly used up in the process of neutralizing and blunting the effects of LDL. Therefore in vivo NO levels do not show consistent rise in preeclampsia in particular and all obstetric vasculopathies in general.

Contrastingly in vitro situation gets changed. This is because the plasma from preeclamptic women used to react against the endothelial cells is diluted (2%).[32] Because of this neutralization, the affectivity and relative concentration of LDLs get reduced. A reduced or muted LDL level is not able to generate the same effects as seen in vivo. By its intrinsic characteristics the lysophosphotidyl choline component of denatured (oxidized) LDL does increase NO synthase (NOS) activity. The result of this is increase in NO release. These NO increase in quantity has a depleted and diluted pool of LDL to neutralize. Thus, fairly large amount of NO is left unutilized. This gets detected on estimation systems. The sum total effect of this is a rise in NO levels detected in vitro when endothelial cells get exposed to the plasma of subject with preeclampsia. This is the basis of the rise in NO levels registered in vitro in preeclampsia and no such rise shown in vivo.

One more important conclusion that emerges from these studies also needs to be understood and appreciated. While plasma from pre-eclamptic subjects showed a rise in NO released from the endothelium, no such rise was shown by the endothelial cells when exposed to the plasma of normal pregnant subjects. This difference is apparently in LDL. Whereas LDL is present in both plasma in equal (though diluted) strength, the LDL of pre-eclamptic subject caused a rise in NO levels from the endothelial cells. The same LDL did not cause any rise when from non-pre-eclamptic subjects. This proves that both LDLs are seemingly making the difference. The difference in LDLs is not in the concentration or density of its particles. This difference is principally in the nature of these LDL molecules. The LDLs from pre-eclamptic subjects are oxidized LDLs. On the other hand in non-preeclamptic plasma no such denaturation occurs. Thus LDL from non-preeclamptic subjects is different from LDL from normal pregnant subjects. While underlining the difference in nature of LDLs from two groups, one still more basic fact gets proved through these observations. Denatured LDLs (peroxidized LDLs) are principle players in causation of obstetric vasculopathy.

PLACENTAL ATHEROSIS IN OBSTETRIC VASCULOPATHY

In some studies the phenomenon of placental atherosis has been demonstrated. This is similar to aging atherosis in human beings.[40] This led to a speculation that obstetric vasculopathy results from the process of atherosis at the fetomaternal interface. It is indeed true that the pathologic lesions of the decidual arterioles bear striking resemblance the atherotic lesions of coronary arteries. Both show fibrinoid necrosis of the vessel wall, aggregation of platelets and accumulation of lipid laden macrophages. It is not specific to preeclampsia. It is also demonstrated in other obstetric vasculopathies like IUGR even in absence of any maternal manifestation.[40] Under light microscopy these changes were limited to registering an excess of villous cytotrophoblasts. But under the electron microscopy these placenta showed villous cytotrophoblastic hyperplasia, focal syncitial necrosis, microvillus abnormalities, reduced syncitial secretory activity, irregular thickening of the trophoblastic basement membrane and the presence of small fetal vessels in the villi.[2]

These changes are due to placental ischemia. This ischemia was the key etiological factor for the proponents of placental ischemia theory in causation of obstetric vasculopathy. However the series of research and observations have shown that this ischemia is just a part of the chain of events that culminate in clinical manifestations of obstetric vasculopathies.

A simplistic conclusion of drawing parallels between the placental atheroma reflecting placental aging and the physical appearance of an IUGR baby ("the old man" look) can be erroneously drawn. It is imperative to understand that these changes of placental aging or atherosis are not extending beyond the placenta. Therefore, simplistically extending the aging process even to the target system, the fetus in this case, would be erroneous.

It would also be interesting to observe that these atheromatous changes in the fetomaternal interface do not extend to the entire maternal vasculature. It may involve some of the vessels and the process is reversible. Therefore, giving a great etiological importance to the process of obstetric vasculopathy may be wrong.

Whilst the basic oxidative stress process is so very well-established in the causation of obstetric vasculopathies, the oxidized products are not demonstrated in maternal vasculature. This is important because it reinforces the confines of the atheromatous process to the maternal and fetal interface. It is, therefore, also clear that the origin of all obstetric vasculopathies occurs at the fetomaternal interface. The maternal vasculature gets secondarily and most of the times reversibly involved.

Interestingly on long-term follow-up of subjects with aPLA syndrome it was found that they have a tendency to develop hypertension later in life. In these subjects, it seems the maternal vasculature have an intrinsic susceptibility to hypertension amplified by antiphospholipid antibodies. On the same lines the higher incidence of myocardial insufficiency reported in subjects of aPLA antibodies is due to the susceptibility of the myocardial vasculature to these changes amplified by aPL antibodies. In all these subjects, aspirin has shown to have a postponing effect for manifestation of the pathology. However, aspirin and heparin will be discussed once again later on in other sections of this work.

EXTRACELLULAR REDUCING SYSTEMS

Having had understood the oxidative stress basis of etiopathology of obstetric vasculopathies it will now be very interesting to study the body reaction to this destructive process. In any live system, whenever a destructive potential is activated the body immediately activates a healing and /or neutralizing systems. A classic example of this is the healing and reparative processes in wounds and incisions. As soon as a cut is made on any live human organ or a tissue including the skin, at that very moment instantaneously the fibroblasts start proliferating to promote healing of that wound. Though clinically the primary healing of any wound may occur within 72 to 96 hours, it is well-known that the first outpour of fibroblasts occur the moment the injury occurs. The body not only activates mechanisms to control blood loss in an injury (platelets and coagulation cascade activation) but it also activates mechanisms to heal concurrently. Similarly as soon as on oxidative denaturation begins, extracellular reducing systems start their process of neutralizing the oxidative injury.

Reducing systems are particles that have an extra unpaired proton. Oxidizing systems are particles that have on extra unpaired electron. As soon as the oxidative injury begins, the extracellular reducing systems start getting liberated in the intercellular matrix. They react with the oxidizing free radicals. In actuality they react much faster with the free radicals than the free radicals reacting with maternal tissues. Therefore, the reducing systems neutralize the oxidative injuries or successfully prevent these injuries from occurring.

Whether a molecule acts an oxidizing substance or a reducing system in any given interaction can often be predicted from tables of standard one-electron reduction potentials.[42] For example, α(x)-tocopherol (X-TOH) slows lipid peroxidation by scavenging lipid peroxyl radicals (LOO*). This breaks the peroxidation chain: LOO*+ X-TOH + X-TOO*. Lipid peroxyl radicals get peroxidized in this reaction to LOOH where the reductant X-TOH provides the hydroxyl radical to complete the reaction. But the radical so formed XTOO* is any day less reactive than the initial peroxyl radical LOO*.

This is just one example of successful neutralization of oxidizing reaction. A series of such reducing systems are naturally active in the extracellular matrix working efficiently and maintaining health of a pregnant subject. However, when the oxidative reactants are more powerful numerous and competent, the maternal reducing systems get overwhelmed. Once overwhelmed, the maternal extracellular reducing systems are unable to stem the oxidative process in the extracellular matrix. Unchecked, the oxidative radicals and the oxidative process successfully overwhelm the lipid moieties that are walking in and out of the matrix and the basic etiopathology of obstetric vasculopathies gets into place.

One classic example of a very competent extracellular reducing system is ascorbic acid. In the reaction described in the preceding paragraphs, ascorbate sustains the continuous supply and regeneration of Xα-TOH by reducing tocopherol radicals in the membranes and lipoproteins at the water lipid interface. Just as the reactive oxygen species (ROS) use the peroxidized lipids to fan out in the fetomaternal interface in particular and in the entire maternal system in general, so do the reducing systems fan out their protection net in the same locations. The reductant change generated by the ascorbate on Xα-TOH is one such classic example. In the maternal systems ascorbate is a super reducing system. There are many other reducing systems working equally competently if not more.

Uric Acid: One of the Most Power House Reductant

Uric acid for generations together has been known to play a cardinal role in disease states. Like ascorbic acid, uric acid or urate is one of the most powerful extracellular reducing systems in the body. It is operational in all human bodies consistently thwarting and neutralizing the disease producing tendencies of oxidative reactions. Interesting average clinicians are used to include estimation of uric acid in the routine list of laboratory investigations list that they request in obstetric vasculopathies. Uric acid levels are, therefore, most consistently requested in preeclampsia and eclampsia. However, a single value of uric acid estimate does not contribute much in assisting the clinician for any form of decision making like any other reducing system, Uric acid is behaving like a policeman when it comes to neutralizing the oxidative reaction. One can understand the role of these reductants better if we visit the policeman to riot model.

Riots—Policemen Model to Understand Uric Acid

If for the sake of understanding one assumes that oxidative stress is a riot and free radicals are rioters, reducing systems are policemen mobilized by the mother to quell these riots. If the rioters are more vitriolic and or more numerous the riots go uncontrolled and a great destruction can ensue. However, if the policemen are competently armed and/or are more in number the riots are quelled from spreading or nipped from the bud. When a clinician requests for a single estimation of uric acid in his practice, it is similar to seeing some policemen at one instance. It only gives an idea that some riot may be on. It does not give any further information. Supernormal levels of uric acid at any one given instance give only this small information that the oxidative riot may be on and so the posse of policemen (uric acid) is present on duty.

However, when one repeats uric acid estimation in any subject in whom the process of obstetric vasculopathy has manifested clinically there are three possibilities:

1. Uric acid levels may not be much different than those values before three weeks. This means that the riot (oxidative process) has not worsened. The policemen have not increased because the riots have not gone out of hand. The prognosis in such cases is not bad through not always favorable.
2. The second possibility is that the subsequent values after three weeks of estimation of the first value the uric acid levels have significantly increased. This is a bad prognosis. In the riot-police model it means that the policemen

have increased in number. Now, when these policemen increase in number it means the rioters are having field day and the riots are not getting quelled. Because the maternal systems are unable to quell the riots (oxidative reactions) more and more policemen are getting mobilized. This is clinically reflected as increasing levels of uric acid. Increasing levels of uric acid indicates that the prognosis is poor. Failure of intrinsic maternal extracellular reducing systems to neutralize the oxidative reaction means the disease process is very active still. In such a situation, the obstetrician needs to intervene or by prepared for an adverse obstetric outcome.

3. The third possibility is that of uric acid levels falling in subsequent estimation. This means the maternal system has successfully thwarted the disease process. The riots have been quelled the policemen have returned home. However, in clinical practice this hardly ever occurs because till the pregnancy is on, the oxidative process is on and so the uric acid levels will not fall.

Thus, both ways uric acid is very critical in obstetric vasculopathies as a strong reducing system in the body and as a sensitive prognosticator for the condition.

Limitations of Reducing Systems

As is so well-known by now, all actions of ROS are not always pathological. There are many vital functions in the body based on oxidative process. In the same way all reducing systems are not necessarily health promoting. Indeed, in the vascular endothelium ROS are disease causing and reducing systems are protective. On the other hand, there are many reductants that also act as oxidizing agents at times. Classic example of this is water soluble Vitamin E analog Trolox C. It shows both, reducing as well as oxidative properties in vitro. Such behaviors of some reductants have made clinicians cautious in recommending universal usage of reducing systems.

It is also very interesting that any drug system which tries to neutralize health promoting or health restoring physiology in the body are met with stiff resistance. The entire system organization of any living body is to preserve and promote life. If any extraneous or to that matter even internal change comes in the way of this orientation of the living system, the latter will make all possible attempts to eliminate it. If total elimination may not be possible from the body system, the body will thwart in or blunt it. This explains why large meta-analysis on efficacy of reducing systems in preventing and/or treating obstetric vasculopathies has not shown consistent results. Not all reducing systems are effective. Also, some reducing systems may be effective partially. Some reducing systems may be effective at some times and ineffective at others. Ascorbic acid for example has been found to be a supreme reductant. This means it is very effective in combating the oxidative process. However, when ascorbic acid is pharmacologically administered it is not found to have equally conspicuous results.

A reducing system can be reductant in one setting and an oxidant in other. Very interesting results emerged in two bioassays which highlighted the inconsistent reductant activities of reducing systems. It is now clear that extracellular iron has a very important amplifying role in the oxidative process. Extracellular iron amplifies the peroxidation process in the intercellular matrix. In the body serum ceruloplasmin and apotransferrin have a very important role to play in eliminating these extracellular oxidized lipid particles in whom extracellular Fe has played an amplification role. In a study by Cranfield et al, a substantial reduction in the serum reducing activity of serum ceruloplasmin and apotransferrin was observed in preeclampsia, relative to normal pregnancy. This was because in preeclampsia the serum apotransferrin levels were decreased. Thus in preeclampsia the elimination of Fe-amplified lipid peroxides is reduced. On the other hand a totally different process occurs concurrently. The reducing system activity (when measured as the ability of the plasma to scavenge water soluble peroxyl radicals) is increased.[41]

Thus on one side in preeclampsia in particular and obstetric vasculopathies in general the ability of the body to eliminate lipid peroxyl particles decreases and on the other, in the same body, in the same disease challenge of obstetric vasculopathy, the scavenging activity of these lipid peroxyl particles is increased. This highlights the consistent inconsistency of the body to respond to an oxidative process. It also shows the inconsistency of body reductants in limiting the oxidant activities. At some level they limit the pathology on other levels they themselves get limited! This provides vital insights into the question of why inconsistent results are observed in the action of reductants when extraneously administered.

Inconsistency of Reducing Systems

The efficacy of reducing systems can be best summarized in one word as "Inconsistent". This is interesting. Simplistically if oxidative process should have such a big role in producing obstetric vasculopathies, reductants must be able to at least prevent if not reverse these conditions. But this does not always happen.

Also on the experimental platforms, reducing systems produce inconsistent changes. In one trial Vitamin E failed to produce a salutary effect on an already established preeclampsia. Also, Vitamin E deficiency is not a characteristic of obstetric vasculopathies. Vitamin E is one of the most popular antioxidant used by clinicians for many (rational and irrational) indications. On the basis of the results that have consistently showed the involvement of oxidative stress in the occurrence of obstetric vasculopathies the first question asked by average clinicians is: can Vitamin E supplementation solve the problem? The answer from the observations of both in vitro and in vivo studies is a big NO.

Thus there was a reduction in a potent reducing system uric acid. There was an increase in the release of Vitamin E which is also an innate reducing system in the human body. On the third side, there was no change in the levels of thiobarbituric acid, indicator of lipid peroxidation activity. Clinically, there was no much difference but a tendency to deliver later. In one word, therefore, if one has to summarize the effect of reductants on obstetric vasculopathy it would be nothing but inconsistent.

As a student of this science one would therefore like to know why the effect of reductants was inconsistent. The answer to this is complex. As has been said in the preceding sections the oxidative changes are sustaining many physiological mechanisms in the human body. Therefore, reducing systems are perceived in the human body as agents of mechanisms that can potentially derail if not completely dysfunction these physiological activities. Human body always resists and tries to neutralize any system that will affect its physiology. Universal reductants like Vitamin E faces a resistance to their activity in the body. Therefore, they get neutralized or are inconsistent in their actions.

On the other hand, the reducing systems themselves have a changing stance as regards their configuration. By this what is meant is there are situations where they behave as reductants as well as oxidative substances. Trolox C, the water soluble Vitamin E an along is a classic example of this.

Thus, besides the blunting by the human body, the reducing systems are themselves by their behavior become inconsistent. The sum total effect therefore is inconsistency in the efficacy of reducing systems to generate effects in obstetric vasculopathies.

The Ideal Reducing System

On the basic of very deep and complicated insights into the etiopathology of obstetric vasculopathies and the role of oxidative stress in the same, one perceives a need for a consistent reducing system. However, this has eluded science. An ideal reducing system therefore would be one which reverses the disease process and/ or prevents their occurrence. At the same time, the reducing system should not alter, hamper or arrest the ongoing physiology in the body that promotes health. As is expected anything ideal is always desirable but not always available. The ideal reducing system, therefore, which will only and selectively prevent or cure obstetric vasculopathies therefore is desirable but not available. Till that time that the ideal reducing system is found, a clinician has to use either less than ideal substances. This goes by the principle if you cannot treat the cause treat the effects.

It also opens up a new concept of desirable and undesirable reducing systems. Undesirable reducing systems would be farthest from the ideal. Desirable reducing systems are those which would be closest to the ideal. The best generator of such desirable reducing systems therefore is the body itself. It is the best organism to judge what can be retained and what can be physiologically detrimental and therefore be eliminated. The latter is undesirable and forms are desirable reducing system. Exercises a physiological and health promoting activity does this very efficiently and classically.

EXERCISE AND PREVENTION OF OBSTETRIC VASCULOPATHIES

Exercises are a natural phenomenon. There is no extraneous drug sent to the body system to manipulate the body mechanisms. Exercises are a form of "healthy stress" electively generated in the body. It will, therefore, be very interesting to study how the body responds to this stress. As exercise is a "physiological stress" the body will respond with distresses that are physiological. They would, therefore, likely to be as close as possible to the "ideal" distresses. If oxidative process is generated during exercise, the reducing systems generated by exercise would be ideal reducing systems neutralizing only the oxidative reaction that produces stress (disease) and not affecting the oxidative reactions that are supporting the physiological processes.

Gavard J A reported a study on effect of exercises on some adverse obstetric outcome including preeclampsia. The purpose of their review was to critically evaluate the scientific literature for the effects of exercise on pregnancy outcome. Maternal outcomes analyzed in this review were gestational diabetes mellitus, preeclampsia and weight gain. Fetal outcomes evaluated were birth weight, time of delivery, and mode of delivery. Despite methodological pitfalls in the studies published, the evidence suggests a benefit of exercise in pregnancy. Exercise in pregnancy could prevent and limit adverse maternal and fetal morbidities and provide a long-term benefit through reduction of maternal weight gain during pregnancy and improvement in cardiovascular fitness. Pregnancy emerges as a unique time for behavior modification.[43] In contrast to this Meher et al while reviewing for Cochrane database found that there is insufficient evidence for reliable conclusions about the effects of exercise on prevention of preeclampsia and its complications.[44]

However, when scientists try to estimate the changes in circulating levels of different substances due to exercises they are likely to err on simplicity. One, two, three or a set of reducing substances that can be assessed by the human experiment conditions are finite in number. Exercises or such physiological stress are causing changes on infinite and therefore a massive number of reductants to increase or change. Many of these may still not be known to science.

There are a series of body reducing systems that may not be increased arithmetically in the body. Instead they simply get activated. This can be similar to activation of a series of cell linings in immunological responses. Many cells get activated by the mother for eliminating the foreign antigen the fetus including the platelets. These platelets do not increase in arithmetic numbers. But they become functionally more active. Similarly, there are a series of reducing systems in the body that simply get activated by the body without arithmetically increasing in circulation. Thus laboratory set-ups can be easily misled into believing that no increase in particular reducing system occurred therefore that reducing system has no role in preventing or reducing obstetric vasculopathies through exercises. In actuality, these are most efficient in reducing the effects of oxidative stress.

Another erroneous behavior is seen in clinical practice by research scientist as well as the clinicians. If any reducing system is shown to be arithmetically increased during exercises, the clinicians will demand that these should be made available in pharmacological forms for clinical administration. This is with a hope that they will bring about exactly the same effects as they do in the human body when physiologically released. The research scientists also would like to generate them pharmacologically to meet this need. But the reducing substances that increase in exercises or any similar physiological stress may not necessarily be primary or most important agent that has increased. It may just be sidekick. The importance of this sidekick became so much pertinent because historically they have been identified and isolated earlier in laboratory condition. This conveniently made the scientists pursue them as most vital leads. On countless occasions scientists have erred in this way in understanding diseases processes and devising treatment.

Chronologically, earlier identified agent may not necessarily be more important in causing or treating the disease. Classical example of this can be found in the discovery of prostaglandins. PG-A was discovered earlier. PG-F was discovered later. It was later proved that PG-A was not necessarily more important in clinical effects as compared to PG-F. Many such historical events and evidences are available in medical science. Therefore, the potential of knowing the useful reducing systems in eliminating the harmful oxidative stresses is immense. There is more that is hidden here than known and this is where a key area of treatment of obstetric vasculopathies is treasured.

TREATMENT BEARINGS

As clinicians one will understandably have a tendency to use these observations for devising treatments to prevent peroxidation of LDLs. If however this is unpreventable, limit these effects by breaking the cycle that supports this process of lipid peroxidation. As a knee-jerk reaction, clinicians and research groups would like to examine the possibility of using pharmacological reducing substances or antioxidants against these LDLs. On the face of it, this seems a sound proposition. But in actual clinical practice dramatic results are not achieved when these reducing systems are administered to pregnant women to prevent or treat the oxidative injury. The reasons of this have been discussed elsewhere in different perspective (P***). However, here one more aspect becomes clear that the reducing substances administered may be able to neutralize the effects of oxidative stress but may not be able to break the ongoing vicious circle. Therefore, their effects may at best be transitory and or inconsistent.

The Beauty of Lysophosphotidyl Choline

With the understanding of lipid peroxidation and its effects on endothelial cell activation, one more intricate but beautiful phenomenon also becomes clear. This phenomenon is that of healing through and by the injuring agents. As is amply evident now the lipid molecules that are peroxidized have two critical bearings in the etiopathology of obstetric vasculopathies. One, direct effect on the vascular smooth muscles through activation of thromboxane prostacyclin imbalance in favor of the former and next, activation of endothelial cells through sublethal injury leading to release of a myriad of substances including endothelin. Whereas the prostaglandin thromboxane generates the vasospasm, much more potent smooth muscle contractors like endothelin maintain and amplify the process.

While this process of injury and disease is ongoing the same peroxidized lipid molecules also concurrently start the healing and neutralizing process. It is now known that lysophosphotidyl choline, a component of oxidatively modified LDL upregulates Nitric Oxide Synthase (NOS).[38] This in simple terms means it enhances the production of NOS. NOS increase leads to increased synthesis of nitric oxide. An enhanced nitric oxide production leads to increased availability of nitric oxide (NO). Now nitric oxide is known to be one of the strongest vasodilators. Thus the sum total effect of peroxidized lipid molecules on vessel wall is vasospasm. But its own compound generates substances that will lead to neutralization of this vasospasm and if possible produce a vasodilatation.

This dichotomy is unique. It gives a very valuable insight into the understanding of the pathophysiology of obstetric vasculopathies. At the same time, it also becomes clear that in the entire gamut of physiology of pregnancy, the fetomaternal interface as well as the mother's body accepts that the processes involved in obstetric vasculopathies are not normal. They are not physiological. As a result these systems generate neutralizing, regulating and even healing processes in response to the pathology.

This can have therapeutic bearing in clinical practice. Methods of neutralizing, masking or suppressing the oxidative phenomenon itself will not give success. Because there are many oxidative processes in the body that support, enhance or generate some physiological process. Thus the human body would try all its might to blunt the effects of any pharmacological agent that would neutralize oxidative processes in general.

Therefore, the need would be for agents which generate, enhance or amplify the production and /or action of molecules like lysophosphotidyl choline. If such substances are generated, the process of oxidative stress would not be arrested but its combative and neutralizing systems would be enhanced. This could be the ideal treatment for obstetric vasculopathies. Such treatment modality would be very close to the ideal reducing system. This means they would not neutralize the physiology but only blunt or combat the pathology. Such agents would have the capacity to reverse the process of obstetric vasculopathy. Therefore, their predominant role would not be in the prevention of these conditions but in reversing and treating them.

Currently, all efforts are confined to use reducing systems to neutralize the oxidative stress and its effects. This has obviously and understandably given limited results. The other set of management strategies for obstetric vasculopathies is by preventing its target effects as the cause could not be neutralized. With such selective mechanisms that generate internal neutralizing systems like lysophosphotidyl choline are produced, the specific pharmacological treatment of obstetric vasculopathies becomes a reality.

REFERENCES

1. Desai P, Rathod S, Garge V, Mansuri Z. Evaluation of pro-oxidants and antioxidants in preeclampsia. *Jr O and G India.* 2003;53 (5): 445-8.
2. Desai P. Reducing systems in preeclampsia In Dasgupta S (ed). *Recent Advances In Obstetrics and Gynecology*-6. Jaypee Publishers, Delhi. 2003;79-98.
3. Neboh E, Emeh J, Aniebue U, Ikekpeazu E, Maduka I, Ezeugwu F. Relationship between lipid and lipoprotein metabolism in trimesters of pregnancy in Nigerian women: Is pregnancy a risk factor, *J Nat Sci Biol Med.* 2012;3(1):32-7.
4. Newbern D, Freemark M. Placental hormones and the control of maternal metabolism and fetal growth. *Curr Opin Endocrinol Diabetes Obes.* 2011;18(6):409-16
5. Mittal P, Hassan S, Espinoza J, Kusanovic J, Edwin S, Gotsch F, et al. The effect of gestational age and labor on placental growth hormone in amniotic fluid. *Growth Horm IGF Res.* 2008;18(2):174-9.
6. Hubel C, McLaughlin M, Evans R, Hauth B, Sims C, Roberts J. Fasting serum triglycerides, free fatty acids, and malanodialdehyde are increased in preeclampsia, are positively correlated, and decrease within 48 hours post partum. *Am J Obstet Gynecol.* 1996;174(3):975-82.
7. Lei Q, Lv L, Zhang B, Wen JY Liu G, Lin X, Niu J. Ante-partum and post-partum markers of metabolic syndrome in preeclampsia. *J Hum Hypertens.* 2011;25(1):11-7.
8. Gosmanov A, Smiley D, Peng L, Siquiera J, Robalino G, Newton C. Vascular effects of intravenous intralipid and dextrose infusions in obese subjects. *Metabolism.* 2012 Apr 5. [Epub ahead of print]

9. Davidson M. Update on CETP inhibition. *J Clin Lipidol.* 2010;4(5):394-8.
10. Czyzewska M, Wolska A, Cwiklińska A, Kortas-Stempak B, Wróblewska M. Disturbances of lipoprotein metabolism in metabolic syndrome. *Postepy Hig Med Dosw.* 2010;64:1-10.
11. Siri-Tarino P, Woods A, Bray G, Krauss R. Reversal of small, dense LDL subclass phenotype by weight loss is associated with impaired fat oxidation. *Obesity.* 2011; 19(1):61-8.
12. Austin M, Edwards K. Small, dense low density lipoproteins, the insulin resistance syndrome and noninsulin-dependent diabetes. *Curr Opin Lipidol.* 1996;7(3):167-71.
13. Shia W, Ku T, Tsao Y, Hsia C, Chang Y, Huang C. Genetic copy number variants in myocardial infarction patients with hyperlipidemia. *BMC Genomics.* 2011;12S(3):S23.
14. Kim O, Chung H, Shin M. Higher levels of serum triglyceride and dietary carbohydrate intake are associated with smaller LDL particle size in healthy Korean women. *Nutr Res Pract.* 2012;6(2):120-5.
15. Miranda Guisado M, Vallejo-Vaz A, García Junco P, Jiménez Jiménez L, García Morillo S, Muñiz Grijalvo O. Abnormal levels of antioxidant defenses in a large sample of patients with hypertensive disorders of pregnancy. *Hypertens Res.* 2012;35(3):274-8.
16. Genc H, Uzun H, Benian A, Simsek G, Gelisgen R, Madazli R. et al. Evaluation of oxidative stress markers in first trimester for assessment of preeclampsia risk. *Arch Gynecol Obstet.* 2011;284(6):1367-73.
17. Desai P, Patel P, Rathod SP, Mahajan S. Selenium levels and glutathione peroxidase activity in spontaneous inevitable abortion. *Jr O and G India.* 2006;56(4); 311-5.
18. Becker B, Massoudy P, Permanetter B, Raschke P, Zahler S. Possible significance of free oxygen radicals for reperfusion injury. *Z Kardiol.* 1993;82(5):49-58.
19. Freeman B, White C, Gutierrez H, Paler-Martínez A, Tarpey M, Rubbo H. Oxygen radical-nitric oxide reactions in vascular diseases. *Adv Pharmacol.* (1995)34:45-69.
20. Urmalia V, Rathod SP Neurological and oxidative stress assessment. Dissertation submitted to Depertment of Pharmacy, MS University of Baroda.
21. Sahlin L, Wang H, Stjernholm Y, Lundberg M, Ekman G, Holmgren A. The expression of glutaredoxin is increased in the human cervix in term pregnancy and immediately post-partum, particularly after prostaglandin-induced delivery. *Mol Hum Reprod.* 2000; 6(12):1147-53.
22. Shibata E, Ejima K, Nanri H, Toki N, Koyama C, Ikeda M, et al. Enhanced protein levels of protein thiol/disulphide oxidoreductases in placentae from pre-eclamptic subjects. *Placenta.* 2001;22(6):566-72.
23. Okatani Y, Wakatsuki A, Shinohara K, Taniguchi K, Fukaya T. Melatonin protects against oxidative mitochondrial damage induced in rat placenta by ischemia and reperfusion. *J Pineal Res.* 2001;31(2):173-8.
24. Twina G, Sheiner E, Shahaf G, Salem S, Madar T, Baron J. Lower Circulation levels and activity of Alpha-1 antitrypsin in pregnant women with severe preeclampsia. *J Matern Fetal Neonatal Med.* 2012.
25. Chakraborty D, Rumi M, Soares M. NK cells, hypoxia and trophoblast cell differentiation. *Cell Cycle.* 2012;11(13).
26. Bussen S, Bussen D. Influence of the vascular endothelial growth factor on the development of severe preeclampsia or HELLP syndrome. *Arch Gynecol Obstet.* 2011; 284(3):551-7.
27. Chaiworapongsa T, Romero R, Kim Y, Kim G, Kim M, Espinoza J, et al. Plasma soluble vascular endothelial growth factor receptor-1 concentration is elevated prior to the clinical diagnosis of preeclampsia. *J Matern Fetal Neonatal Med.* 2005;17(1):3-18.
28. Akolekar R, de Cruz J, Foidart J, Munaut C, Nicolaides K. Maternal plasma soluble fms-like tyrosine kinase-1 and free vascular endothelial growth factor at 11 to 13 weeks

of gestation in preeclampsia. *Prenat Diagn.* 2010;30(3):191-7.

29. Hoffmann P, Saoudi Y, Benharouga M, Graham CH, Schaal JP, Mazouni C, et al. Role of EG-VEGF in human placentation: Physiological and pathological implications. *J Cell Mol Med.* 2009;13(8B):2224-35.
30. Di Paolo S, Volpe P, Grandaliano G, Stallone G, Schena A, Greco P, et al. Increased placental expression of tissue factor is associated with abnormal uterine and umbilical Doppler waveforms in severe preeclampsia with fetal growth restriction. *J Nephrol* 2003;16(5):650-7.
31. Cho E, Park M, Kim S, Kang G, Choi S, Lee Y, et al. Vasorelaxing Activity of Ulmus davidiana Ethanol Extracts in Rats: Activation of Endothelial Nitric Oxide Synthase. *Korean J Physiol Pharmacol.* 2011;15(6):339-44.
32. Taylor R, Roberts J. Endothelial Cell Dysfunction. In: Lindheimer M, Roberts J, Cunningham F, (eds). *Chesley's Hypertensive Disorders of Pregnancy.* Stamford, Appleton and Lange. 2nd edn, Pg 395-430.
33. López-Jaramillo P, Arenas W, García R, Rincon M, López M. The role of the L-arginine-nitric oxide pathway in preeclampsia. *Ther Adv Cardiovasc Dis.* 2008;2(4):261-75.
34. Bernardi F, Constantino L, Machado R, Petronilho F, Dal-Pizzol F. Plasma nitric oxide, endothelin-1, arginase and superoxide dismutase in pre-eclamptic women. *J Obstet Gynaecol Res.* 2008;34(6):957-63.
35. Teran E, Chedraui P, Vivero S, Villena F, Duchicela F, Nacevilla L. Plasma and placental nitric oxide levels in women with and without preeclampsia living at different altitudes. *Int J Gynaecol Obstet.* 2009;104(2):140-2.
36. Baker P, Krasnow J, Roberts J, Yeo K. Elevated serum levels of vascular endothelial growth factor in patients with preeclampsia. *Obstet Gynecol.* 1995;86(5):815-21.
37. Davidge S, Signorella A, Hubel C, Lykins D, Roberts J. Distinct factors in plasma of preeclamptic women increase endothelial nitric oxide or prostacyclin. *Hypertension.* 1996;28(5):758-64.
38. Hirata K, Miki N, Kuroda Y, Sakoda T, Kawashima S, Yokoyama M. Low concentration of oxidized low-density lipoprotein and lysophosphatidylcholine upregulate constitutive nitric oxide synthase mRNA expression in bovine aortic endothelial cells. *Circ Res.* 1995;76(6):958-62.
39. Rubbo H, Freeman BA. Nitric oxide regulation of lipid oxidation reactions: formation and analysis of nitrogen-containing oxidized lipid derivatives. *Methods Enzymol.* 1996;269:385-94.
40. Sheppard BL, Bonnar J. An ultrastructural study of uteroplacental spiral arteries in hypertensive and normotensive pregnancy and fetal growth retardation. *Br J Obstet Gynecol.* 1981;88(7):695-705.
41. Cranfield L, Gollan J, White A, Dormandy T. Serum antioxidant activity in normal and abnormal subjects. *Ann Clin Biochem.* 1979;16(6):299-306.
42. Pierucci F, Piazze Garnica J, Cosmi E, Anceschi M. Oxidability of low density lipoproteins in pregnancy-induced hypertension. *Br J Obstet Gynecol.* 1996;103(11):1159-61.
43. Gavard JA, Artal R. Effect of exercise on pregnancy outcome. *Clin Obstet Gynecol.* 51 2008;(2):467-80.
44. Meher S, Duley L. Exercise or other physical activity for preventing preeclampsia and its complications. *Cochrane Database Syst Rev.* 2006;(2):CD005942.

CHAPTER

6

The Placenta, Trophoblasts and Obstetric Vasculopathies

CHAPTER OUTLINE

- Basic Process of Normal Placenta and Placentation
- Oxygenation and Trophoblastic Differentiation
- Faults in Fetomaternal Linkage at Placenta and Obstetric Vasculopathy
- Maternal Environment Preventing Trophoblastic Invasion

BASIC PROCESS OF NORMAL PLACENTA AND PLACENTATION

In earliest stages of normal human pregnancy when the embryo comes in contact of the maternal decidual surface, the process of placentation begins. This process has two fundamental functions to accomplish:

1. To affix and anchor the placenta to the maternal surface and
2. To establish vascular contacts with maternal system.

The first process of anchorage has a very simple and easily understandable function. This is to ensure the physical fixing of the placenta in the uterus. Without anchorage the placenta can't stay there in the uterus. However, this basic anchorage does not have any modulatary role. The second process is most complex. This is the process by which the fetus establishes contacts with the maternal vasculature and the entire fetomaternal exchange mechanism gets established. This function brings about the growth and nourishment of the fetus.

The entire process of anchorage and establishment of functional and robust vascular contacts with the mother is brought about principally by differentiation of the epithelial stem cells of the placenta termed as cytotrophoblasts. How these cytotrophoblasts differentiate will determine whether the functional units of the placenta the chorionic villi, will anchor the conceptus to the placental wall or will float into the maternal vascular system.

During the process of anchorage many cytotrophoblasts fuse to form syncitiotrophoblasts. These syncitiotrophoblasts are very specialized cells. They have the most critical function to play in the fetal withstanding of maternal rejection process. They also have other functions including bringing about oxygen transport from the maternal blood to the fetal blood. They seem to function like the alveoli of the lungs. During the anchorage process most of the cytotrophoblasts by and large do not fuse. They retain their cell wall. They detach from their cell membranes and form columns of cells.

It is of intrigue to know that the vascular invasion confines itself by and large to the arterioles sparing the venules. The venous invasion remains superficial and seems of little consequence. By late second trimester the entire spiral vasculature gets lined by the trophoblasts exclusively. This process has many sonological images and also a great clinical bearing. In the process of vascular invasion, the maternal spiral arterioles lose their muscular layer. This makes the maternal bed at this level a pool of low-resistance vascular flow. It also shields off the fetomaternal interface from the changes taking place in the maternal system. As a result the vasodilatory and vasoconstrictive substances circulating in the maternal system do not affect the fetomaternal blood circulation. This makes the fetomaternal vascular circulation autonomous.

Role of Oxygen Tension in Trophoblastic Invasion

In normal pregnancy, the cytotrophoblasts invade the larger arterioles (spiral arterioles) and are bathed by a well-oxygenated maternal blood. Nevertheless in obstetric vasculopathy, the invading cytotrophoblasts are relatively hypoxic. *In vitro* experiments have provided vital leads to the understanding of cytotrophoblastic invasion. One study in this aspect of obstetric vasculopathy studied the impairment of trophoblast invasion associated with preeclampsia. For this they studied if adenosine (A3) receptors modulate matrix metalloproteinase (MMP) secretion in villous explants from preeclamptic pregnancies. This was with the basis that the impairment of trophoblast invasion associated with preeclampsia may involve MMP. A3 receptors expression in trophoblast is upregulated in preeclampsia. Villous explants from normal and preeclamptic pregnancies were cultured at 20% and 3% oxygen. There were significantly increased A3 receptor and reduced MMP-2/-9 expression at low oxygen level in normal and preeclamptic explants. Interestingly, in preeclamptic explants, after high oxygen culture, the expression of MMP-2/-9 was recovered to almost same level of those in normal explants. This study indicated that trophoblastic adenosine A3 receptors are 1) modulated by oxygen tension, and 2) regulate MMP-2/-9 expression.[1]

There are many situations in medical science in particular and in general biological science where the cause-effect relationships between two events fail to get obvious. Whether event A is the cause of event, B or is it vice versa. Same seems to be occurring for oxygen tension and trophoblastic invasion. It is true that the oxygen pressure in the intervillous space is estimated to be approximately 18 mm of Hg and 40 mm of Hg, respectively at 8 to 10 weeks gestation. The two points where these pressures were estimated respectively at the uterine surface and within the endometrium.[2] Afterward at midtrimester when the trophoblastic proliferation and invasion of the endovascular space occurs, the pressure is as high as 90 to100 mm of Hg. These enticed scientists into believing that oxygen tension might regulate cytotrophoblastic proliferation and differentiation along the invasive pathway.[3]

On the other hand, it seems that oxygen tension is more an effect rather than the cause of endovascular invasion of trophoblasts. Trophoblasts themselves are autonomous and very critical cell lining which save the fetus from maternal rejection. Besides this it has got many critical functions of transport of gasses, nutrients, and elimination of waste. Chronologically their first function is anchorage of the placenta to the maternal tissue.

In obstetric vasculopathy, a consistent feature that has been observed is defective endovascular invasion of the trophoblasts. In common parlance trophoblastic invasions have been interpreted to be occurring as two waves. The first wave is for anchorage and is complete by 8 to 10 weeks. The second wave is related to endovascular invasion and is complete by midtrimester.

To what extent does oxygen gradient influence or is the result of endovascular invasion of trophoblasts is a matter of great interest. Trophoblasts are autonomous cell linings. By and large, they self-regulate their growth and functions. They are in a position to sense that the oxygen tension is enough for its sustenance, growth and functioning at the fetomaternal interface. If they sense that this gradient is not enough, they will seek to neutralize this crisis by invading smaller spiral arterioles. Thus invasion of smaller arterioles in obstetric vasculopathy seems to be a result to generate oxygen sufficient states. If they are not able to get sufficient oxygenation from large bore vessels, they try to neutralize this lack of oxygen gradient by proliferating and invading into smaller vessels.

Oxygen gradient has got a very important role to play in deciding where and in what will the trophoblasts invade into. *In vitro* experiments have proved this hypothesis of oxygen gradient playing an important role in deciding the completeness and efficiency of trophoblastic invasion in work done by Genbacev et al.[4] They showed that when trophoblasts both the anchoring as well as the endovascular invading trophoblasts were subjected to hypoxic environment, they proliferated both in size well as in numbers. Up to three times the number of columns were generated of these cell linings when the oxygen tension was low.

Thus, maternal low oxygen gradient seems to be a very important event in bringing about a trophoblastic invasion. By increasing their numbers, trophoblasts in hypoxic environments tend to compensate for low oxygenation. They also try to seek oxygen from the smaller spiral arterioles. This leads to very interesting clinical effects. If the proliferating and invading trophoblasts find that at the potential fetomaternal interface where the oxygen gradient is sufficient they invade large bore spiral arterioles. Their oxygenation requirements are taken care of and so they do not need to proliferate into any other vessels further. Clinically these subjects will not develop any features of obstetric vasculopathy.

However, if the proliferating trophoblasts sensing a hypoxic environment at the potential fetomaternal interface, they would invade into medium bore arterioles. Their oxygen requirements would be met with and again clinical expression of obstetric vasculopathies would not occur. On the other hand, when the hypoxic environment at the potential fetomaternal interface is such that even the invasion into middle bore vessels of the trophoblasts is unable to neutralize, the proliferation now spreads to small bore spiral arterioles. Nevertheless these arterioles are unable to provide for the oxygen gradient that is deficit. In such cases full blown manifestations of obstetric vasculopathies occur clinically.

Even when the trophoblasts need to proliferate into the mid-size spiral arterioles some milder clinical manifestations of obstetric vasculopathies can occur. But these would never be very severe and complicating. The entire process of cytotrophoblastic proliferation and invasion into the spiral arterioles both have been independently studied in reference to oxygen gradient. Studies carried out by Genbacev, et al.[4,5] showed that when cytotrophoblasts were incubated in 20% oxygen they undergo cell cycle arrest whereas culturing them in 2% oxygen induces them to undergo mitosis. This means hypoxic environments not only affect the invasion of arterioles but also lead to further proliferation of these cell lining. An average clinician would try to take a simplistic view of this suggesting that if by some means of drugs the uterine oxygen environment in early days of pregnancy can be manipulated, the causation and outcome of obstetric vasculopathies can be influenced. This needs to be examined.

OXYGENATION AND TROPHOBLASTIC DIFFERENTIATION

One aspect where oxygen tension is important vis-à-vis trophoblastic activity is in the differentiation process of the latter. It is found that under normal oxygen tension trophoblasts express different stage specific antigens. Some of these antigens are expressed at the stage of trophoblastic adhesion and invasion of uterine decidua. Others are expressed at the stage of trophoblastic invasion of vascular channels. Antigen-like Integrin ITGA-1 is expressed by the trophoblasts at the stage of decidual invasion. This expression does not occur in hypoxic conditions. This reduction of expression of antigens is not universal. This means all antigens are not reduced or ameliorated in expression. Antigens like HLA-G and integrin ITGB-5 do not change. It would therefore be important to deduce that those antigens which have critical stage specific function get modulated in expression as a response to lowered oxygen tension.

This has a direct bearing on the quality of placentation. The process of placentation needs qualitative and quantitative optimum activity of trophoblastic tissue. Any suboptimal expression of any of these will affect both the qualitative and quantitative function of trophoblasts, which will have a direct bearing on placentation. Obstetric vasculopathies are essentially a result of defective placentation. Alterations in oxygen tension leading to defective quantitative and qualitative expression of trophoblastic activities leads to defective placentation causing obstetric vasculopathies.

One more interesting aspect that has been added to the understanding of trophoblastic invasion is the fact that it is also a function of oxygen tension. It has been found that at lowered oxygenation the depth of trophoblastic invasion also gets affected. This means at lowered oxygen tension the trophoblasts invade suboptimally, both qualitatively and quantitatively. They also invade superficially. Superficial invasion by trophoblasts leads to defective anchorage. Defective anchorage can directly result in abruption of the placenta causing the clinical condition of accidental hemorrhage. It therefore seems that the entire plethora of conditions that are included under the head of obstetric vasculopathies get explained by the explanations for defective trophoblastic activity. All defects qualitative, quantitative as well as functional of trophoblasts singly or in different combinations together produce obstetric vasculopathies.

FAULTS IN FETOMATERNAL LINKAGE AT PLACENTA AND OBSTETRIC VASCULOPATHY

It is now well proved that a faulty and therefore shallow cytotrophoblastic invasion is seen in preeclampsia and intrauterine growth retardation. Taking this concept further, it is now clear that cytotrophoblasts that are invading the maternal vasculature are actually undergoing a simultaneous differentiation of its phenotypic characteristics. In this, these cytotrophoblasts assume attributes of the maternal endothelium that they replace in the spiral arterioles.

The spiral arterioles are indeed vascular channels that do not change their function fundamentally on being invaded by the cytotrophoblasts. In such an event it becomes imperative upon the cytotrophoblasts to transform themselves into the characteristics of the maternal spiral arterioles which they are invading. If this does not occur the spiral arterioles would cease to function as maternal vascular channels and instead get clogged up. Albeit, the spiral arterioles do get metamorphosed structurally losing their muscular layer and becomes a low-resistance vessel pool. This differentiation of the cytotrophoblasts into maternal vascular characteristics is therefore critical. Defective differentiation of cytotrophoblasts is very important in causation of obstetric vasculopathies.

The fetus and the mother therefore should link up properly at the fetomaternal interface. If this linkage is suboptimal, the result will be obstetric vasculopathy. Interestingly, this linkage should occur at both the placental component and the maternal component. If the cytotrophoblasts fail to differentiate and assume maternal phenotypic vascular function early, they result in spontaneous missed abortion. (This term is now replaced by embryonic or fetal demise as per the duration of pregnancy.) This is the earliest manifestation of obstetric vasculopathy.

This opens up two very important new areas. First, a chromosomal defect has an obstetric vasculopathy type of basis in some situations. Second, the phenotypic differentiation of the cytotrophoblasts in the maternal vascular channels can be variable quantitatively as well as qualitatively. If the phenotypic differentiation is less, quantitatively the results will be an IUGR. If the failure of phenotypic differentiation is massive, it leads to a fetal demise. This leads to spontaneous miscarriage.

MATERNAL ENVIRONMENT PREVENTING TROPHOBLASTIC INVASION

In the successful and robust linkage that occurs between the placenta and the fetus, the cytotrophoblasts can fail to phenotypically differentiate into maternal vascular phenotypic characteristics. Similarly, it is possible that the maternal systems too may resist this differentiation. This is found in conditions like lupus, diabetes mellitus and in some cases of maternal obesity where adverse obstetric outcomes are known.

The concept that there is a failure of trophoblastic invasion in obstetric vasculopathies now has been further elaborated. It is therefore clear that cytotrophoblastic invasion failure may be a qualitative failure. This means that the cytotrophoblasts for whatever reason are failing to phenotypically differentiate into maternal vascular endothelium. Thus, the maternal vascular system fails to metamorphose to the requirements of a healthy pregnancy need of effective linkage between the placental and maternal system. This is defective placentation of obstetric vasculopathy.

The impression for many years is that in failure of trophoblastic invasion the cytotrophoblasts simply fail to physically invade the maternal vascular channels. This may not be the whole story. The cytotrophoblasts do invade but functional invasion fails. This introduces a totally new concept of functional invasion of maternal vascular system. If the cytotrophoblasts structurally invade the maternal spiral arterioles they would clog up the maternal vascular blood supply in the placenta. Therefore after physical invasion the trophoblasts have to change. They have to differentiate. They have to become phenotypically like the maternal vascular endothelium. This is critical.

Phenotypic differentiation of the trophoblasts into maternal endothelium serves two functions. It keeps the maternal vascular bed perfusing the placenta, open. At the same time, it is also able to mold the vascular bed to its own requirement of converting it into a low-resistance vessel pool. This is effectively done by destroying the vascular muscular lining.

Thus, fetomaternal vascular linkage becomes the key to the etiopathology of obstetric vasculopathies. Once these connections are clearly understood, it will be possible to devise methods for early diagnosis and even treatment as well as reversing the pathology of obstetric vasculopathies.

REFERENCES

1. Kim Y, Hwang H, Kim Y, Kim H, Park Y. Modulation of matrix metalloproteinase secretion by adenosine A_3 receptor in preeclamptic villous explants. *Reprod Sci.* 2008; 15(9):939-49.
2. Rodesch F, Simon P, Donner C, Jauniaux E. Oxygen measurements in endometrial and trophoblastic tissues during early pregnancy. *Obstet Gynecol.* 1992;80(2):283-5.
3. Torry D, Mukherjea D, Arroyo J, Torry R. Expression and function of placenta growth factor: implications for abnormal placentation. *J Soc Gynecol Investig.* 2003;10(4):178-88.
4. Genbacev O, Zhou Y, Ludlow J, Fisher S. Regulation of human placental development by oxygen tension. *Science.* 1997;12;277(5332):1669-72.
5. Genbacev O, Joslin R, Damsky C, Polliotti B, Fisher S. Hypoxia alters early gestation human cytotrophoblast differentiation/invasion in vitro and models the placental defects that occur in preeclampsia. *J Clin Invest.* 1996;97(2):540-50.

CHAPTER

7

The Genetics of Obstetrics Vasculopathies

CHAPTER OUTLINE

- Basis for Reviewing the Role of Genetics in Obstetric Vasculopathies
- Challenges to the Genetic Studies in Obstetric Vasculopathies
- Mammalian Studies
- Application of Genetic Models
- Examining Associations
- Fetal Contributions: Any?
- Reverse Associations
- Immunology and Genetics
- Inputs from Animal Models
- Epigenetic Features in Preeclampsia

BASIS FOR REVIEWING THE ROLE OF GENETICS IN OBSTETRIC VASCULOPATHIES

For quite some time now, scientists have tried to find out if there are some aspects of genetics involved in the process of obstetric vasculopathies. Merely on basis of observational studies in an epic work, Leon Chesley[1] suggested that preeclampsia had some strange tendency to run into families. However, efforts to identify a single and specific gene that produces preeclampsia or other vasculopathies remain unproductive. Also, preeclampsia is not a disease of polygenic origin. This means that there is no particular genotype specific to any of the obstetric vasculopathies.

In absence of any genotype particular to obstetric vasculopathy, the case for genetic basis becomes all the more queer. It is now believed that one or more relatively common alleles act as "major genes" conferring susceptibility to preeclampsia. They act as susceptibility loci. They lower a women's threshold for developing preeclampsia.[2] What holds true for preeclampsia in particular seems to be holding true for obstetric vasculopathies in general. Therefore, the basis of genetics which operates for preeclampsia seems to be acting for other obstetric vasculopathies as well.

Angiotensin-converting enzyme (ACE) plays a vital role in the renin-angiotensin system (RAS) which regulates blood pressure by converting angiotensin-1 into a powerful vasoconstrictor angiotensin-2. On the presumption that placental, immune and genetic factors play an important role in preeclampsia

(PE)'s pathophysiology, one study was investigated the association between angiotensin-converting enzyme (ACE) insertion/deletion (I/D) polymorphism and preeclampsia. It concluded that there was significant difference in genotype distribution between preeclampsia and controls.[3] In another study, a role of single nucleotide polymorphism in the risk of severe fetal growth restriction complicated preeclampsia has been suggested.[4]

However, one study ruled out the association of gene mutations with adverse obstetric outcomes of preeclampsia. The purpose of this study was to determine whether maternal or fetal genotype frequencies of the inherited thrombophilic gene mutation (F V Leiden, F II) are altered in adverse pregnancy outcomes like severe preeclampsia, IUGR, abruption of placenta and stillbirth. They found that Factor V Leiden and prothrombin gene mutations did not seem play a significant role in adverse pregnancy outcome in our population.[5]

In such a confusing picture it seems that the entire plethora of activities at fetomaternal interface and maternal vasculature response may be under some genetic control. These genes may be maternal or fetal. The process of generation of ROS, denaturation of lipid molecules, activation of endothelium and generation of vasospasm seem to have a genetic basis. Yet the major point that needs to be understood is the question as to whether the genetic basis causes the entire process or only one of the initiating events. It is possible that once the key event is initiated, the entire process may be self-maintained through its cyclic and interdependent character.

On the other hand, it is very much possible that the entire process at every step may be under the genetic control. One principle basis for this thinking is that the neutralizing and protective responses of the mother are very powerful. Intrinsically unsupported and non-amplifying processes would be instantly neutralized and eliminated from the system. If the initiation of the process only would have a genetic oversee and control the process would never become clinically obvious. Therefore to sustain and amplify the pathology of obstetric vasculopathy at every step it has to be supported and enhanced. It therefore seems that the genetic basis of obstetric vasculopathies is far more extensive than mere trigger for the process.

CHALLENGES TO THE GENETIC STUDIES IN OBSTETRIC VASCULOPATHIES

It is a very queer fact that many loose criteria have been clubbed together to call a condition as preeclampsia. Hypertension seems to be the most consistent clinical feature of all what is labeled as preeclampsia. There remain other associates to this so-called critical feature of hypertension like proteinuric hypertension, gestational hypertension or preeclamptic hypertension superimposed on an under running chronic hypertension. Similarly, other clinical features which can be called as phenotypes are also inconsistent and heterogeneous. These include edema, proteinuria, renal changes described as glomeruloendotheliosis, hepatic changes, ocular changes and so many others. While one subject may have one set of phenotypes, the other subject labeled as preeclampsia may just give one or most of this amiss. This proves a big challenge for the geneticist. Which phenotype should be ascribed to the genetic basis is just a very difficult act to do. Also, inconsistency in their occurrence as well as inconsistency in their intensity of occurrence makes the going very challenging for the geneticist.

This would become clear if an attempt to understand this process is made by some model. Here, the easiest model could be T21 or mongolism as it is known as in lay parlance. The phenotypes of T21 are consistent and regular. The facial features and mental challenges found in the subjects with T21 are found in all its subjects albeit with different intensity. Therefore, it becomes easy for a geneticist to associate T21 genotype with the phenotype of mongolism. This consistency is completely lacking in preeclampsia in particular and more so if other obstetric vasculopathies are also considered. Hypertension which is most consistent and supposed to be most critical too is inconsistent in its manifestation.

One more challenge for the geneticist in assigning phenotypes to a genetic basis of preeclampsia is the fact that all of these are occurring in relation to pregnancy. Pregnancy is obviously a sex-limited trait. What role do the males therefore have in this condition is also a matter to be understood.

MAMMALIAN STUDIES

Many interesting studies based on records of mothers, daughters, sisters and even granddaughters of indexed subjects who had preeclampsia were undertaken at different instances of time. The principle results of these studies were:

- *Humphries J:* Preeclampsia occurred in 28% of daughters of mothers who had preeclampsia. This incidence was 13% in controls[6]
- *Chesley:* Rate of preeclampsia was higher in mothers, sisters, daughters and granddaughters of subjects who had preeclampsia[1]
- *Studies from Aberdeen:* Different studies were undertaken. It was found that sisters of preeclamptic women had a 2.1 to 3.4 fold increase in the rate of preeclampsia. Mothers of subjects who had preeclampsia showed four times higher incidence of the condition compared to mothers of non-preeclamptic controls[7,8]
- *Arngrimsson*: The recurrence risk for preeclampsia in the daughters of eclamptic and preeclamptic subjects was in the range of 20–40%, for sisters this was 11–37%[9]
- *Procopciuc LM:* In preeclampsia, both maternal and newborn genetic variations implicated in blood pressure regulation are important.[10]

In absence of any identifiable gene and a set genotype, these studies throw some very important light on the familial behavior of preeclampsia. Though there are hardly any studies on this matter on other obstetric vasculopathies, these studies may open a window to the chromosomal basis of these conditions. It becomes obvious from these analytical studies that there is some familial link in preeclampsia. This link does not seem to be based on food, living styles or any such confounding variable. This is so because by three to four generations, food habits or to that matter all other similar extraneous factors undergo a sea of change. Therefore the only link that binds these subjects is genes. Also, the fact that these subjects who showed higher incidence of preeclampsia were essentially blood relatives and not related through marriage eliminates the extraneous factors on one hand and reasserts the possible genetic basis on the other.

Nonetheless, it is also of importance to note that the inheritance is not following any set pattern. There is no mathematical model applicable to the pattern of inheritance unlike that seen in autosomal dominant and recessive conditions. This also means that there may not be one single gene responsible for preeclampsia or to that matter all obstetric vasculopathies in general. So as to get further insight into the possible genetic factor responsible, behavior of preeclampsia in multiple pregnancies could have provided vital leads. Yet in absence of any good quality study in this, no worthy leads emerge here from. Another possible area that could give leads in patterns of inheritance is consanguineous marriages. Here too hardly any good quality studies are available which can give worthwhile leads in the matter. Therefore, the possibility of genetic basis in preeclampsia remained by and large amorphous but possible.

APPLICATION OF GENETIC MODELS

As has been described in the previous sections, no set pattern of inheritance appears in preeclampsia in these studies of the families. Expectedly therefore all sorts of inheritance patterns have been suggested. There are some who have suggested a recessive pattern of inheritance. There are others who have also suggested a polygenic origin. Lack of consistency in these results confirms that though there is some genetic factor that is indeed playing a role in inheritance this role is at best amorphous. However, obstetric vasculopathies being autosomal dominant condition is ruled out.

On the basis of all these studies at this stage, it appears that the genetic factor that contribute to preeclampsia is at best increasing the susceptibility of a woman to preeclampsia. Also, it seems that the maternal genetic configuration has a bigger role than the fetal genetic configuration through the fetomaternal interface plays a crucial role in occurrence of obstetric vasculopathies.

EXAMINING ASSOCIATIONS

In some strange ways in clinical practice, one finds some apparent association of obstetric vasculopathies with some genetic conditions. Thus includes conditions like Beckwith-Wiedemann syndrome, trisomy-13 and some triploids if at all the pregnancy lasts that long. But these have at best remained associations not maturing to any cause-effect relationships.

FETAL CONTRIBUTIONS: ANY?

The fetomaternal interface seems to have a big role to play in the etiopathology of obstetric vasculopathies. It is therefore of interest to study the role of fetal genetic contribution in obstetric vasculopathies. For this one has to assess the role of the father. This is because the genetic contribution of the mother in the fetus is similar to her. Therefore, the expression in the fetus would also be similar to the mother. The difference in fetal genetic makeup therefore is only that from the father. Therefore, the paternal genetic component has to be assessed if one wants to study the role of the fetus in the genetic basis of obstetric vasculopathies.

On pure clinical observational classic study one is made aware of very early in his career as a medical graduate, is by a gentleman in Utah. It was reported that he lost two of his wives to eclampsia. His third wife also developed severe preeclampsia.[11] Another study concluded that short duration of exposure to sperm was more common in women with preeclampsia compared with controls.[12]

Arngrimsson study[9] also hinted at some interesting observation. It hinted at the possibility of daughter-in-law of preeclamptic subjects having a small but distinct chance of developing preeclampsia. This needs to be closely examined and peacefully understood. The fetus in question sired by the daughter-in-law has genetic contributions from four sources; One her father, two her own mother, three her husband's father and four her husband's mother. Thus, the father-in-law has indeed a small but distinct genetic contribution in building the fetus being sired by the daughter-in-law of the subjects who had preeclampsia. When Arngrimsson et al found that there is some association between the history of preeclampsia in subjects and their daughters-in-law developing this condition, the association too was very weak but distinct.[9] This also means that the subjects did develop preeclampsia but did not follow any set genetic model of inheritance.

This weakness in association could be attributable to the dilution of paternal genetic material that occurs in the fetus sired that occurs in the fetus sired by the daughter-in-law to one-fourth. This weakness is further supported by the fact that as such the contribution of genetic factors in etiopathology of preeclampsia is amorphous. In the light of such amorphous association in the basic, even if Arngrimsson et al[9] could find some association with preeclampsia, in itself is very important and noteworthy.

Another important phenomenon in abnormal pregnancy condition is molar pregnancy. For decades together if not more, scientists and clinicians have found that subjects with vesicular mole have a higher chance of developing preeclampsia. This higher chance strongly hints at a paternal contribution. Vesicular mole has two sets of paternal chromosomes, the maternal chromosomes being absent. This absence of maternal chromosomal contribution is because the ovum fertilized in vesicular mole is a "ghost ovum". This means it lacks chromosomal contribution. Herein only paternal chromosomal contribution exists and these subjects develop preeclampsia with a much higher and furious intensity. Similar associations have been identified with conditions like Beckwith-Wiedemann syndrome and Trisomy-13. In all these conditions, mothers siring pregnancies have a higher chance of developing preeclampsia.

In all these conditions the defect in genetic contribution, is paternal. Therefore, it is well understandable that the father through the fetus and fetomaternal interface has a small but important contribution to make in the etiopathology of preeclampsia. Such associations with other obstetric vasculopathies have not been reported because they have probably not been studied. The question being considered is mother-in-law who has preeclampsia have a small – but distinct higher chance of having daughters-in-law who develop preeclampsia. This could be due to the father of the fetus who sired it. He carries his mother's genes (besides that of his father). Thus, the paternal genes indirectly pass down the susceptibility to preeclampsia down to this baby.

REVERSE ASSOCIATIONS

By and large in the preceding pages attempts have been made to assess the possibility of some genes singly or in combination being directly responsible for the etiopathology of obstetric vasculopathies. Nevertheless in clinical practice there are some clinical conditions occurring due to genetic disorders having an association with preeclampsia. For such associations hardly any studies have been done for other obstetric vasculopathies. If attempts are made in future to identify these associations, IUGR would be able to reveal these relatively easily.

Coming back to reverse associations, in clinical practice there are some genetic conditions that show some association with preeclampsia. Principle amongst these are factor V Leiden mutation, angiotensinogen genetic variations and the like. These subjects have a higher chance of developing preeclampsia. Therefore, it seems that there exist some association between preeclampsia and the genes.

IMMUNOLOGY AND GENETICS

Immunology has been accepted to play a very big role in the occurrence of obstetric vasculopathies. The fetus is now accepted as an allograft that has a tendency to get rejected by the mother. This is due to the distinctly different antigenicity of the mother and the fetus. There seems to be a constant struggle between the survival efforts of the fetus and the destructive effects of the mother. In preventing and protecting the fetus from rejection and destruction, the trophoblasts play a very important role. It has been found that if the fetus and the mother share histocompatability antigens, there is a distinct chance of rejection. The reasons for this have been elaborated elsewhere in this work (Chapter 3). However the interesting fact is that the sharing of antigens, Major Histocompatability Antigens (MHC Class 1) or Minor Histocompatability Antigens (MHC Class-2) is strongly genetic based.

The classic MHC 1 most studied and documented is HLA (Human Leucocyte Antigen). It is well known that mother and the fetus share HLA larger the sharing higher the chance of rejection. These HLA antigens are shared through common alleles. Thus there is a strong genetic basis for the expression and activation of the entire immunological process. Queerly this does not get expressed strongly in inheritance. This means that the mother and the fetus share the alleles and loci of the MHC 1 and MHC 2 antigens. But they do not follow any inheritance pattern. Therefore, the genetic inheritance model is not seen so distinctly. Instead the expression becomes operational at the fetomaternal interface of the indexed pregnancy. Hence, it would futile to seek mothers who have obstetric vasculopathies having babies having obstetric vasculopathies immunologically. This genetic interplay is confined to one indexed pregnancy.

One interesting study will not be out of place to quote in this regard. Data from Danish women (1996 to 2002) with single live-birth pregnancies complicated by severe preeclampsia/eclampsia were compared to women with term pregnancies uncomplicated by hypertension. HLA A, B, and DR types were resolved at the intermediate-level typing (antigen). The odds ratios of preeclampsia/eclampsia in mothers sharing both HLA antigens with their infants were 1.19 (95% confidence interval: 0.81–1.76) for HLA A, 0.91 (0.59–1.42) for HLA B, and 1.05 (0.5–1.59) for HLA DR antigens. No specific HLA antigens in either mother or infant appeared important after Bonferroni correction, except possibly DR01 in mothers (protective). Thus, it was concluded that this is not the basis for the mother developing preeclampsia/eclampsia.[13]

INPUTS FROM ANIMAL MODELS

For such profound and devastating conditions as obstetric vasculopathies, animal experiments and models if any could prove of great help. Human experiments have ethical and legal concerns. On the other hand, animal experiments face most serious challenge from reproducibility. Still, there are certain common factors that have been identified between human and animal physiology and pathologies that can serve as vital basis for understanding the pathophysiology of obstetric vasculopathies. The commonest animals that have been used in laboratories for studying this phenomenon are dogs, rabbits, sheep and primates like monkeys and baboons.[14] The principle reasons of popularity of these animals are a series of similarities of changes that take place in them with human pregnancy. As regards the physiologic changes in human pregnancy and pregnancy in these animals, the commonest is a tendency to lowering of blood pressure in both during pregnancy. Interesting while this phenomenon is seen in both nearly all throughout pregnancy it becomes most obvious at mid-pregnancy. Therefore in human pregnancy at midtrimester fall in BP is a well-known phenomena.

EPIGENETIC FEATURES IN PREECLAMPSIA

On basis of a mouse model, some workers have indicated that there may be a role of epigenetics in preeclampsia. Epigenetics incidentally is the study of heritable changes in gene expression or cellular phenotype caused by mechanisms other than changes in the underlying DNA sequence. Development of the trophoblast lineage is mediated by interactions between genetic and epigenetic factors. Insights have been gained from analysis of mouse models into the epigenetic mechanisms that are required for the early establishment of the trophoblast lineage and for the development of specialized cell types of the fetal placenta. These insights are beginning to be extended toward human studies and initial results suggest that the causes and consequences of a variety of placental pathologies are related to epigenetic processes. Furthermore, the epigenetic landscape that regulates trophoblast cells seems to be particularly vulnerable to perturbation during development. The placenta is required for the growth and survival of the fetus during pregnancy. In particular, epigenetic processes, which determine how genes are switched on and off, are necessary for the early establishment of the placental lineage and also for the development of specialized cell types within the mature placenta. These crucial and recent insights form the basis for suggesting some epigenetic basis for preeclampsia and extended to other vasculopathies.

Initial results suggest that the causes and consequences of a variety of placental pathologies are related to epigenetic pathways.[15]

Other such physiological changes especially of interest are changes in cardiovascular system. The changes include increased cardiac output lowered resistance in the renovascular system and a relative refractoriness of the vascular system to extraneously administered pressure substances.[2] It is understandable that the focus of scientists working in this field confines itself to those systems and organs that get affected by obstetric vasculopathies. These therefore include besides the cardiovascular system the renal system, the hepatic system and the brain.

Renal System

The importance of renal system in obstetric vasculopathies is indeed high. However with advances in complex immunology and understanding of the etiopathology, it won't be wrong to state that the renal system involvement in this process in overhyped. It seems that the renal system does not play so much of a role in etiopathology but gets involved in the pathophysiology. The reason why the renal system got so much importance was probably the relative ease with which the scientists could access the system. Assessment and examination of urine reflected the changes in the renal system both in animal and human studies. Urine examination is relatively cheap and easily available. This got correlated with the changes documented in renal function like increase in glomerular filtration rate the like. Also the relative ease with which the renal system like the hepatic system can be biopsied also made it a popular locus for study in both animal and human experiments.

One of the most consistent and at times dubbed as pathognomonic feature of obstetric vasculopathies is fibrin deposits in the glomeruli. Though subsequent understanding of the complex etiopathology revealed that this deposit is a part of a generalized immunological challenge that occurs as fibrin deposition was also found in the endothelial bed. Vascular changes were also demonstrated in the liver of animal experiments. This is not to deny the fact that animal experiments revealing different physiological and pathological changes did provide a valuable insight into the pathophysiology of this condition.

However, there are many understandable limitations of animal studies. Besides the species specific limitations, neither rabbits nor rats show an increase in gestation induced increased renal blood flow in contrast to human pregnancies.[16] Still a consistent increase in GFR has been registered. Through renal catheterization and similar procedures it was found that the blood supply to the kidney did not significantly increase but the renal vascular resistance declined significantly. This led to the understanding of the reasons for GFR increase without a significant rise in renal vascular flow.

On the basis of these facts, one can infer that animal experiments by and large reveal more of physiological changes that pathological in pregnancy. Most animals do not register any condition exactly similar to obstetric vasculopathies. Therefore, the animal experiments especially those from the renal system are by and large helpful albeit in limited way.

REFERENCES

1. Chesley L. Hypertension in pregnancy: definitions, familial factor, and remote prognosis. *Kidney Int.*1980;18(2):234-40.
2. Ward K, Lindheimer M, Roberts J. Endothelial Cell Dysfunction. In: Lindheimer M, Roberts J, Cunningham F, editors: Chesley's Hypertensive Disorders of Pregnancy Stamford. Appleton and Lange. 2nd edn 1999;431-452.
3. Bereketoğlu C, Kasap M, Pazarbaşı A. Studies on angiotensin-converting enzyme insertion/deletion polymorphism and genotype distributions in Turkish preeclampsia patients. *J Pregnancy.* 2012:108206, 2012. Epub 2012 Mar 25.
4. Rosta K, Molvarec A, Enzsöly A, Nagy B, Rónai Z, Fekete A, et al. Association of extracellular superoxide dismutase (SOD3) Ala40Thr gene polymorphism with preeclampsia complicated by severe fetal growth restriction. *Eur J Obstet Gynecol Reprod Biol.* 2009;142(2):134-8.
5. Vavrinková B, Binder T, Hadacová I, Hrachovinová I, Salaj P, Hruda M. Thrombophilic mutation by women with serious pregnancy complications. *Ceska Gynekol.* 2012; 77(2):171-4.
6. Humphries J. Occurrence of hypertensive toxemia of pregnancy. *Obstet Gynecol.* 1960; 107:271-7.
7. Adams E, Finlayson A. Familial aspects of preeclampsia and hypertension in pregnancy. *Lancet.* 1961;(7217):1375-8.
8. Cooper D, Liston W. Genetic control of severe preeclampsia. *J Med Gen.* 1979;16:409-416.
9. Arngrimsson R, Bjornson S, Geirsson R, et al. Genetic and familial predisposition to eclampsia and preeclampsia in a defined population. *Br J Obstet Gynecol.* 1990;97, 762-9.
10. Procopciuc L, Caracostea G, Zaharie G, Puscas M, Iordache G, Popa M, et al. Olteanu I, Stamatian F: Maternal/newborn genotype contribution of the renin-angiotensin system (Met235Thr, Thr174Met, I/D-ACE, A2350G-ACE, A1166C-AT2R1, C3123A- AT2R2, 83A/G-REN) to the risk of preeclampsia: a Romanian study. *J Renin Angiotensin Aldosterone Syst.* 2011;12(4):539-48.
11. Astin M, Scott J, Worley R. Preeclampsia: eclampsia: the fatal father factor. *Lancet.* 1981;5;2(8245):533.
12. Sadat Z, Abedzadeh Kalahroudi M, Saberi F. The effect of short duration sperm exposure on development of preeclampsia in primigravid women. *Iran Red Crescent Med J.* 2012; 14(1):20-4.
13. Biggar R, Poulsen G, Ng J, Melbye M, Boyd H. HLA antigen sharing between mother and fetus as a risk factor for eclampsia and preeclampsia. *Hum Immunol.* 2010;71(3):263-7.
14. McArdle A, Roberts C, Maduwegedera D, Flower R, Denton K. Chronic maternal hypertension characterized by renal dysfunction is associated with reduced placental blood flow during late gestation in rabbits. *Am J Physiol Regul Integr Comp Physiol.* 2010;298(4):R1043-9.
15. Rugg-Gunn P. Epigenetic features of the mouse trophoblast. *Reprod Biomed Online* 2012;25(1):21-30.
16. O'Hagan K, Alberts J. Uterine artery blood flow and renal sympathetic nerve activity during exercise in rabbit pregnancy. *Am J Physiol Regul Integr Comp Physiol.* 2003; 285(5):R1135-44.

CHAPTER

8

Obstetric Vasculopathies and their Effects on Heart

CHAPTER OUTLINE

- Hemodynamics in Normal Pregnancy and During Obstetric Vasculopathies
- Effect of Preeclampsia on the Offspring—Any?

INTRODUCTION

The hallmark pathology of obstetric vasculopathy is vasospasm. This is coupled by endothelial activation and oxidative stress. Along with these, maternal reducing systems also come into play as protective mechanisms. The vicious cycle of vasospasm and reperfusion damage that occurs can affect a series of body organs and systems. The main hub of these changes is located at the fetomaternal interface. However, it can easily spread and involve the entire maternal vasculature and as a consequence all critical body systems of the pregnant woman get affected. At the other end of the fetomaternal interface, lies the fetus. It too gets affected profoundly at times compromising it to the state of its death. Being a disorder of vascular basis, it would be worthwhile examining changes in blood and blood delivery systems first. Such an understanding can make understanding of other systemic involvements a little easier.

HEMODYNAMICS IN NORMAL PREGNANCY AND DURING OBSTETRIC VASCULOPATHIES

In normal pregnancy not complicated by preeclampsia, the tendency of the cardiovascular system of the pregnant subject is to ensure a low resistant flow throughout the body system of the gravida. All critical organ systems in particular and the entire body in general have more blood supply flowing with less resistance. The body efficiently ensures this by bringing about a series of changes. Critical in this is the increase in cardiac output and significant increase in the blood volume in the pregnant woman. Also the vascular channels through which this increased body of blood reaches the organs and systems including the placenta have a tendency to remain dilated and reduced in counter resistance to the flow. This latter effect is brought about by the sum total effect of thromboxane prostacyclin balance being shifted in favor of prostacyclin. This prostacyclin (PGE_2) has a vasodilatory tendency. Some good quality work in this regards has been reported by Clark et al. It was found that women in normal late pregnancy have a decreased systemic vascular resistance (21%), pulmonary vascular resistance (34%) and increase in pulse rate as well as up to 40% (precisely 43%) increase in cardiac output.[1]

One more interesting is the Left Ventricular Stroke Work Index. This index reflects the work to do to maintain the circulation. In comparative terms, LVSWI is increased if blood circulation faces a resistance when compared to blood circulation of a normal healthy pregnant subject. Vassar and Wallenberg have shown that in preeclampsia the LVSWI is markedly increased. This means that the heart has to work significantly more to maintain blood supply to vital organs and systems of the body of a pregnant gravida.[2]

The results so obtained by Vassar and Wallenberg are absolutely on the expected lines.[2] They are a result of vasospasm that is universally observed in preeclampsia. This resists the blood flow and so as to overcome this resistance, the heart especially the left ventricle has to work more. This increase in LVSWI could be as high as double the healthy pregnant subject. The clinical effect of this is a ready tendency of the heart pump to fail and a back pressure pulmonary edema in preeclampsia – one of the most dangerous and dreaded complications. While preeclampsia remains an important cause of hypertensive acute pulmonary edema in pregnancy and preventive strategies include close clinical monitoring and restricted fluid administration.[3]

It is worth nothing here that all obstetric vasculopathies do not show such extensive changes and complications. The epicenter of complex changes in all obstetric vasculopathies is the fetomaternal interface. However in preeclampsia, besides the fetomaternal interface, the entire maternal vasculature gets involved. As a result the hemodynamic changes are much more extensive and profound compared to other obstetric vasculopathies.

It is interesting to know that though dreaded, pulmonary edema doesn't occur as easily as it is expected to be in preeclampsia. This is because the increase in LVSWI efficiently compensates for the peripheral resistance that the heart faces while pumping the blood. But the power of cardiac muscle contractility does not significantly alter. The muscles remain agile and efficient. Any situation which increases the load so much on the heart that the LVSWI or its efforts can't match, the heart starts failing. This readily occurs if indiscriminate attempts are undertaken to cause volume expansion by aggressive infusion of volume expanders. It is therefore advisable to keep a preeclamptic subject a little under-infused than over-infused.

The other situation where the heart can fail is when the cardiac musculature is overstretched for a long duration of time. A fatigued cardiac musculature readily fails as soon as a little more load is inflicted on it. This occurs in a chronically hypertensive subject with preeclampsia superimposed over it. A cardiac failure leads to smudging of blood in the "back-waters" or the pulmonary circulation. The slowed and lowered bloodstream leads pulmonary edema which ultimately proves fatal.

In clinical practice only two situations in preeclampsia produce pulmonary edema: 1) Indiscriminate transfusion of volume expanders, and 2) Superimposed preeclampsia in a pregnant subject who is chronically hypertensive. In all other subjects by and large pulmonary edema does not occur. The cardiac musculature is agile enough to maintain the heavier load of work that it has to do.

EFFECT OF PREECLAMPSIA ON THE OFFSPRING—ANY?

Interesting insights have developed to reveal that preeclampsia in particular can alter the cardiovascular phenotype of the fetus. While it was found that women who have had a pregnancy complicated by preeclampsia have a 4-fold increased risk of later cardiovascular disease. Intriguingly, the offspring of affected pregnancies also have an increased risk of higher blood pressure and almost double the risk of stroke in later life.[4] Interestingly, children born after preeclampsia may show effects of a negative impact on the heart already at the age of 5 to 8 years.[5]

REFERENCES

1. Clark S, Cotton D, Wesley L. Central hemodynamic assessment of normal term pregnancy. *Am J Obstet Gynecol.* 1989;161:1439-42.
2. Vassar W, Wallenberg H. Central hemodynamic observations in untreated preeclamptic patients. *Hypertension*. 1991;17:1072-77.
3. Dennis A, Solnordal C. Acute pulmonary oedema in pregnant women. *Anaesthesia.* 2012;67(6):646-59.
4. Davis E, Newton L, Lewandowski A, Lazdam M, Kelly B, Kyriakou T, et al. preeclampsia and offspring cardiovascular health: mechanistic insights from experimental studies. *Clin Sci.* 2012;123(2):53-72.
5. Fugelseth D, Ramstad H, Kvehaugen A, Nestaas E, Støylen A, Staff A. Myocardial function in offspring 5–8 years after pregnancy complicated by preeclampsia. *Early Hum Dev.* 2011;87(8):531-5.

CHAPTER

9

Obstetric Vasculopathies and their Effects on the Renal System

CHAPTER OUTLINE

- Vulnerability of Renal System
- Special Features of Renal Failure in Obstetric Vasculopathies
- Kidney Lesions
- Renal Function Alterations in Preeclampsia

VULNERABILITY OF RENAL SYSTEM

For some reasons known and unknown renal system bears a unique challenge in obstetric vasculopathies. One very well-known but undocumented quiz question is "What should the registrar of the unit check in the subject the day after she had an abruptio placenta?" The answer expected is "Urine Output". This underlines the importance of renal system in these conditions. In normal pregnancy, as is so well known, the glomerular filtration rate (GFR) is increased. This leads to a series of changes including the most obvious increase in urine output. Why should this occur is not known. However the mechanism is understandable. Increase in blood volume common to pregnancy and increase in renal circulation are both contributing to increased urine output. There is more blood to be filtered in pregnancy therefore the renal system goes into an unstressed overdrive.

During obstetric vasculopathies this entire competent system seems to be getting derailed. During preeclampsia, the blood volume that is increased in pregnancy is either annulled or constricted. Also, in preeclampsia the renal vascular system undergoes vasoconstriction as does the entire vascular system of the pregnant mother. This produces a big challenge. The renal system which is all geared up to handle the increased load actually faces a reduced load (lowered blood volume and vasoconstriction). As a result it gets precariously poised and has a tendency to get dried up. The intensity and frequency with which this occurs depends on the severity of obstetric vasculopathy. It also depends on the intrinsic robustness of the renal system to bear the alterations.

Once the precarious balance of blood supply to the renal system is understood, one can understand the grave complications of obstetric vasculopathy more easily. In conditions like abruptio placenta with preeclampsia, the renal system gets further impoverished of its blood supply. This is like pushing someone who is about to fall. With the added insult of accidental hemorrhage the kidneys may not be able to bear it any further and at times renal failure occurs. This explains the answer to the question raised at the commencement of this section "What should the registrar of the unit which has handled a subject with abruptio placentae check for on the next day morning." The answer to this was given as "Urine Output".

In most subjects the intrinsic reserve of these systems is able to withstand the changes to a great extent. Therefore, a total renal shut down is not seen so often. However, oliguria is definitely more commonly seen in preeclampsia as the pathology increases in severity.

This brings up one more challenge in managing the fluid and electrolyte balance in subjects of obstetric vasculopathy especially severe preeclampsia and accidental hemorrhage. It has been found that when infusions are given to preeclamptic subjects the heart goes quickly into an overdrive. It increases the cardiac output by increasing the LVSWI. This means the left ventricle is forced to pump out more blood. However, the heart is already facing stiff resistance from narrowed blood vessels through which it tries to push the blood through. In such a situation attempts to increase the renal perfusion by increasing the fluid and electrolytes by infusing them can cause the heart pump to falter. This results in pulmonary edema. Thus managing oliguria in preeclampsia is very challenging.

One more common "shortcut" applied in clinical practice to combat the renal slowdown resulting in oliguria in preeclampsia is with diuretics. This can also be dangerous if done indiscriminately. This is because the diuretics will increase the blood supply to the kidneys forcibly. A system which is already impoverished of blood supply is forced to divert blood to the renal system which is not desirable. The heart would pump still faster and fail much more readily as a result. It would therefore, be imperative for a clinician who is battling a renal compromise in severe preeclampsia to put a central venous pressure line to get an idea of how much to give and when not to give.

SPECIAL FEATURES OF RENAL FAILURE IN OBSTETRIC VASCULOPATHIES

The renal failure mentioned above in reference to accidental hemorrhage complicating preeclampsia is also worth examining closely. While the pathophysiology is already seen what is of interest is the fact that usually this failure is a result of tubular necrosis and less of cortical necrosis. Usually thus is in a ratio of 80:20 for tubular to cortical insult. If prompt and adequate blood transfusion is given to such subjects of preeclampsia complicated by accidental hemorrhage, renal failure can be reversed or altogether prevented. Resultant long term effects on the renal system are very few.

It is relevant to note here that accidental hemorrhage has a notorious habit to recur. It is also true that if the previous pregnancy severe preeclampsia got complicated by accidental hemorrhage leading to a renal shut down, it can recur notoriously consistently in the next pregnancy as well. However, with better monitoring facilities available and better neonatal intensive care facility obstetricians tend to intervene and end such pregnancies with past history of torrid adverse outcome, much earlier. This has changed the profile of clinical practice. If the obstetric team is not vigilant or if the subject is unable to get quality antenatal care, recurrent renal failure with poor outcome can still occur.

In 20% subjects in whom the cortical necrosis becomes predominant, renal failure is irreversible warranting a renal transplant and dialysis. In subjects with persistent albuminuria in severe preeclampsia there is an increased tendency to renal failure. However, presence of albuminuria may not be indicative of an impending renal shut down. It in actuality reflects the compromised renal function the consequence of which is a renal shut down. Thus proteinuria is not the cause of renal compromise and renal failure but in actuality it is a marker of the underlying pathology.

A word about uric acid estimation for assessing renal function in preeclampsia will not be out of place. This matter has been broached in previous sections however in greater details. While many biochemical markers have been used to assess renal function in non-pregnant subjects many of them as seen above become incompetent in pregnancy more so in preeclampsia. Uric acid assessment in preeclampsia has been done by different workers at different times to assess renal function. Plasma uric acid has been reported by them in preeclampsia.[1] But over the period of time it has been recognized that uric acid is a strong reducing substance in the body. It has therefore a very limited role in reflecting the renal function in a preeclamptic subject. Thus when one assesses uric acid level he/she is assessing the state of oxidative stress in the pregnant subject. No wonder, Salako BL et al found uric acid to be unreliable for assessing renal function in pregnancy.[2] This mater has been dealt with in much larger details elsewhere.

While accidental hemorrhage is one situation where renal failure is a grave but distinct possibility, one more such association is found with the clinical condition of HELLP syndrome. HELLP is the acronym for elevated hepatic enzymes, low platelets and hemolysis. Some workers have shown that HELLP syndrome can also occur in absence of preeclampsia. But its most consistent association is with hypertensive disorders of pregnancy. When HELLP syndrome is associated with preeclampsia, renal failure if it occurs, will be stormy and can be irreversible. This is because in such combinations, acute cortical necrosis gets precipitated. This is irreversible form of renal failure. A combination of comorbidities like accidental hemorrhage and preeclampsia and HELLP syndrome and preeclampsia together account for upto 80% of subjects with pregnancy related irreversible renal failure.[3,4]

One more point that needs to be noted here while on renal function alterations in preeclampsia and other obstetric vasculopathies is the fact related to postpartum hemorrhage. In this regards it must be added that if any of the severe forms of preeclampsia and/or accidental hemorrhage are complicated by postpartum hemorrhage, renal function gets readily compromised. Therefore, this combination with postpartum hemorrhage can prove to be lethal for renal functioning.

One obstetric vasculopathy that has no bearing on maternal renal functioning is intrauterine growth retardation (IUGR). It seems that when the vasculopathy process is confined to the fetomaternal interface and has fetal effects like IUGR, still births or recurrent miscarriages following fetal demise, renal function compromise is not known to occur. However, if any of these fetal complications occur along with preeclampsia and or accidental hemorrhage renal compromise can occur.

KIDNEY LESIONS

Pathological changes in the kidneys occur principally in two obstetric vasculopathies: preeclampsia and accidental hemorrhage. In the former the changes are due to vasospasm and in the latter due to acute blood loss. While one is examining the pathological changes that are taking place in the kidneys –one cannot help but salute the pioneering work done by Sheehan and his team in the same. This group diligently studied and documented renal changes in subjects who died in pregnancy on postmortem. They compared 112 non-preeclamptic subjects who died of preeclampsia/eclampsia with those who died of some other cause. They performed postmortems in these subjects within two hours of death. In this way, they successfully reduced the changes occurring as an aftermath of death. Thus their results were very accurate. The accuracy in their results could be understood from the fact that modern imaging technologies have also corroborated with the changes described by Sheehan and colleagues. Therefore, even to date no discussion and pathology of preeclampsia/eclampsia gets complete without taking into account the description of these workers. The entire compilation of their work has been published in details in a book by Sheehan and Lynch.[5]

Doubts on Veracity of Pathognomonic Lesions

In some other sections of this monogram a short reference has been made regarding why the renal lesions may have been overhyped. It will now be worthwhile to study this aspect in greater details. While one must accept that the kidneys do bear a very heavy brunt of the disease of preeclampsia, they are not the game-changers in the entire etiopathology of preeclampsia. This is very important to understand from various angles.

Access to the renal system is relatively easy. Also, renal systems can be easily focused through urine examination so easy to obtain and equally easy to test. Renal system changes can be relatively easily viewed as kidney biopsies are not very difficult. Resident doctors relatively junior in experience can perform renal biopsies with some training and expertise. All this gave the kidneys an advantage of getting studied extensively and with great ease. No doubt, kidneys do get involved in preeclamptic process of obstetric vasculopathy with great consistency. However, the ease of access to kidneys led scientists to give excessive importance to renal changes in obstetric vasculopathy. So much so that renal changes were described as pathognomonic of preeclampsia. Also, there were suggestions that the etiopathology of preeclampsia and its complications lies in the kidneys. In short renal changes seem to have got overhyped.

In accidental hemorrhage too the renal system suffers due to blood loss. II seems the body of the pregnant subject is very efficient in prioritizing. It seems to give lowest priority to the fetus (placenta) and then to the kidneys. This means that while the body preserving mechanisms tend to preserve the functioning of the liver, the heart and the brain in crisis, it may do so at the cost of the fetus and the placenta. It is, therefore, understandable that even in accidental hemorrhage profound changes in the kidneys are known to occur. Tubular necrosis and in some unfortunate subjects even cortical necrosis can occur.

It is now obvious that it is not the kidneys but the fetomaternal interface that is at the basis of all etiopathology in obstetric vasculopathies. Changes emanating here involve other organs and systems in their processes secondarily. Involvement of the kidneys therefore, though extensive is by and large secondary to changes at the fetomaternal interface. The principle reason why kidneys got noticed has been described in preceding pages **(P···)**. However science did not have accurate and reliable means to know what is happening at the fetomaternal interface. Undoubtedly therefore kidneys the easiest accessible to study got studied extensively and others just followed. With the advent of ultrasonography in general and colour Doppler in particular, imaging of what is happening at the fetomaternal interface become possible.

Scientists had long since known that vasospasm is the basic pathology in obstetric vasculopathies. But they could access only the kidney and to some extent the liver to study the effects of vasospasm easily. On the other hand, as soon as color Doppler studies become available reports of renal changes in preeclampsia got few and far between. Currently hardly any research papers are seen which deals with renal changes in obstetric vasculopathies vis-à-vis etiopathology of obstetric vasculopathies in general and preeclampsia in particular.

One reason why papers related to renal biopsies have become few and far between is the fact that there are now stringent guidelines for doing renal biopsies in pregnancy. This could be due to many reasons including possible grave complications like hemorrhage which can occur while biopsying kidneys in pregnancy. Renal biopsies in pregnancy have become rare also because the need to biopsy kidneys has become rare. This brings out an obvious fact that kidneys get involved in the changes of preeclampsia and accidental hemorrhage like many other systems getting involved. But the renal system being low on priority of the maternal protecting systems when faced with crisis of survival bears a brunt of the pathology.

Gross Changes in the Kidneys

While examining the pathology it can be traditionally divided into gross appearance and microscopic appearance. Microscopic appearance can be further divided into light microscopic appearance and appearance under electron microscopic appearance. As regards gross appearance of kidneys in preeclampsia, there is an insignificant increase in size of the kidneys. On cut section the kidneys appear pale and have a relatively enlarged cortex. However, compared to gross changes, microscopic changes are for more extensive.

On Microscopy

The glomeruli are enlarged and solidified ("bloodless"), as a result of narrowed or occluded capillary lumens that are the result of swelling of the native endothelial cells and, to a lesser extent, mesangial cells. Glomerular volume is increased and correlates with the severity of the disease.[6] Thrombosis by light microscopy is decidedly unusual, although fibrin can be detected by immunofluorescence in glomeruli. In marked contrast, in non-preeclamptic thrombotic microangiopathies (TMA), thrombosis of vessels and/or glomeruli is a central finding. TMA is a term used to describe a group of clinically diverse entities, such as hemolytic uremic syndrome and malignant hypertension, among others, that are defined by a primary locus of injury—the endothelium—and the ensuing thrombosis and vascular injury. Their similar pathologic expression has led nephropathologists to adopt the term TMA to describe them all.

These lesions of preeclampsia share some similarities with and intriguing differences from those of non-preeclamptic TMA, likely owing to their differing pathogenesis.[7] The immunofluorescence findings are somewhat variable with fibrin deposition often being a prominent feature. The low-level glomerular Ig deposition in severe preeclampsia, reported by some, probably represents nonimmunologic insudation. This conclusion is supported by the ultrastructural observation that electron-dense deposits are inconspicuous. Its chief diagnostic role lies in excluding an immune complex glomerulonephritis, such as lupus nephritis, which often flares during pregnancy.[7]

Some tend to call these changes as glomerular nephropathy. This is typically characterized by glomerular hypertrophy and decreased glomerular space as a result of swelling of glomerular endothelium and increased capillary wall thickness without significant changes in glomerular cellularity. From the description of Sheehan et al it seems that increase in glomerular size could be a result of a response to falling renal circulation due to vasospasm in preeclampsia.[5] While the blood supply reduces, kidneys make internal arrangements to make their working more competent.

As regards the cellular alterations here too attempts are made by the kidneys to improve their functioning in face of impoverished blood supply. This gets reflected in terms of increased proliferation of the mesangial cells and endothelial cells that are the dominant changes as regards the cellularity of the renal system in preeclampsia.[8] Though these cells have been shown to proliferate, the increase in cellularity is at most very mild, numerically. There are some reports of increased cellularity of the glomeruli in preeclampsia but these seem to be based on general impression of the examiner while evaluating the sections under microscope rather than based on some objective criteria.

One of the characteristic features of preeclampsia is what is described as "bloodless glomeruli". These are obstructed hypovascular appearance of the glomeruli tufts. Narrowing of the glomerular capillary loops reflecting the generalized process of vasospasm is also consistently found. Endothelial hypertrophy a characteristic feature of the microvascular pathology of preeclampsia is partly responsible for the compromise of the vascular spaces in the glomeruli.[9]

The etiopathology of these changes specifically in the kidneys has been described by Obeidat M et al.[10] The glomerular capillary endothelium seems to be a highly specialized to support the selective filtration of massive volumes of plasma. Glomerular endothelial cells are extremely flat and perforated by dense arrays of transcellular pores, the fenestrae. This phenotype is critical for the high glomerular water permeability and depends on podocyte-derived VEGF, as well as TGF-β. In preeclampsia, inhibition of the VEGF and TGF-β signaling pathways leads to endothelial swelling and loss of fenestrae, reducing the glomerular filtration rate. Similarly, in the thrombotic microangiopathies, glomerular endothelial cell injury coupled with inappropriate VWF activation leads to intracapillary platelet aggregation and loss of the flat, fenestrated phenotype, thus reducing the glomerular filtration rate. Normally, a remarkably small fraction of albumin and other large plasma proteins passes across the glomerular capillary wall despite the massive filtration of water and small solutes. An elaborate glycocalyx, which covers glomerular endothelial cells and their fenestrae, forms an impressive barrier that, together with other components of the glomerular capillary wall, prevents loss of plasma proteins into the urine. Indeed, microalbuminuria is a marker for endothelial glycocalyx disruption, and most forms of glomerular endothelial cell injury including preeclampsia and thrombotic microangiopathies can cause proteinuria.

One more feature ascribed to preeclampsia in the kidneys is the presence of "foam cells". This so called foamy appearance of some cells is a reflection of characteristic alterations in the cytoplasm showing the presence of clear vacuoles and lipid droplets. When the cytoplasm is displaced by massive intracellular lipid deposits, the cells acquire a foamy appearance and so they are called as "foam cells".[11]

Mobilization of fat to enter the cytoplasm and generation of foam cells is likely to be a marker of grave crisis. It indicates that the organ or the system is gravely challenged and its very own harmony or even existence is at-risk. Thus demonstration of foam cells in the kidneys can similarly be a reflection of grave challenge to the renal system. This was the belief when electron microscopy had still not made its appearance. However with electron microscopic studies becoming available, a more sensitive and minute pictures became available to science. It was now possible to detect even tiny amounts of fat mobilization and deposition on the glomeruli. It became evident that presence of intraglomerular foam cells does not necessarily represent a terminal event. It just shows the in evolutional stage of the disease.

The reported frequency of intraglomerular foam cells is quite variable. It can vary between 4 to 35% depending on the timing of the biopsy, method of tissue processing and staining, and the sensitivity of the technique used to detect the presence of intraglomerular fat cells.[11,12]

One more change reported from studies of renal biopsies that have created lots of confusion and debate is the presence of capillary wall thickening in the tuft of glomerular capillaries. This was wrongly labeled as "membranous glomerulonephritis". However with the technological advances, it was found that presence of capillary wall thickening in the glomeruli is a reflection of the severity of the disease and nothing beyond. The empty bloodless glomerular tufts with obstructed loops of the capillaries dominate the pathology of Preeclampsia.[13]

There are other capillary loop pathologies that have also been described in literature. These include the so called "cigar shaped" loops, "ballooned loops", "Pouting", etc. These appear in some references at different period of time. However, their clinical bearing as well as bearings on understanding of etiopathology is at the most limited.

Sheehan has described classical changes in glomerular mesangium in preeclampsia. He has described it as a peculiar change in the mesangium, commonly associated with the healing stage of the disease. It is characterized by vacuolation of the mesangial stalks resembling a "string of beads".[12] In the same reference, Sheehan has further qualified that the various mesangial lesions described are usually focal in nature. However, approximately 8% of the subjects associated with severe form of the disease manifest a generalized dilatation of the mesangium and distortion of capillary loops, Sheehan adds.

While there is a general deprivation for renal tissue of blood supply due to vasospasm shown by the classical empty bloodless glomerular tufts, there can also be focal ischemia. This ischemia can be patchy and localized to different areas of the kidney. It gets represented as epithelial crescents.[14] Gabel et al (1998) have further qualified that infarcted or preinfarcted glomeruli are not common. But if found, they recommend that like the finding of glomerular thrombi, one should exclude the presence of lupus anticoagulant or coagulopathy associated with HELLP syndrome.[15]

Two more lesions that have been described in the kidneys of patients effected by preeclampsia are focal segmental glomerular sclerosis (FSGS) and its variants described as early cellular lesions or glomerular tip lesions. The clinical bearing of these lesions is unknown and therefore they remain by and large confined to the realms of pathology books of the disease. The scientists who tried to study the clinicopathological correlation between FSGS and preeclampsia basically tried to study the clinical course of the disease, resolution and long-term consequences in subjects with FSGS. No such correlation has been found. It seems that subjects with FSGS are not having a more severe form of the disease, they do not have poorer or better obstetric outcome and they tend to reverse the changes of preeclampsia as early or as late as those subjects who do not show FSGS. However there is one study that FSGS to confuse the picture. It showed that there indeed was a poorer outcome in subjects who showed these lesions. But these subjects have persistent or recurrent hypertension and proteinuria, frequent relapses with subsequent pregnancies and eventual progression to chronic renal insufficiency in majority of patients that they studied.[16] In a more recent study such a risk has been restressed. This study suggested that preeclampsia triggered metabolic stress may cause vascular injury, thus contributing to the development of cardiovascular disease and/or chronic kidney disease in the future. This risk appears to be increased especially in women with a history of recurrent, severe preeclampsia and eclampsia. The investigation of a history of preeclampsia may assist in assessing the future risk of cardiovascular disease and or chronic kidney disease, their prevention and early diagnosis.[17]

Gabel et al beautifully summarized this entire controversy regarding the clinical importance if any related to FSGS. They state that localized lesions resembling those of FSGS are identified in approximately 20% subjects, who have clinical diagnosis of preeclampsia. To date as stated by them, there is no evidence that this subset of patients will have long-term renal dysfunction albeit they may present with atypical or severe preeclampsia.[15]

As regards the vascular changes in the renal system including the juxta-glomerular apparatus, it is found that these changes are more of functional than structural. This could well be expected as the entire process of preeclampsia is vascular in basis. Alterations in vascular function are responsible principally for the profound effects of preeclampsia. Therefore, when attempts to study renovascular structural changes were undertaken they were not found to be contributory.

Preeclampsia—A Renal Pathogenic Model for Understanding other forms of Hypertension

Hypertension is in 85 to 90% of cases of unknown etiology, in spite of efforts undertaken by modern medicine to elucidate it. Numerous experimental studies were conducted in order to explain the pathogenesis of this disease. Recent observations revealed that during therapy with anti-VEGF medication, used in treating different forms of cancer, hypertension and proteinuria occur, and at kidney level endothelial injuries appear similar to pregnancy related hypertension. Antiangiogenic factors, such as sFlt-1, are produced during pregnancy induced hypertension, especially in preeclampsia. They block the circulating VEGF. Consequently, proteinuria, and sometimes edema occur together with hypertension. Renal injuries are of glomerular endotheliosis type. It is appreciated that one can draw a parallel between these pathologic situations, as is ablative treatment of antiangiogenic medication (anti-VEGF) and pregnancy induced hypertension, preeclampsia, respectively.

The main pathogenic mechanism of pregnancy induced hypertension that causes the disease is placental ischemia. This is followed by the placental release of pressor substances that are involved both in generalized endotheliosis that characterizes the disease, and in hypertension. The prototype hypertension caused by renal ischemia is renal artery stenosis. Both pregnancy induced hypertension and hypertension in renal artery stenosis have a similar factor in their pathogenesis that is organ ischemia with production of consecutive pressor substances. Since this ischemic factor can intervene in other forms of hypertension, its characterization becomes of importance at present. Thus, pregnancy induced hypertension in pregnancy can represent a real pathogenic model of hypertension that is reflected in non-pregnancy hypertension.[18]

George M et al have studied renal thrombotic microangiopathy in mice. On the basis of Eps15 Homology Domain-containing 3 (EHD3), a member of the EHD protein family that regulates endocytic recycling, being the first protein reported to be specifically expressed in the glomerular endothelium in the kidney; they generated Ehd3 (–/–) mice and studied renal development and pathology. Ehd3 (–/–) animals showed no overt defects, and exhibited no proteinuria or glomerular pathology. However, as the expression of Ehd4, a related family member, was elevated in the glomerular endothelium of Ehd3 (–/–) mice and suggested functional compensation, they generated and analyzed Ehd3 (–/–); Ehd4 (–/–) mice. These mice were smaller, possessed smaller and paler kidneys, were proteinuric and died between 3 to 24 weeks of age. Detailed analyses of Ehd3 (–/–); Ehd4 (–/–) kidneys demonstrated thrombotic microangiopathy (TMA)-like glomerular lesions including thickening and duplication of glomerular basement membrane, endothelial swelling and loss of fenestrations. Other changes included segmental podocyte foot process effacement, mesangial interposition, and abnormal podocytic and mesangial marker expression. The glomerular lesions observed were strikingly similar to those seen in human Preeclampsia and mouse models of reduced VEGF expression.[19]

RENAL FUNCTION ALTERATIONS IN PREECLAMPSIA

As has been made amply clear alterations in renal function are profound in preeclampsia. Also, renal system is not on a priority list of the pregnant subject when it faces a crisis. Therefore, pathological alterations get all the more amplified. Compensatory processes in renal systems for crisis are present but once they crash the renal systems get handsomely beaten up. Besides these, renal system is relatively easily accessible to the investigating scientific community. Urine is easy to procure and profusely available. Also renal biopsy is easily doable with some experience. Thus functional and structural alterations can be studied with relative ease. By 1998, 23 groups had already published their studies on renal changes in preeclampsia as has been catalogued tabularly by Conrad and Lindheimer in 1998.[20]

Glomerular filtration rate and renal plasma flow increase by 40 to 65% and 50 to 85%, respectively, during normal pregnancy in women.[21] The most consistent physiological alteration reported in most of the studies is the significant reduction in the glomerular filtration rate (GFR) and effective renal plasma flow (ERPF) are reduced in preeclampsia.[22,23]

All possible biases that can affect the GFR and ERPF have been eliminated to come to this conclusion of a consistent reduction of GFR and ERPF in preeclampsia. This includes a possible reduction in renal flow by the position of the gravida. A supine gravida has her uterus on the great vessels. This can possibly alter the GFR. This bias was eliminated by measuring indicators of GFR and ERPF in lateral positions. In all of these studies about 30 to 35% reduction in these two parameters emerges consistently.

Methods to accurately assess GFR alterations in preeclampsia continue to be looked for so that biases get progressively eliminated. One such attempt has been through assessing serum cystatin C (Cys – C) to assess alterations in renal function in preeclampsia. It seems serum Cys-C seems to reflect the GFR precisely in women with severe preeclampsia and can be a good marker to monitor the renal function from antepartum to postpartum.[24]

Basically, these changes should not come as a big surprise. Vasospasm which has been stressed, restressed and probably overstressed in these pages understandably leads to reduction in blood flow of the renal system. Also the blood volume in a preeclamptic pregnant subject is constricted in comparison to the pregnant non-preeclamptic subject at same pregnancy duration. Both of these produce a reduction in an effective blood flow through the kidneys. This in turn leads to reduction in physiologies on which the kidney function is based like the GFR and ERPF.

Indeed other mechanisms also contribute to the alterations like the vascular endothelial damage that occurs in preeclampsia. However, this and allied glomerular dysfunctions reported are also a result of organ hypoperfusion found in preeclampsia and therefore subsequent effects.

As regards the recovery of renal function it has been found that the GFR improves most consistently within the first week to ten days postpartum. In this postpartum, phase the recovery of functions is much faster than the structural recovery. Though GFR recovery is most notable, ERPF recovery occurs little sluggishly. This means the renal system regains it competence much beyond the functioning and structural recovery from and importance of organ, tissue and cellular competence has been continuously stressed in these pages. Thus even if the structural recovery may not occur so fast (as reflected in changes in renal biopsy) or functioning may not recover as fast (as reflected in ERPF) but the kidneys regain their competence much faster as if there is no time to waste! This is reflected through the recovery in GFR outstripping the recovery in ERPF which in turn is outstripping the recovery on renal biopsy changes.

Renal Handling of Proteins in Preeclampsia

There are two features of preeclampsia in clinical practice which makes one inquisitive to know how the kidneys handle proteins in preeclampsia. These two features are albuminuria and edema. Both of these have a direct relation to how the kidneys handle proteins in preeclampsia. The intravascular mass of albumin showed no change between non-pregnant, 7 and 12 weeks values but there was a significant rise of 19.5 g between 12 and 28 weeks of gestation, an overall increase of 19%. However, the extravascular albumin mass tends to decline.[25] The net effect of this is that fluid tends to get held back in the intravascular channels. Any alteration in this relationship between intravascular albumin mass and its extra-vascular distribution tends to release the fluids held on by the albumin and a result edema occurs. It is possible that estradiol and/or progesterone together may mediate in the reduced synthesis of albumin.

Urinary protein excretion is increased during normal pregnancy as has been widely known. Workers have studied this aspect in great details using different positions occupied by the gravida as well as the timing of the day like urinary protein excretion in night compared with excretion during the day. It is also of interest to note that the alteration in this urinary function of protein excretion is not restored to pre-pregnant stage till upto 16 weeks to 1 year postpartum. However, in most subjects it restores by 16 weeks. Only rarely it may go on upto one year.

Similarly, other proteins like low-molecular proteins and enzymes are also excreted in increased amount in normal pregnancy. Also the proximate tubular resorption is also reduced in normal pregnancy. This restores faster after pregnancy compared to the excretory changes.

Handling of Urinary Excretion of Proteins in Preeclampsia

Serum albumin as well as low molecular weight proteins like IgG are decreased in circulation in preeclampsia as has been shown in many studies.[26] Going in further details Honger found that serum concentrations of albumin, intravascular mass of albumin as well as the total exchangeable mass of albumin are all reduced in preeclampsia.[25] It seems that the overall disposition of the kidneys is such that in preeclampsia there is an increased loss of proteins especially albumin. This is coupled by incompetent resorption of excreted proteins through the glomerular membrane. It seems that the electronic disposition of the glomerular membrane also plays an important role in these changes which ultimately predisposes a preeclamptic pregnant subject to develop albuminuria. When and at what stage of pregnancy this excretion becomes obvious on laboratory reports is difficult to predict. However, by the rule of thumb it appears that the increasing severity of preeclampsia makes albumin and other proteins more easily apparent in urine of preeclamptic subjects.

Renin-Angiotensin System in Preeclampsia

While on kidneys it is worthwhile briefly visiting this aspect of obstetric vasculopathies as well. It has been postulated that angiotensin II may be playing an essential role in the pathogenesis of preeclampsia; however, the beneficial effect of the suppression of RAS has not yet been fully explained. In a transgenic mouse model developed pregnancy associated hypertension (PAH) by the overproduction of Angiotensin II in maternal circulation during late pregnancy. In addition, mice with PAH exhibited maternal and fetal abnormalities, such as proteinuria, cardiac hypertrophy, placental morphological changes and IUGR. In one study, to attenuate the activity of redundant renin angiotensin system during the advanced stages of PAH, olmesartan an angiotensin receptor blocker was administered and captopril, an angiotensin converting enzyme inhibitor, from 17 to 19 days of gestation, and evaluated its effect on cardiac and placental abnormalities and fetal growth. Olmesartan and captopril administration lowered the blood pressure of mice with PAH, and placental histological change and severe IUGR were markedly ameliorated in both groups. On the contrary, olmesartan or captopril treatment had little effect on cardiac remodeling during the advanced stages of PAH. These findings highlight a variety of therapeutic actions of renin angiotensin system repression on the progressive pathology of PAH in mice.[27]

REFERENCES

1. Wakwe V, Abudu O. Estimation of plasma uric acid in pregnancy induced hypertension (PIH). Is the test still relevant? *Afr J Med Med Sci.* 1999;28(3-4):155-8.
2. Salako B, Odukogbe A, Olayemi O, Adedapo K, Aimakhu C, Alu F, et al. Serum albumin, creatinine, uric acid and hypertensive disorders of pregnancy. *East Afr Med J.* 2003;80(8):424-8.
3. Gurrieri C, Garovic VD, Gullo A, Bojanić K, Sprung J, Narr B, et al. Kidney injury during pregnancy: associated comorbid conditions and outcomes. *Arch Gynecol Obstet.* 2012;286(3):567-73.
4. Ahonen J, Nuutila M. HELLP syndrome—severe complication during pregnancy. *Duodecim.* 2012;128(6):569-77.
5. Sheehan H, Lynch J. Pathology of toxemia of pregnancy. Baltimore, Williams and Wilkins. 1973, 807.
6. Tsokos M, Longauer F, Kardosová V, Gavel A, Anders S, Schulz F. Maternal death in pregnancy from HELLP syndrome. A report of three medico-legal autopsy cases with special reference to distinctive histopathological alterations. *Int J Legal Med.* 2002;116(1):50-3.

7. Stillman I, Karumanchi S. The glomerular injury of preeclampsia. *J Am Soc Nephrol.* 2007;18(8):2281-4.
8. Naicker T, Randeree I, Moodley J, Khedun S, Ramsaroop R, Seedat Y. Correlation between histological changes and loss of anionic charge of the glomerular basement membrane in early-onset preeclampsia. *Nephron.* 1997;75(2):201-7.
9. Eremina V, Sood M, Haigh J, Nagy A, Lajoie G, Ferrara N et al. Glomerular-specific alterations of VEGF-A expression lead to distinct congenital and acquired renal diseases. *J Clin Invest.* 2003;111(5):707-16.
10. Obeidat M, Obeidat M, Ballermann B. Glomerular endothelium: a porous sieve and formidable barrier. *Exp Cell Res.* 2012,15;318(9):964-72.
11. Ogino S. An electron microscopic study of the glomerular alterations of pure-preeclampsia. *Nihon Jinzo Gakkai Shi.* 1999;41(4):413-29.
12. Sheehan H. Renal morphology in preeclampsia. *Kidney Int.* 1980;18, 241-52.
13. Geber L, Lindheimer M. In: Hypertensive disorders of pregnancy. Lindheimer M, Roberts J, Cunningham F (eds). 2nd edn Stamford: Appleton and Lange. 1998; Page 238.
14. Kharfi A, Giguère Y, Sapin V, Massé J, Dastugue B, Forest J. Trophoblastic remodeling in normal and preeclamptic pregnancies: implication of cytokines. *Clin Biochem.* 2003;36(5):323-31.
15. Gabel L, Spargo B, Lindheimer M. The nephrology of preeclampsia. In: Renal Pathology, Tisher C, Brenner B, (eds), Philadelphia. Lippincott. 2nd edn 1994, 419-41.
16. Lee H, Kim T. A morphometric study of preeclamptic nephropathy with focal segmental glomerulosclerosis. *Clin. Nephrol.* 1995;25:116-25.
17. Facca T, Kirsztajn G, Sass N. Preeclampsia (marker of chronic kidney disease): from genesis to future risks. J *Bras Nefrol* 2012;34(1):87-93.
18. Gluhovschi G, Gluhovschi A, Petrica L, Anastasiu D, Gluhovschi C, Velciov S. Pregnancy induced hypertension—a particular pathogenic model, similarities with other forms of arterial hypertension. *Rom J Intern Med;* 2012;50(1):71-81.
19. George M, Rainey M, Naramura M, Foster K, Holzapfel M, Willoughby, et al. Renal thrombotic microangiopathy in mice with combined deletion of endocytic recycling regulators EHD3 and EHD4, *PLoS One.* 2011;9:6(3).
20. Conrad K, Lindheimer M. Renal and cardiovascular abnormalities. In: Hypertensive disorders of pregnancy. Lindheimer M, Roberts J, Cunningham F, (eds): Chesley's. 2nd edn Stamford, Connecticut Appleton and Lange. 1998, Page 280.
21. Jeyabalan A, Conrad K. Renal function during normal pregnancy and preeclampsia. *Front Biosci.* 2007;12:2425-37.
22. Liu X, Zhou Z, Cao Y, Wang B, Xu G. Contributions of blood pressure to proteinuria and renal function in the puerperium. *Blood Press.* 2009;18(6):362-6.
23. Lafayette R, Druzin M, Sibley R, Derby G, Malik T, Huie P, et al. Nature of glomerular dysfunction in preeclampsia. *Kidney Int.* 1998;54(4):1240-9.
24. Guo H, Wang C, Li Z, Gong S, Zhou Z, Leng L. The application of serum cystatin C in estimating the renal function in women with preeclampsia. *Reprod Sci.* 2012;19(7):712-7.
25. Whittaker PG, Lind T. The intravascular mass of albumin during human pregnancy: a serial study in normal and diabetic women. *Br J Obstet Gynaecol.* 1993;100(6):587-92.
26. Benoit J, Rey É. Preeclampsia: should plasma albumin level be a criterion for severity? *J Obstet Gynaecol Can.* 2011;33(9):922-6.
27. Ishimaru T, Ishida J, Nakamura S, Hashimoto M, Matsukura T, Nakamura A. Short-term suppression of the renin-angiotensin system in mice associated with hypertension during pregnancy. *Mol Med Report.* 2012;6(1):28-32.

CHAPTER

10

Obstetric Vasculopathies and their Effects on the Central Nervous System

CHAPTER OUTLINE

- The Privileged Status of Central Nervous System (CNS)
- Pathological Lesions in Preeclampsia
- Psychiatric Complications Following Obstetric Vasculopathies: Any Correlation?

THE PRIVILEGED STATUS OF CENTRAL NERVOUS SYSTEM (CNS)

Amongst the critical involvements of different systems and organs, CNS involvement seems to be more covert than overt. It is relevant to note that the central nervous system seems to have a privileged status. Human body seems to be programmed in such a way that the blood supply and oxygenation of the CNS is maintained efficiently. This can occur even at the cost of other systems. Therefore CNS gets affected in the onslaught of preeclampsia only after other systems are affected. This is the usual picture. Never the less in some pregnant subjects CNS may be more readily affected.

This type of privileged status of CNS can also be seen in the fetus. In states of chronic hypoxia like IUGR, oxygenation of the fetal brain is affected only as a terminal event. This is a well-observed phenomenon on color Doppler studies where the umbilical artery flows and flows of major vessels get so adjusted in states of hypoxia that the fetal CNS oxygenation is maintained till the end. Once fetal CNS oxygenation gets affected, the fetus is at a grave risk of death.

The most dreaded clinical feature of CNS changes of preeclampsia is eclampsia. In this grandmal epiletiform seizures occur. These are usually neglected or fast deteriorating preeclampsia subjects. However, even before the subject develops an eclamptic convulsion subjects who have headache in severe preeclampsia have been found to have an abnormal cerebral perfusion. This was shown through color Doppler studies.[1] This type of abnormal perfusion shown is a result of vasospasm. Such vasospasm is also coupled by passive over distention of these vessels due to failure of autoregulation of vascular caliber. Interestingly this abnormally of central circulation seems to get reversed on administration of magnesium sulfate as has been observed in clinical practice.

Some pregnant subjects develop eclampsia readily when compared to others. Interestingly Sibbai et al demonstrated that changes on electroencephalogram (EEG) shown in eclamptic subjects may even be found sometimes in the family members. This suggests that some pregnant subjects have a familial predisposition to eclampsia.[2] While this familial susceptibility to eclampsia may also account for increased vulnerability of CNS manifestations this is indeed rare. While still on EEG changes it is found that a correlation between EEG abnormalities and MR findings exists. The combined use of MR and EEG may help to determine the prognosis for these patients, but the interictal EEG findings recorded in eclampsia were nonspecific.[3]

PATHOLOGICAL LESIONS IN PREECLAMPSIA

The classical description of pathological features of CNS changes in preeclampsia includes ischemic lesions, edema, and perivascular microhemorrhage.[4] These changes are typical of vasospasm and subsequent reperfusion damage that occurs in obstetric vasculopathies. Extensive documentations of CNS changes in preeclampsia eclampsia have been done by Sheehan and Lynch.[5] Their classic work in this area is still quoted even decades after they first published it. They showed 76 types of lesions in 48 subjects on postmortem who died of eclampsia. Of these the most common were piaarachnoid hemorrhages, cortical patechiae, subcortical patechiae and multiple small focal softening or patechiae in white matter or midbrain.

Their descriptions are admirably detailed and they vividly fit into one common explanation *reperfusion damage* of obstetric vasculopathies. Many other workers have documented these or similar changes in severe preeclamptic or eclamptic subjects who were alive. There are a few additions on those described by Sheehan and Lynch[5] as technology advanced and CNS imaging became easier. However these just complete the list but do not add significantly to our understanding of the disease process.

Brain

On gross examination, edema is found postconvulsion which means that cerebral edema is not the cause of convulsions but the effect of the same. Administration of mannitol may reduce this edema. However mannitol can produce severe complications like pulmonary edema and volume overload in a strained cardiovascular system of on eclamptic subject. This could even prove fatal. Therefore it is no more used in modern obstetrics.

As regards those capillaries that did not break, they show evidence of stasis of circulation. This was indicated by fibrin deposition. Once again this is a manifestation of vasospasm. It is possible that this stasis may not be confined to the capillaries but also to the pre-capillary segments of vessels wherein too this type of fibrin deposition may extend to. Stasis following vasospasm and then after a reperfusion damage produces fibrin deposition in close proximity to petechial hemorrhages.

PSYCHIATRIC COMPLICATIONS FOLLOWING OBSTETRIC VASCULOPATHIES: ANY CORRELATION?

Epidemiological studies have provided some evidence that exposure to obstetric complications is associated with an increased risk for later development of schizophrenia.[6] Preti A et al.[7] carried out an interesting study on this aspect. The goal of this study was to determine whether cases with schizophrenia or related disorders show a history of obstetric complications significantly more often than control subjects and, if so, whether the enhanced risk of a negative pregnancy outcome also extends to the non-schizophrenic offspring of cases. Data based on the obstetric birth case-notes of patients with diagnosed schizophrenia or related disorders were compared to those of normal 'healthy' control subjects; each case/control pair was individually matched by gender, time and parity of birth, maternal age and marital status. It was found that severe, brain-damaging obstetric complications would seem to be a possible antecedent to a diagnosis of schizophrenia or a related disorder in adulthood. Indeed, some early onset cases may be accounted for by prenatal brain lesions. The authors feel that this enhanced risk of negative pregnancy outcome may be under genetic control, contributing to the persistence of schizophrenia in the general population. But the sample size limits the statistical power of calculations and therefore further studies are required to draw the final conclusions on this matter.

REFERENCES

1. Marsál K. Association of cerebral perfusion pressure with headache in women with preeclampsia. *BJOG.* 2001;108(1):126-7.
2. Sibbai B, Spinnato J, Watson D. Eclampsia IV. Neurological findings and future outcome. *Am J Obstet Gynecol.* 1985;152:184-92.
3. Osmanağaoğlu M, Dinç G, Osmanağaoğlu S, Dinç H, Bozkaya H. Comparison of cerebral magnetic resonance and electroencephalogram findings in pre-eclamptic and eclamptic women. *Aust N Z J Obstet Gynaecol.* 2005;45(5):384-90.
4. Topuz S, Kalelioğlu I, Iyibozkurt A, Akhan S, Has R, Tunaci M, Ibrahimoğlu L. Cranial imaging spectrum in hypertensive disease of pregnancy. *Clin Exp Obstet Gynecol.* 2008;35(3):194-7.
5. Sheehan H, Lynch J. Cerebral lesions. In: pathology of toxemia of pregnancy. Baltimore, Williams and Wilkins. 1973, Chapt 32.
6. Boksa P. Animal models of obstetric complications in relation to schizophrenia. *Brain Res Rev.* 2004;45(1):1-17.
7. Preti A, Cardascia L, Zen T, Marchetti M, Favaretto G, Miotto P. Risk for obstetric complications and schizophrenia. *Psychiatry Res.* 2000, 30;96(2):127-39.

CHAPTER

11

Obstetric Vasculopathies and their Effects on Hematological System

CHAPTER OUTLINE

- Alteration in Coagulation Factors (other than Platelets) and Procoagulants
- Alteration in other Cellular Components of Blood
- Review of Coagulation Alterations in Obstetric Vasculopathies

INTRODUCTION

Widespread hematological changes have been demonstrated in obstetric vasculopathies. Before going into details of these hematological changes, it should indeed be qualified that all subjects do not show these changes. Also, all changes are not seen in one subject. Nevertheless, hematological changes are not as rare as ophthalmic changes. The commonest of these and most consistent is development of thrombocytopenia.

ALTERATION IN COAGULATION FACTORS (OTHER THAN PLATELETS) AND PROCOAGULANTS

While thrombocytopenia is one major contributor to hypocoagubility in preeclampsia there are many other factors that add up to this state. One principle contributor to this is fibrinogen. In normal pregnancies uncomplicated by any obstetric vasculopathy body fibrinogen levels rise steeply. These can reach up to 800 mg /dl. However with development of preeclampsia and accidental hemorrhage these levels tend to fall. In preeclampsia, the entire maternal vasculature has fibrin deposition all along its endothelial surface. This is a result of an immunological process leading to massive consumption of fibrinogen which ultimately gets converted to fibrin. This low-key but extensive coagulation process that is found in the entire maternal vasculature leads to hypofibrinogenemia.

One more aspect of hypofibrinogenemia needs to be understood here: normal pregnancy is a hypercoagulable state. Besides many changes that occur in the coagulation system of the pregnant subject, rise in fibrinogen level is one of them. While normally in non pregnant states fibrinogen can rise up to 400 mg/

dl, in pregnancy these levels can rise up to 800 mg/dL. This is where clinical decision-making can get wrongly influenced. It is the order of routine teaching that fibrinogen levels less than 200 mg ms/dL should be viewed with great caution. Levels less than 150 mg/dL can invite clinical manifestation of bleeding and levels less than 100 mg/dL announces a state of crisis, warranting energetic treatment. However, these absolute mathematical levels can be very tricky. If a subject who had her pregnancy levels of fibrinogen rising up to 800 gm/dL, waiting for 200 mg/dL could be very dangerous. If levels of fibrinogen before the onset of obstetric vasculopathies are known it is wise to consider halving of levels as hypofibrinogenemia. In that case 400 mg/dL which is a normal value at the highest point of fibrinogen levels becomes a cutout for calling a state as hypofibrinogenemia. There is lots of pragmatism and wisdom in adopting such a policy as bleeding due to coagulation failure is not only very challenging to handle but can also invite very serious complications.

ALTERATION IN OTHER CELLULAR COMPONENTS OF BLOOD

When hematological changes are being reviewed in the light of obstetric vasculopathies, it will be in the fitness of things to consider other changes which are relevant. Some of these changes can be on a simple peripheral smear examination of blood. A series of seemingly bizarre shape changes have been found in the peripheral smears of affected women. The peripheral smear can show cells like schizocytes, spherocytes, reticulocytes, etc. These changes may also be associated with hemoglobinuria and hemoglobinemia.

One more peculiar cell that has been described in peripheral smear of subjects with ongoing vasculopathy is *Barr Cell*. These too are erythrocytes which show presence of changes that make them appear like wheels with spokes. This spoke-wheel appearance bearing cells are extremely fragile and if present indicate the ongoing process of hemolysis. It is believed that the entire spectrum of changes in RBCs is as a result of their circulating through vascular channels lined with fibrin complexes. This eosinophilic material lining the vascular channels in preeclampsia in particular is believed to be immune complexes. When blood circulates through the vascular channels, the RBCs seemingly wriggle through the narrowed vascular space due to vasospasm. While the RBCs are wriggling though these vessels, the fibrin gets deposited in the cells. As a result their fragility increases and they develops these bizarre shapes. Bar cells that show spoke-wheel appearance is precisely due to this fibrin getting deposited in the cells. While fibrin deposition produces increased fragility of RBCs, Barr cells are a peripheral smear marker of this phenomenon.

Presence of hemoglobinuria and occasional hemoglobinemia also is a result of the RBCs that have become fragile and are therefore quickly breaking down. One more feature of ongoing hemolysis is development of jaundice. It is very interesting to note that while hemolysis is relatively more common in subjects of obstetric vasculopathy especially preeclampsia, jaundice does not appear so readily. The only explanation for this is the fact that hepatic function tends to remain unaffected to a considerable degree in preeclampsia. Therefore, the liver is able to handle the increased load of metabolites resulting from hemolysis. As the disease process advances and the maternal condition rapidly deteriorate, the liver competence also breaks down and jaundice appears. As expected, the rise in prehepatic component of bilirubinemia will be more as it is not being metabolized and eliminated effectively by the sick liver cells. One possible reason of the liver being able to handle the increased load of hemolysis could be the anatomical double blood supply that the liver has. Very few body organs have double blood supply in the human body. Consequently, in spite of vasospasm and consequent challenge to the organ systems that occurs in preeclampsia, liver is able to handle the load much more efficiently.

REVIEW OF COAGULATION ALTERATIONS IN OBSTETRIC VASCULOPATHIES

It is very well known that the entire coagulation process gets greatly challenged in obstetric vasculopathies especially in preeclampsia. The other obstetric vasculopathy where coagulation system gets challenged is accidental hemorrhage. Normal uncomplicated human pregnancy is a procoagulant state. Blood tends to coagulate more readily. This is achieved through a series of cellular and noncellular changes that take place in pregnancy. Basically, it is a protective change. Every pregnant woman is likely to bleed in variable amounts during the process of parturition. This is feebly but notably countered by such attempts of the body systems of the pregnant subject.

It is also necessary to note at this stage that the challenge to body procoagulant disposition is quite resilient. This is proved by the fact that very few subjects with preeclampsia actually develop coagulation dysfunction in clinical practice.

Platelets in Normal and Preeclamptic Pregnancies

Platelets levels are hardly affected in normal pregnancy. Thrombocytopenia if at all it occurs is seen as the severity of the disease that is increasing. It is also noteworthy that even if the circulating platelet counts get reduced in pregnancy, the neonatal circulating platelets remain by and large unaffected.

One very interesting observation was made by Redman et al (1978). They found that circulating platelet levels fell in early stage of clinical manifestation of the disease of preeclampsia. This was concurrently matched with a rise in uric acid levels in the body of the subject. This observation was unique because it establishes one very important correlation.[1] In the preceding sections, it has been made amply clear that uric acid levels in the body reflect an oxidative stress. Uric acid is known to be one of the strongest reducing systems in the body. Rising levels of uric acid means an ongoing and even an accelerated phenomenon of oxidative stress in the body. When this is coupled with falling levels of platelets the correlation can be well understood. Platelets are known to undergo a process of activation. This process of platelet activation is critical and precedes the clinical manifestations of preeclampsia. Therefore rising levels of urate getting coupled with falling levels of platelets indicates that the two, oxidative stress and platelet activation are coupled in the etiopathology of preeclampsia.

One more interesting observation has been found regarding platelets and clinical manifestations of coagulation abnormalities. This is an important observation. Many obstetricians who deal with high-risk obstetric patients have a routine to get a coagulation profile done in subjects with preeclampsia eclampsia. This seems to be an overdoing. Tests like estimation of Prothrombin Time (PT) and Activated Partial Thromboplastin Time (APTT) should be confined to only those subjects who have platelet counts less than 1,00,000/dL. Till the platelet counts fall to at or below this level, other coagulation indices will not alter. Thus estimation of these indices is futile. Also, a coagulation profile that does not include a platelet count is fractured or invalid.

It has also been found that the size of the platelets in circulation during the process of severe preeclampsia/eclampsia is larger. The mean platelet volume increases gradually in pregnant women affected by preeclampsia compared to women with normal pregnancies.[2] This increase in size of platelets seems to be occurring irrespective of numerical alterations. It is therefore possible that this is one of the reflections of the process of platelet mobilization occurring at a much faster pace in preeclampsia. Mobilizations following an enhanced production of all cell lines from megakaryocytes reflect a faster production of that cell line. It also reflects the fact that younger cells are getting mobilized in that disease process.

One more change that has been well documented in preeclampsia and hints strongly at the process of platelet activation occurring in preeclampsia is degranulation. It has been found that before the clinical manifestations of preeclampsia there is a rise in circulating levels of β-thromboglobulin by about four weeks.[3] Endothelial damage and platelet releasing reaction detected by β-thromboglobulin may be significantly more enhanced in women with severe preeclampsia than in women with mild preeclampsia.[4] There is a direct correlation between rise in β-thromboglobulin levels and degranulation of platelets. Also, platelet degranulation suggests an ongoing process of platelet activation. This process begins very early in preeclampsia. It may occur even before clinical manifestations of even milder forms of the disease getting manifested.

Also, neonatal thrombocytopenia is sometimes reported in babies born to mothers with preeclampsia.[5] with an associated risk of neonatal bleeding.[6] But this has not been consistently found. Nevertheless if there is maternal thrombocytopenia, there is a risk of neonatal thrombocytopenia requiring a control of the blood count for the baby at birth and within 5 days, newborns have to be treated if the platelet count is less than 20×10^9/L.[7]

Concept of Competence Alteration (Efficiency) of Platelets

One interesting feature of thrombocytopenia in pregnancy was demonstrated by Kelton et al.[8] This group has demonstrated that in subjects with severe preeclampsia even if thrombolytic levels are normal, bleeding time gets prolonged. This is very interesting. Though they have not tried to explain, it seems this is a matter of efficiency of platelets.

Modern medical science by and large bases its interpretations of results of markers of different processes on arithmetic correlation. By this it is meant that a linear rise in neutrophils indicates an acute infection. Similarly, a linear rise in levels of transaminases indicates deteriorating liver function. But modern medical science misses a very vital component of these indicators and that is the markers of competence. While rising neutrophils indicates a higher mobilization of these leukocytes in presence of acute infections it is indeed also happening that then neutrophils become more efficient in their working. It is quite likely that increase in the number and competence both are essential for combating the acute infection. A raised count of neutrophil to 13.000 per dl of blood may be shooting up to 20,000 to 25000 had their competence too not improved concurrently. Modern medical science hardly tries to explore this aspect.

Studies of Kelton et al[8] could be a pointer to this phenomenon albeit in a negative way. Rise in bleeding time in absence of significant fall in circulating levels of thrombocytes indicates that in presence of obstetric vasculopathies the competence of platelets gets compromised. As a result their levels on hematological investigations do not reduce but bleeding time increases. This concept of competence evaluation and competence alteration opens up many exciting possibilities of understanding disease processes and their laboratory parameters in totally different light.

Although laboratory parameters peg a level of 150,000/dl to be at the lower limit of normal, most pregnant subjects do not bleed till the platelet levels sink to less than 50,000/dl. A study by Laskin et al showed that abnormal coagulation occurred in 105 of 1405 eligible women (7.5%). The odds of having abnormal coagulation were increased for women with platelet counts $< 50 \times 10^9$/L and between 50 and 99 $\times 10^9$/L compared with women who had platelet counts above 150 $\times 10^9$/L. Platelet counts $< 100 \times 10^9$/L were associated with significantly increased odds of adverse maternal outcomes, most specifically blood transfusion. A platelet count of $< 100 \times 10^9$/L had good specificity in identifying abnormal coagulation and adverse maternal outcomes, but poor sensitivity.[9] It is possible that in states of sinking levels of platelets in preeclampsia, their competence improves. Therefore with lesser number of platelets, the functioning result of hemostasis is maintained.

Platelet Activation and Thromboxane A2 Production

While explaining the etiopathogenesis of obstetric vasculopathies in general and preeclampsia in particular it has been stressed that an unabated oxidative process leads to series of cascading changes which subsequently lead to vasospasm. This vasospasm has been stressed as the main villain inviting organ and systemic manifestations of the disease process. One link that was hitherto missing was in the last step. This is the step of alteration in thromboxane prostacyclin balance in favor of thromboxane. This thromboxane is a vasoconstrictor. It produces a vasospasm by a direct effect on vascular smooth muscles. It does so by mobilization of column into the smooth muscle cells to produce muscular activity of constriction.

The answer is evident now. It is principally occurring due to increase in thromboxane production. This increase in thromboxane production is due to platelet activation. This increased thromboxane biosynthesis seems to be derived from platelets. Thus, the activated platelets lead to increase in thromboxane production. This ultimately tilts the balance in favor of thromboxane, in the thromboxane prostacyclin imbalance.

Prior to this increased thromboxane production there is a reduction in prostacyclin production also. This reduction in production is coupled with reduction in sensitivity to prostacyclin. This reduction in sensitivity is coupled through messengers like cAMP (Cyclic Adenosine Mono Phosphate). So the production as well as the sensitivity of vascular endothelium to prostacyclin is also reduced. This leads to platelet activation or at least promotes platelet activation. It is of interest to note that both the aims of the balance between thromboxane prostacyclin are altered in favor of thromboxane which leads to a series of changes to produce a vasospasm.

Platelets are known to have quite a few structural and biochemical characteristics of smooth muscle cells.[10] There seems to be a great similarity between smooth muscles and platelets in behaviors and vascular tone. This similarity is very important to acknowledge and understand. Therefore, it shows that what is true for platelet behavior is also true for smooth muscle responses. Therefore, this explains the similarity in response to prostacyclin thromboxane imbalance leading to platelet aggregation and activation as well as increase in smooth muscle vascular tone. Thus, platelet aggregation and activation and smooth muscle contraction are not disjointed events. They are two manifestations of the same event. Understanding this is very important because it will explain critical events in the etiopathogenesis of preeclampsia in particular and other obstetric vasculopathies in general.

REFERENCES

1. Redman C, Bonnar J. Plasma urate changes in pre-eclampsia. *Br Med J.* 1978; 1(6125):1484-5.
2. Dundar O, Yoruk P, Tutuncu L, Erikci A, Muhcu M, Ergur A, et al. Longitudinal study of platelet size changes in gestation and predictive power of elevated MPV in development of preeclampsia. *Prenat Diagn.* 2008;28(11):1052-6.
3. Belleges V, Spitz B, De Baene L. Platelet activation and vascular damage in gestational hypertension. *Am J Obstet Gynecol.* 1992;166:629-33.
4. Hayashi M, Inoue T, Hoshimoto K, Negishi H, Ohkura T, Inaba N. Characterization of five marker levels of the hemostatic system and endothelial status in normotensive pregnancy and preeclampsia. *Eur J Haematol.* 2002;69(5-6):297-302.
5. Chen Z, Liang M, Wang J. Etiology and clinical characteristics of pregnancy-emerged thrombocytopenia. *Zhonghua Fu Chan Ke Za Zhi.* 2011;46(11):834-9.
6. Kadir R, McLintock C. Thrombocytopenia and disorders of platelet function in pregnancy. *Semin Thromb Hemost.* 2011;37(6):640-52.
7. Khellaf M, Loustau V, Bierling P, Michel M, Godeau B. Thrombocytopenia and pregnancy. *Rev Med Interne.* 2012;33(8):446-52.
8. Kelton J, Hunter D, Naema P. A platelet function defect in preeclampsia. *Obstet Gynecol.* 1995;65:107-9.
9. Laskin S, Payne B, Hutcheon J, Qu Z, Douglas M, Ford J, et al. The role of platelet counts in the assessment of inpatient women with preeclampsia. *J Obstet Gynaecol Can.* 2011;33(9):900-8.
10. Baker P, Cunningham F. In: Lindheimer M, Roberts J, Cunningham F (Eds). Chesley's Hypertensive disorders of pregnancy. 2nd edn. Stamford: Appleton and Lange. 1998. p.357.

CHAPTER

12

Obstetric Vasculopathies and their Effects on the Liver

CHAPTER OUTLINE

- Pathological Changes in the Liver
- Liver in Hemolysis Elevated Liver Enzymes Low Platelets (HELLP) Syndrome

INTRODUCTION

One more vital organ system that bears a heavy brunt of obstetric vasculopathies is the hepatic system. A student of obstetrics gets introduced to hepatic involvement in preeclampsia in very early days of his career. One of the commonest questions he/she is asked as a student of the subject is related to differentiating mild preeclampsia from severe preeclampsia (or what is also called as impending eclampsia). The answer expected besides others is epigastric pain. This epigastric pain in worsening preeclampsia is possibly due to hepatic capsule getting stretched and/or hepatic edema in severe preeclampsia. It could be due to hepatocellular edema and/or hepatic cellular necrosis and/or stretching of the Gilson capsule. Sometimes, this pain has also been attributed to a varied amount of subcapsular hemorrhage with worsening preeclampsia.

Another interesting but probably overhyped complication of preeclampsia is capsular rupture of the liver. The most common clinical feature of this condition is upper quadrant or epigastric pain. Many other more severe consequences of this condition have also been reported. Grand'Maison S, et al reviewed 9 cases of rupture of hepatic hematoma associated with hemolysis, elevated liver enzymes, and low platelets. They suggested use of hepatic artery embolization to help minimize morbidity and maternal mortality in such subjects.[1] However in actual clinical practice this complication of preeclampsia is rarely seen. Even an obstetrician working in a high-risk obstetric unit may get one case if at all in his/her entire life.

Another feature of worsening preeclampsia is a rise in hepatic enzymes. This has been attributed to periportal hemorrhagic necrosis by some workers.[2] With the advent of ultrasound such an association between rising liver enzymes and periportal hepatic hemorrhage has not been consistently reported. Hepatic periportal hemorrhagic necrosis is one of the features of preeclampsia leading to elevated liver enzymes. Another intriguing but challenging association of preeclampsia that has elevated liver enzymes is HELLP syndrome.

PATHOLOGICAL CHANGES IN THE LIVER

It is of interest to know that clinical evidence of liver involvement in preeclampsia is not very commonly found. Subclinical involvement may be much more. It is known that the liver, heart and the brain are preferred over other systems in the body of a pregnant human female. This is more so when the body faces a crisis as in severe preeclampsia or eclampsia. While it is relatively common to see a compromise in placental and renal functioning in these crisis states, liver function hardly ever gets clinically compromised. It seems that the liver functioning is given a priority by the double blood supply that this organ has. Consequently in spite of a compromise in vascularity of all organs in preeclampsia, liver is able to withstand this impoverishment much more easily. The heart and the brain have their own unique systems for achieving this priority.

One of the common changes demonstrated in livers of preeclamptic subjects is the presence of subcapsular hemorrhage and hematoma. This has been covered in clinical features extensively correlating it with epigastric or upper abdominal pain in subjects worsening from mild preeclampsia to severe preeclampsia or imminent eclampsia. Some workers have estimated that there changes are present in as high as 45% of the subjects.[3] However, clinical manifestations of these changes are limited to very few.

As regards the gross changes in liver petechial hemorrhages, subcapsular hematoma and ischemia have been consistently found. Their frequency varies from one study to the other. In fact these are demonstrations of the vasospasm-reperfusion damage that occurs as the main pathogenesis of preeclampsia and its complications. Failure of the hepatic vessels to withstand the pressure of reperfusion leads to their breaking of the vessel walls. This may cause patechiae, subcapsular hematoma and other hemorrhages in the liver. The extent to which a vessel can withstand the force of the blood depends on its intrinsic capacity. It varies from individual to individual and even in the same individual it may vary from one vessel to the other. Concurrently with the reperfusion is the occurrence of vasospasm. This explains the hepatic ischemia seen on descriptions related to microscopic changes seen in preeclampsia.

The hemorrhages could be pinpoint petechial hemorrhages or if large vessels have been disrupted there could be confluence of hematomas and hemorrhagic areas. On gross examination besides these changes, liver remains unaffected. As regards the microscopic changes manifestations of deprivation of blood supply occurs very late in the liver. This is in contrast to the kidneys where the so-called "bloodless glomeruli" was a very consistent feature at all stages of the disease. In liver, changes of necrosis appear in very severe form of the disease like subjects dying of eclampsia. Infarction and necrosis being not so common in liver in spite of vasospasm shows the efficiency with which double blood supply of liver is able to handle this deprivation.

Contrastingly however, instead of vasospasm damages, liver shows evidence of reperfusion damages much more consistently. Sheehan and Lynch described hemorrhage in hepatic cellular columns at the periportal bases where the hepatocytes get pushed up in their stromal sleeves.[4] In most of the descriptions of liver changes in preeclampsia/eclampsia hemorrhage is found to be the most consistent finding.

One more interesting observation found was that most of the times the severity and extent of lesions did not match with the severity of clinical conditions. This was more so in mild and moderate forms of the disease in clinical practice. This reflects the capacity of the liver to handle the deprivation of blood supply.

Description of pathology of preeclampsia would not be complete if fatty changes in the liver are not touched upon. Vigil-de Gracia P and Montufar-Rueda al describe an 'AFLP-Triad' in women with acute fatty liver of pregnancy. This triad included three set of features. First (symptoms): nausea/vomiting, jaundice, epigastric pain; second (laboratory): results indicated renal dysfunction, coagulopathy, liver function abnormalities, low glycemia, and third (complications): renal failure, coagulopathy, ascites, and encephalopathy.[5] In clinical practice acute fatty liver is diagnosed by a severe and sudden deterioration in clinical condition of the subject. This is coupled by rapid rise in liver enzyme levels and ultrasonographic evidence of acute fatty liver changes. Though these manifestations are consistently found is severe and deteriorating forms of the disease, they are not found in all subjects with such severe stages of preeclampsia. Clinically, acute fatty liver of pregnancy is more fatal than eclampsia. So when present, it kills decisively.

LIVER IN HEMOLYSIS ELEVATED LIVER ENZYMES LOW PLATELETS (HELLP) SYNDROME

Most consistently associated with preeclampsia but reportedly occurring even without it, HELLP syndrome as is well known by now is the acronym for Hemolysis, Elevated Liver Enzymes, Low Platelets. This is notoriously associated with other critical organs system involvements and can be potentially fatal. It is known to have vicious associations including those with other obstetric vasculopathies like accidental hemorrhage. It readily invites renal failure, pulmonary edema and subcapsular hemorrhage in the liver, the kidneys and the cardiovascular systems get readily involved in HELLP syndrome.

In most instances delivery is known to ameliorate the condition. Nevertheless there are a small but sizable percentage of subjects where the situation may worsen postpartum. Therefore, obstetric management of these subjects becomes very challenging. A rapid delivery through cesarean section is understandably readily resorted to. But this too is fraught with dangers of wound hematoma and intraoperative ooze.

HELLP syndrome has a distinct risk of recurrence. Leeners et al has pegged the recurrence rate at 12.8%.[6] Some workers have suggested an autoimmune etiology for its occurrence. The immunological basis for HELLP syndrome can be considered as there is associated IUGR, accidental hemorrhage, stillbirths and preterm deliveries in subsequent pregnancies. Most of these are known major manifestation of obstetric vasculopathies and have a known strong immunological basis.

By and large the hepatobiliary system is not affected in a very big way compared to the renal, cardiovascular and central nervous system in obstetric vasculopathies. It is possible that hepatobiliary involvement if occurs will readily get manifested into HELLP syndrome. One missing link however remains here. This missing link is the association between hemolysis and hepatic involvement. Also thrombocytopenia and elevated liver enzymes becomes a little difficult to explain. A simplistic looking explanation to this could be the hemopoietic system involvement in the immunological process. However, this needs more research.

REFERENCES

1. Grand'Maison S, Sauvé N, Weber F, Dagenais M, Durand M, Mahone M. Hepatic rupture in hemolysis, elevated liver enzymes, low platelets syndrome. *Obstet Gynecol.* 2012;119(3):617-25.
2. E Knox TA, Olans LB. Liver disease in pregnancy. N Engl J. Med. 1996;335:569-76.
3. Mamouni N, Derkaoui A, Bougern H, Bouchikhi C, Chaara H, Banani A, et al. Subcapsular hematoma of the liver complicating preeclampsia: about 6 cases. *Pan Afr Med J.* 2011;9:47.
4. Sheehan H, Lynch J. Pathology of toxemia of pregnancy. Baltimore: Williams and Wilkins. 1973, 807.
5. Vigil-de Gracia P, Montufar-Rueda C. Acute fatty liver of pregnancy: diagnosis, treatment, and outcome based on 35 consecutive cases. *J Matern Fetal Neo Med.* 2011;24(9):1143-6.
6. Leeners B, Neumaier-Wagner P, Kuse S, Mütze S, Rudnik-Schöneborn S, Zerres K, et al. Recurrence risks of hypertensive diseases in pregnancy after HELLP syndrome. *J Perinat Med.* 2011;39(6):673-8.

CHAPTER

13

Ophthalmic Features in Obstetric Vasculopathy

CHAPTER OUTLINE

- Retinal Edema
- Central and Peripheral Cause of Visual Alterations

INTRODUCTION

It was not uncommon to find subjects presenting in emergency of an obstetric unit with complaints of dimness of vision and epigastric pain in or after midtrimester of pregnancy who hardly took antenatal care. In all of them, severe preeclampsia or worsening preeclampsia is a consistent feature. There is also a possibility of dimness of vision progressing to frank blindness. Also it has a tendency to recur regularly in subsequent pregnancy. Dimness of vision therefore can be grouped as a feature of severe preeclampsia and/or imminent eclampsia. Established ophthalmic entities associated with (pre) eclampsia are cortical blindness, serous retinal detachment, Purtscher-like retinopathy, central retinal vein occlusions, and retinal or vitreous hemorrhages. Ensuing visual symptoms include blurry vision, diplopia, amaurosis fugax, photopsia, and scotomata, including homonymous hemianopsia.[1] The pathogenesis of the Purtscher retinopathy is the embolism of the retinal arterioles, by leukocytic aggregation, as a response to the activation of the complement.[2]

There are multiple explanations for this ophthalmic feature. One of these is peripheral. By peripheral it is meant that the cause is in the retina. The exudative retinal detachment is a rare cause (under 1%) of visual loss in preeclampsia/eclampsia, being produced by the involvement of the choroidal vascularization.[2] As is well known, the human retina is a multilayered tissue. The deepest layer of the retina continues as optic nerve. In normal non-diseased situations an image focused on the superficial layer of the retina, transmits an electronic impulse down the subsequent layers to the optic nerve. This nerve carries the impulse to the brain. Here, the impulse gets processed and flipped by 90° and the human being "sees".

RETINAL EDEMA

In severe preeclampsia, in susceptible subjects, there occurs a process of retinal edema. This is a direct result of vasospasm locally followed by reperfusion damage and incompetence of vessel walls. Retinal edema leads to diffuse separation of retinal layers. This distances the most superficial layer of the retina from the deepest layer. In retinal edema of severe preeclampsia, the image formed does send the signal to the deeper layer. But due to edema this impulse gets diluted and fuzzy. Also the distance between the layers gets increased. As a result of this the optic nerve gets a weak signal. This depleted or weakened signal leads to perception of dimness of vision by the subject. The separation of retinal layers could be more severe. In such a situation, though the image does form on the superficial layer, deep down the impulse just fails to reach the optic nerve. Result of this is a blackout or blindness.

However, these peripheral causes are by and large completely reversible. This is because once the subject delivers, the retinal edema is reversed. Once the edema reverses all layers of the retina falls back to their original state. They are again in close approximation with each other. So the image formed on the superficial layer once again quickly sends the impulse to the optic nerve and the subject stats "seeing" again. Also, the reversal of edema prevents distortion and dilution of the image formed. Result of this a reperception of sharp and crisp image.

CENTRAL AND PERIPHERAL CAUSE OF VISUAL ALTERATIONS

There are some subjects in whom the visual disturbance does not get completely reversed. These are subjects who have a central cause of visual disturbance. Optic nerve fibers once emerging from the deep layer of the retina go to the optic chiasma. From the optic chiasma these fibers pass to the occipital lobe from where they are directed to the anterior brain. In subjects with central cause of visual disturbances, the cause of visual disturbance is at the occipital lobe. This usually results in a permanent damage to nerve fibers here. In such a situation there is hardly any local or peripheral cause of visual disturbances. Unluckily this central cause does not reverse as the damage is permanent. The subject in such situation may not get the complete restoration of her visual faculty. This is due to central nervous system having an inherent inability to regenerate and repair once injured or destroyed. Though the percentage of such subjects having a permanently disabled or disturbed visual function is very less, it is debilitating.

Visual Alterations of Special Mention—Recurrent and Unilateral

Another feature of these visual disturbances in subjects with imminent eclampsia is recurrence. In some this is notoriously recurrent. It is not uncommon to find such subjects reporting themselves with first signs of visual alterations to the emergency obstetric care units seeking help. In these subjects retinal vasculature has an inherent propensity to develop edema and subsequent changes. As a result they develop these features every time there is preeclampsia. Indeed in these subjects preeclampsia is also recurrent. However, visual disturbances can occur much earlier and in more severe forms with each subsequent pregnancy.

One more interesting aspect of blindness in preeclampsia is the fact that in some subjects this visual handicap develops unilaterally. Usually these are retinal in origin as described above **(P···)** and reversible. As regards the cortical origin of visual disturbance that is seen in some subjects of preeclampsia, it has been found that occipital lobe gets principally involved.[3]

While on ophthalmic changes in severe preeclampsia eclampsia, it is worthwhile revisiting the fundoscopic changes in this condition. Metaphorically, it has been stated that retinal vessels reflect the changes in renal and intracranial vessels. It has also been show that the severity of retinopathy in preeclampsia is directly related to the level of placental insufficiency and intrauterine growth retardation. The severity of retinopathy might be independent of systemic BP.[4] However there are three points where fundoscopic examination does help in division making in clinical practice:

- Firstly it helps to differentiate between a chronic hypertensive subjects developing a superimposed preeclampsia over non hypertensive subjects
- Secondly, worsening changes a fundoscopy if serially done in clinical practice helps decide in favor of early intervention
- Finally, presence of papilledema at any stage of pregnancy, in a subject with preeclampsia is an indication for immediate intervention.

In modern times with the advent of color Doppler fundoscopy has lost its value. Color Doppler is any day better and more versatile help in decision making in obstetric vasculopathies in general and preeclampsia in particular.

REFERENCES

1. Roos N, Wiegman M, Jansonius N, Zeeman G. Visual disturbances in (pre) eclampsia. *Obstet Gynecol Surv.* 2012;67(4):242-50.
2. Mihu D, Mihu C, Tălu S, Costin N, Ciuchină S, Măluţan A. Ocular changes in preeclampsia. *Oftalmologia.* 2008;52(2):16-22.
3. Swende T, Abwa T. Reversible blindness in fulminating preeclampsia. *Ann Afr Med.* 2009;8(3):189-91.
4. Gupta A, Kaliaperumal S, Setia S, Suchi S, Rao V. Retinopathy in preeclampsia: Association with birth weight and uric acid level. *Retina.* 2008;28(8):1104-10.

CHAPTER

14

Vascular Responses in Obstetric Vasculopathy

CHAPTER OUTLINE

- Blunted Vascular Response
- Placental Ischemia
- Animal Experiments
- Hard Facts Emerging from Animal Experiments

BLUNTED VASCULAR RESPONSE

Some peculiar historical series of events have for quite some time a semiguided the scientists. The initial experiments of Abdul-Carim and Assali need a mention as a benchmark.[1] These scientists showed that during pregnancy the sensitivity of the maternal vascular system in animals was reduced to pressure substance angiotensinogen. As a result, reduced or blunted response to angiotensin-angiotensinogen was extensively studied. It was even demonstrated that those animals (and humans) who did not show a blunted response to these substances had a higher chance of developing preeclampsia in particular and probably other obstetric vasculopathies in general. Efforts were then after made to identify genes that mediated this response. However as time passed it was revealed that angiotensin-angiotensinogen do not have any great privileged status. In reality the maternal vascular system was blunted in response to nearly all pressor substances. Those that got added to this list included vasopressin and norepinephrin.[2] Leaving aside the importance that angiotensin received, one glaring fact became obvious that maternal vascular system in uncomplicated pregnancies resist the pressure substances from generating a vasospasm and a subsequent preeclampsia.

However there were some profound changes that are occurring in some subjects, which annul this bluntness. As a result, the vascular system becomes highly responsive to the circulating pressure substances. This peculiar vascular reactivity difference in complicated and uncomplicated pregnant subjects opened up an environment for the potent vasoconstrictors like thromboxane A2 and endothelin to act. At this stage, cutting the story short, one can accept that animal experiment of vascular system gave vital insights into the prevention of vasospasm in normal subjects and its occurrence in subjects with vasculopathies.

PLACENTAL ISCHEMIA

As regards the etiopathology of obstetric vasculopathies placental ischemia has been found to have an important role. Leads into this happening came from studies in animals. These experiments have been considered in these pages. It is therefore necessary to include even seemingly "old" references for a comprehensive perspective of the matter. There were animal studies where uterine ischemia was surgically produced by clipping the uterine arteries in rabbits. Strangely there was no effect in the blood pressure of these animals. Usually rabbits were used for these experiments. Subsequently, they produced placental ischemia in these animals by applying the so-called Z-stitch in the placenta. It was found that the blood pressure of the animal shot up expeditiously.[3] This led to the conclusion that it is not the uterine ischemia but placental ischemia that results in preeclampsia.

Subsequently another set of experiments were conducted to see the effect of "chronic" ischemia. These experiments were confined to the dogs. In nonpregnant state their utero-ovarian vessels were ligated. It was found that there was no change in the blood pressure of the dogs. However, when the dogs became pregnant, its blood pressure showed a distinct and significant rise.[4]

These experiments showed vital leads for understanding the pathophysiology of preeclampsia. Uterine ischemia generated by banding or clipping failed to show any significant change in the blood pressure of the animal. This is also seen in human beings in a totally different perspective. For decades, uterine artery, utero-ovarian arteries and internal iliac arteries have been ligated in human beings for treatment of postpartum hemorrhage. Internal iliacs have also been legated for treatment of intractable or uncontrollable bleeding during OBGYN surgery in human females. Prophylactic anterior division of internal iliac has been ligated in gynecological surgeries where bleeding is expected to be more. In none of these subjects any adverse effects of any type have been found in human being following devascularization procedures. Interestingly, there have been countless pregnancies reported in these subjects with hypovascularized or so-called "devascularized" uterus. But no rise in any adverse obstetric outcomes has been reported.

In the initial days of advent of these surgeries to prevent and/or treat hemorrhage apprehensions have been expressed about the possibility of such uteri developing gangrenes or atrophies. These apprehensions did not prove to be true. Subsequent vascular studies including angiography of these uteri revealed that efficient collaterals took over the function of providing blood to uteri preventing any devascularizing injuries.

ANIMAL EXPERIMENTS

Some explanation can be forwarded for the hypertension that developed in those dogs in which vascular supply to their uteri was impeded, once they became pregnant. The most likely explanation for this goes thus: in nonpregnant states the collaterals efficiently take over the vascular supply to the uterus experimentally devascularized. This could be akin to what happens in human females. As soon as the added stress or demand of pregnancy is added on the uterus the collaterals fail to cope up. In the initial days of pregnancy (up to about 7 weeks) there was no change in BP of dogs. However as the demand of the placenta increased the collaterals failed to provide with this increased demand which resulted in placental ischemia and rise in blood pressure producing a clinical situation similar to preeclampsia. Human clinical experience therefore helps to explain phenomenon found in experimental animals. Clinical situations where results of animal experiments are applied to human beings are phrased as results expanded to human beings. In this matter therefore clinical happenings in human beings can be "constricted"to explain observations in animal experiments.

Experiments by Abitbol[5] respectively in rabbits and in dogs were interesting. These groups of workers clipped the aorta of the experimental animals below the levels of renal vessels. All these were pregnant animals. It was found that these animals developed rise in BP and even proteinuria consistently. It was also found that in both the species, the kidneys developed profound changes similar to "glomeruloendotheliosis" of PIH. It is indeed a fact that these experiments opened up a consistent feature that vascular resistance is critical in developing preeclampsia. However what was challenged in Abitbol's experiment was the fact that by clipping the aorta distal to the renal vessels, the entire distal body vascularity is compromised. This does not leave the exclusivity of the uterus in developing an ischemia. Technically this is not ideal for reproducing or expanding the results to human conditions. One more objection to studies of Abitbol was that the dogs were anesthetized which itself can have profound effect on BP of the body. However, one has to grant the fact that these experiments did provide a very vital lead in understanding of placental ischemia as a key event in development of obstetric vasculopathies. Subsequent advances in technology and techniques helped scientist perform these animal experiments without having the need to continuously anesthetize them. Baboons and rhesus monkeys the two species that are considered closest to humans were used.[6] Even the need for surgery could be eliminated and longitudinal studies could be undertaken satisfactorily.

With these refined techniques and pain free experiments the experimental animals were subjected to minimal or no pain. However, there were no starting or so called "game changer" results that emerged. All these studies pointed to the fact that increased vascular resistance led to rise in blood pressure and affects a series of organs and tissues. Proteinuria and renal changes as described under "glomerular endotheliosis" were all resulting from this increased vascular resistance. These were already shown in animal experiments on rabbits and dogs earlier.

However there were certain limitations of these studies, both technical and interpretative. Some of these included a sudden appearance of clinical features like hypertension does not occur usually in human pregnancy. In the latter, the rise in BP is usually gradual and less sudden. One more objection raised to these was the fact that thus hypertension so registered was not sustainable at times, proteinuria inconsistently occurring and renal dysfunction not always found. All these were hampering the growth of drawing very reliable conclusions from animal experiments. However, some workers have suggested that Placental ischemia is a consequence rather than a cause of preeclampsia.[7] Without muddying waters further the matter is left as it is.

In human beings the entire mischief takes place with the arrival of the placenta at the fetomaternal interface. When confined to this small locus, clinical conditions like IUGR, abruptio placenta and stillbirths occur. However, when it involves the entire maternal vasculature the mother develops preeclampsia.

Dietary Deficiency and Animal Experiments

While one huge set of animal experiments concentrated on generating preeclampsia-like conditions in experimental animals through increase in vascular resistance, another set of animal experiments tried to correlate dietary manipulations with preeclampsia.[8] While these experiments were by and large confined to generation of artificial general nutritional deficiencies by fasting these animals, others studied effect of deficiency of specific nutrients. The concept that a single nutrient deficiency produced preeclampsia was not acceptable to scientists.[9]

However, one deficiency that gained some importance and popularity was deficiency of calcium. Work done by Prada et al[10] showed that calcium deficiency specifically generated preeclampsia like features in pregnant ewes. Since calcium was known to control vascular tone thereby influencing BP[11], these experiments became interesting. Later on in some studies it was found that calcium deficiency has some role in preeclampsia.[12] Studies by Bucher et al[13] showed that calcium supplements in pregnancy reduced the chances of preeclampsia. Therefore work of Karenja N[13] and similar on animals did gain some credibility and popularity. However, later on when large bodies of evidence was examined through meta-analysis it was found that calcium deficiency did not universally produce preeclampsia. It was found that calcium deficiency may be associated with preeclampsia only in those subjects in whom there was dietary deficiency of calcium.

This once again confirmed the understanding that dietary deficiencies of single agents have a very limited role if at all any in producing preeclampsia. When these studies are examined with the larger clinical scenario they show very inconsistent and contradictory results. Calcium supplementation is a routine and universal in clinical practice. In spite of this preeclampsia and other obstetric vasculopathies developed with equal impunity. Also if generalized nutritional deficiencies are to be examined in larger clinical scenario, it has been seen that obstetric vasculopathies occur in nutritionally sufficient subjects with nearly the same frequency as it occurs in subjects from poor socioeconomic backgrounds with generalized nutritional deficiency states.

Though there is a large body of animal experiments with nutritional factorization in preeclampsia, the results emerging from them are at best inconsistent. Also, when evaluated in the light of clinical scenario on a large canvas, it was found that nutrition and deficiency or sufficiency of nutritional compounds have a very limited role in causation and/or progress of preeclampsia in particular and other obstetric vasculopathies in general.

Quantification of Fetomaternal Interface Vascular Activity

All throughout it has been maintained that the initiation of etiopathology of obstetric vasculopathies occurs at the fetomaternal interface. It may then after confine itself to this interface or may involve the entire maternal vasculature. It would therefore be of great importance to access the fetomaternal interface in whatever way possible. Due to invasiveness of these attempts, trying to gain an access to this interface is a big challenge in human beings. Information gained is therefore indirect and at times circumstantial. While color Doppler is a boon to a clinician monitoring these pregnancies, to a research scientist it has limitations. Color Doppler is always indirect and is done externally not accessing the fetomaternal interface directly. Therefore, its results have innate limitations for a research scientist.

In this aspect, animal experiments score. It is possible to access the fetomaternal interface directly and record events there with much more accuracy in animals. For this radiolabel lead microspheres escaping from the target organ especially the highly vascular fetomaternal interface have been used.[14] In these experiments radiolabeled spheres are transferred into the left ventricle of experimental animals. From here they are pumped out by the heart and dissipated to the entire body. This enables the animal experiment performing scientists to study the cardiac output as well as the blood flow through the organs, tissues and interfaces in the body. However for this the animal needs to be sacrificed and the organ understudy removed. It is then acid washed in the laboratory helping to accurately measure the microspheres trapped in that organ. On the basis of results so obtained one can deduce about the blood flow through the isolated organ. On the basis of these animal experiments it was accurately shown that blood flow at the fetomaternal interface (the uteroplacental blood flow) is greatly reduced in obstetric vasculopathies. These were some of the most accurate and direct observations.

With the advancement in technology, the direct access to fetomaternal interface became easier through placement of fine color Doppler probes directly at the fetomaternal interface. This needed to reversibly anesthetize the animal at the time of probe placement. Once the probes were in place, the animal need not be anesthetized any more. Blood flow can then be studied continuously and directly giving an accurate idea of what is happening within. Also with modern microprobes and cordless technology becoming very popular and accessible there would be still more accurate and easy accessibility to uteroplacental circulation possible. These are exciting areas in current animal experiments.

Salient Results Emerging from Animal Experiments

On basis of all these body of experiments certain salient and irrefutable results emerge which provide vital leads in understanding the etiopathology and pathogenesis of obstetric vasculopathies.

- Endothelial cell activation occurs very consistently and critically
- Uteroplacental blood flow if diminished leads to hypertension and complications
- Nitric oxide and allied vasodilators have a very important role to play in combating the vasoconstrictive effects of changes taking place at fetomaternal interface.

In uncomplicated pregnancies, maternal vasculature is refractory to constrictive effects of pressor substances. However, this refractoriness is abolished completely or partially in complicated pregnancies. This makes the maternal vasculature susceptible to circulating pressor substances in these pregnancies. The balance of thromboxane to prostacyclin is in favor of the vasodilatory prostacyclin in normal pregnancy. This balance gets reversed. In pregnancies susceptible to preeclampsia the balance shifts in favor of thromboxane. This leads to vasoconstrictive tendency in obstetric vasculopathy. Vasoconstrictive orientation in pregnancy invites a series of changes protective and destructive. The maternal system senses that there is resistance to blood flow. So as to compensate for this and neutralize the resistance, the blood pressure of the mother raises thereby leading to development of preeclampsia and its complications.

It must be acknowledged that obstetric vasculopathy in its pure form is confined to only the human species. Therefore drawing conclusions from animal experiments will have its limitations. Nevertheless, they do provide vital insights into what is happening in the mother's system during these pathological states.

Some Intriguing Observations from Animal Experiments

There are some intriguing observations from animal experiments that need to be taken cognizance of when on the subject.

Preeclampsia: A Price for Two Legged Humans?

There are many aspects of comparative medicine in general and comparative obstetrics and gynecology in particular that are attributed to the conversion of humans into two-legged animals from four-legged evolutionary predecessors. Classic example of this is the J-shaped pelvic pathway in human pelvis. This turn of the angle that takes place approximately at the level of ischial spines leads to human labor process becoming difficult and obstruction susceptible. These types of problems that a human childbirth faces are not found in four-legged animals. Even the extreme forms of obstetric disasters like ruptured uterus due to obstructed labor are thought to be unique to human pregnancy and not heard of in four-legged animals like ewes, cows and buffaloes.

The process of preeclampsia is found to be unique to human pregnancy. It has not been found to occur in lower animals are two legged. On the basis of this Enhorning G[15] suggested that due to two-legged walking style, the gravid uterus produces pressure on the ureters. This pressure is intermittent and leads to what is described as physiological hydronephrosis and hydroureter of pregnancy. Enhorning produced intermittent pressure on the ureters of pregnant sheep to study its effects. It was found that these sheep developed hypertension when subjected to intermittent obstruction of the ureters. On the basis of these results Enhorning suggested that a human gravida exerts pressure intermittently on the ureters through its gravid uterus. This pressure is by and large occurring when the woman is walking standing or lying supine. However, this pressure is not exerted when the pregnant human gravida is lying on the sides. It is a very well-know clinical fact that when a pregnant gravida lies at her side her BP goes down.

Enhorning used three points to prove that preeclampsia is the price paid by human beings for their conversion from four-legged animals to two-legged animals: (1) the observation of development of physiological hydronephrosis and hydroureter in pregnancy due to pressure of gravid uterus; (2) the observation that the BP lowers in lateral positions of resting human females; and (3) the animal experiment of intermittent urteric obstruction that he conducted showing a rise in BP

Though these observations may appear very sound there are some subtle but very important features that cannot be explained. Preeclampsia is now accepted as one of the manifestation of obstetric vasculopathies. Other notable amongst obstetric vasculopathies is the phenomenon of IUGR. It has been found that some lower animals do register the occurrence of IUGR in them. This is described as "runting" in lower animals especially mammals. The phenomenon of preeclampsia (hypertension) may be explained by Enhorning's theory of it being a disease of two-legged humans. However, it doesn't explain the process of IUGR or abruptio placenta. The latter two were not found and so not explainable by Enhorning's theory. It therefore appears that his explanation for preeclampsia is apparently too simplistic.

Gene Variation and Preeclampsia, One More Intrigue

One intriguing observation in genetics has rekindled interest in renin-angiotensin mechanism of preeclampsia. Ward K et al[16] have shown that women who express a molecular variant of angiotensinogen have a much higher preeclampsia rate as compared to those who do not express this variation. Interestingly Morgan T et al[17] have shown that the expression of molecular variant of angiotensinogen T235 was elevated in decidual spiral arteries of women. This led this group to suggest that the abnormal activation of renin-angiotensin system due to genetic difference leads to atherotic changes in the vessels. However, the matter of intrigue in this set of experiments based on animal models suggests a revival of interest in renin-angiotensin system in etiopathology of preeclampsia. Also, the demonstration of their variant of genetic expression in the spiral arterioles brings the focus back at the level of fetomaternal interface. It is apparent that this is the focal point in the etiopathology of obstetric vasculopathies. Concurrently these studies also open up a possibility of using genetic engineering to manipulate this genetic variation. This could lead to correction of genetic structure and thereby prevent obstetric vasculopathies from occurring. While this is exciting, it is also very intriguing.

The Exclusivity of Human Pregnancy

One basic fact that emerges from all animal experiments is the fact that preeclampsia is a disease of human pregnancy. In lower animals hypertension and/or proteinuria can be generated in experimental conditions. But in none of them could exact preeclampsia, its effects on many systems and organs as well as its complications all could be generated. This proved the basic simple fact that preeclampsia is a disease of human pregnancy. Amongst the most prominent clinical features of preeclampsia, hypertension and proteinuria are two that are most prominent and objectively and easily demonstrable. As a result, these were studied maximally. Also, proteinuria led scientists to study kidney involvements. Therefore after hypertension and proteinuria, renal changes were maximally studied. However these were inconsistent and could never be generated in all attempts with equal regularity. This too leads one to conclude that preeclampsia is a disease of human pregnancy only.

HARD FACTS EMERGING FROM ANIMAL EXPERIMENTS

If one reviews the large body of animal experiments and their sound results the biggest fact that emerges is of course the fact that preeclampsia is a disease of human pregnancy. Two other basic facts also emerge. One there is placental hypoperfusion and two, its interlinked activation of endothelial cells are hallmarks in the etiopathology of preeclampsia in particular and obstetric vasculopathies in general. While preeclampsia is acknowledged as the disease of human pregnancy, it is not the price that we pay for being converted by the evolution process from four-legged animals to two-legged animals.

Finally the last hard fact that emerges is a sort of warning. Extrapolating animal experiments to human pregnancies is wrought with great dangers. The results of animal experiments are species specific. Also, none of the animals ever had preeclampsia. Thus applying results that can be patchy and inexact may drive the scientific world to a completely false destination. This is more so when these are times of evidence based medicine.

Very high level of discretionary mental faculty is needed in those who want to evaluate and apply results of animal experiments in human beings. Many studies can on the face of it appear sound and scientific. Therefore, their results could be easily passed off as evidence of high quality. This could prove hasty and erroneous. The entire understanding of the etiopathology and consequent possible treatments could be just a sham. Therefore, the scientific world has to be cautious in handling the so called evidence emerging from animal experiments for preeclampsia.

REFERENCES

1. Abdul-Karim R, Assali NS. Renal function in human pregnancy. V. Effects of oxytocin on renal hemodynamics and water and electrolyte excretion. *J Lab Clin Med.* 1961; 57:522-32.
2. Wedel Jones C, Mandala M, Barron C, Bernstein I, Osol G. Mechanisms underlying maternal venous adaptation in pregnancy. *Reprod Sci.* 2009;16(6):596-604.
3. Berger M, Cavanagh D. Toxemia of pregnancy—the hypertensive effect of acute experimental placental ischemia. *Am J Obstet Gynecol.* 1963;87:293-305.
4. Hodari AA. Chronic uterine ischemia and reversible experimental "toxemia of pregnancy". *Am J Obstet Gynecol.* 1967;97(5):597-607.
5. Abitbol M, Pirani C, Ober W, Driscoll S, Cohen M. Production of experimental toxemia in the pregnant dog. *Obstet Gynecol.* 1976;48(5):537-48.

6. Combs C, Katz MA Kitzmiller J, Brescia R. Experimental preeclampsia produced by chronic constriction of the lower aorta: validation with longitudinal blood pressure measurements in conscious rhesus monkeys. *Am J Obstet Gynecol.* 1993;169(1):215-23.
7. Ayuk P, Matijevic R. Placental ischemia is a consequence rather than a cause of preeclampsia. *Med Hypotheses.* 2006;67(4):792-5.
8. Thatcher C, Keith J Jr. Pregnancy-induced hypertension: development of a model in the pregnant sheep. *Am J Obstet Gynecol.* 1986;155(1):201-7.
9. Chesley L. False starts in the study of preeclampsia-eclampsia. *Obstet Gynecol Annu.* 1976;5:177-87.
10. Prada J, Ross R, Clark K. Effect of atrial natriuretic peptide and other vasoactive compounds on the uterine vascular bed of the nonpregnant sheep. *Proc Soc Exp Biol Med.* 1992;201(3):261-6.
11. Karanja N, McCarron D. Calcium and hypertension: A review. *Annu Rev Nutr.* 1986; 6:475-94.
12. Belizán J, Campodónico L. Calcium supplementation and toxemia of pregnancy. *Gynecol Obstet Invest.* 1988;26(4):341-2.
13. Bucher H, Guyatt G, Cook R, Hatala R, Cook D, Lang J, et al. Effects of dietary calcium supplementation on blood pressure: A meta-analysis of randomized controlled trials. *JAMA.* 1996;275(13):1016-22.
14. Venuto R, Donker A. Prostaglandin E2, plasma renin activity, and renal function throughout rabbit pregnancy. *J Lab Clin Med.* 1982;99(2):239-46.
15. Enhorning G. Pre-eclampsia. a hypothesis for its pathogenesis. *Acta Obstet Gynecol Scand Suppl.* 1984;118:7-11.
16. Ward K, Hata A, Jeunemaitre X, Helin C, Nelson L, Namikawa C, et al. A molecular variant of angiotensinogen associated with preeclampsia. *Nat Genet.* 1993;4(1):59-61.
17. Morgan T, Craven C, Nelson L, Lalouel J, Ward K. Angiotensinogen T235 expression is elevated in decidual spiral arteries. *J Clin Invest* 15. 1997;100(6):1406-15.

CHAPTER

15

Clinical Profile of Obstetric Vasculopathies

CHAPTER OUTLINE

- Hypertension
- Proteinuria
- Edema
- Other Laboratory Parameters

INTRODUCTION

An obstetrician's nightmare, a delight for a research scientist and potentially lethal, the clinical spectrum of obstetric vasculopathies can be diverse and having a vast spectrum. The multisystem involvement of the pregnant female further enlarges the clinical profile of these conditions. The complex pathophysiology leads to inconsistency in presence of many features. Therefore profiling the clinical spectrum of obstetric vasculopathies is in itself a challenge if not exactly a nightmare. Many times clinical teachers of the subject have tried to divide the spectrum of clinical features into major features, minor features and features of associates and complications. Though, this type of grouping is clinically helpful it may not remain watertight as there can be a considerable overlap from one group to the other.

HYPERTENSION

Hypertension is the cardinal or major clinical feature of obstetric vasculopathies. While acknowledging the fact that hypertension is consistently present, it is not a must. There are many clinical situations where an obstetric vasculopathy may occur without the subject registering hypertension. IUGR is one such manifestation of obstetric vasculopathy which occurs quite often without hypertension. Abruptio placenta can similarly occur without hypertension.

In fact bleeding in early pregnancy may be one of the important and early signals of obstetric vasculopathy. 264 cases with history of bleeding per vaginum in 1 trimester and who continued their pregnancies were analyzed. They were found to have higher incidence of placenta previa and preeclampsia in the mothers.

Babies born to such mothers had higher incidence of IUGR preterm labor and Apgar less than 6 at 1 minute. A strong possibility of immunological basis linking up some of these events becomes obvious in these results.[1]

What BP is Hypertension?

It is by and large agreed that any subject who registers a BP of 130 systolic and/or 90 diastolic in pregnancy taken on two consecutive readings six hours apart after adequate rest of at least half an hour is hypertensive. While this definition uses both systolic as well as diastolic BP mean arterial pressure (MAP) is considered to make things easy. MAP is calculated with both these indices together. As is well-known, MAP is diastolic pressure plus one-third the pulse pressure. MAP of 103 and above once again taken after adequate bed rest (of at least half an hour) on two consecutive readings at least six hours apart is considered as indicative of hypertension.

It is very amusing to note that as soon as one defines any feature – clinical or investigative in obstetric vasculopathies, controversies, different viewpoints and inconsistencies start pouring in. The multiplicity of constituent conditions, the variations involved and its intrinsically dynamic pathophysiology involved in obstetric vasculopathies cause these controversies. To a research scientists who has gone deep into the etiopathology however, such inconsistencies, controversies and variations in clinical features is more a beauty of obstetric vasculopathy if not anything else.

In labeling a subject as hypertensive in pregnancy such controversies do arise. One big such controversy is the cutout of 130/90 BP. At times it does happen that a subject may show changes of hypertension well before the levels of 130/90 are reached. This happens usually in petite subjects whose basal BP itself is very low. Their so-called "rheostats" are set at a much lower basal BP. Many Indian pregnant subjects have their normal systolic BP hovering around 100 and diastolic BP hovering around 64 to 70. In them, to wait for the BP to reach the threshold of 130/90 may be late and even dangerous. Also, a subject usually shows a fall in B.P. during midtrimester. This can further reduce an already low set BP of a pregnant subject. It is not unusual to find subjects with a normal basal BP of 90/65 (average) at midtrimester in India.

Does this require redefining hypertension? The answer to this is negative. It is not necessary to redefine hypertension but add a further specification which makes situations easy and broadly encompassing to handle. It is, therefore, added that if any pregnant subject registers a rise of 30 mm Hg in her systolic and/or 15 mm Hg in her diastolic BP to her known basal BP she is labeled as hypertensive. The rider BP recorded after adequate bed rest of at least half an hour holds for all. Also the rider that these BP readings should be taken at least at a gap of six hours too holds. Thus, if a subject has a basal BP set at 94/68 in a given situation, for her BP of 124/83 and above becomes hypertension.

This addition can act as a double-edged sword. It can prove to be an advantage for the fact that many subjects who may be missed as hypertensive can be brought under care. On the flip side of it, however, is the fact that if the basal BP of the subject is not known, this definition may become inapplicable. Yet there will still be 5% or less subjects at maximum who may be under or over diagnosed as hypertensive with these two definition facets. Therefore, for a clinician most of the times 130/90 BP (MAP: 103) and /or a rise in 30 mm Hg systolic and/or 15 mm Hg diastolic should suffice to label as hypertension in a pregnant subject.

When one is examining obstetric vasculopathies so comprehensively, it is worth while understanding the pathophysiology that can render these definitions sometimes ineffective or inadequate. Obstetric vasculopathies are a result of a very dynamic process. There is a continuous process of destruction, reconstruction and opposition to destruction occurring in the body of the pregnant female. It is, therefore possible that when the pathology supervenes, the subject may register hypertension. On the other hand, if her preventive and health preserving mechanisms supervene the subject will not register clinical hypertension. What however of complexity is the fact that a subject may not render her vasculature clinically hypertensive but her response and reparative mechanisms may not be completely competent. They may be able to prevent the destruction to the level of registering a clinical hypertension but at the same time can produce some vascular changes that cause complications of hypertension. It is this dynamic state of the pathophysiology of hypertensive disorders of pregnancy in particular and obstetric vasculopathies in general which renders all definitions of clinical manifestation handicapped at one or other instance. Acknowledgement of this fact will make a student of the subject more clear in his perception and understanding rather than confused.

One more complexity of hypertension that needs to be understood here is the fact that some subject register complications far too disproportionate to actual clinical hypertension that she register. By and large the complications of preeclampsia are linked to the severity of hypertension. Complications like eclampsia, renal failure and coagulation failure occur as BP increases. In clinical practice preeclampsia is many times graded as mild preeclampsia, severe preeclampsia and imminent eclampsia. This gradation depends greatly on the severity of hypertension. However every clinician is also aware of the fact that eclampsia can occur in some unfortunate subjects at much lower BP. This was believed to be due to the central nervous system being intrinsically susceptible to rise in BP much earlier.

This may be only part of the complete picture. If one recalls the intricacies of pathophysiology of preeclampsia discussed in great lengths elsewhere (Chapters 4, 5 and 14), it is known that the entire conglomeration of changes depends greatly on profound destructive process generated in the mother's body due to the presence of fetus. Correspondingly, the maternal system also generates protective responses to these changes. It seems that there is a continuous conflict between the maternal rejection systems and the fetal preservation systems. By and large these are confined at the fetomaternal interface. However, in obstetric vasculopathies like preeclampsia they involve the entire maternal vasculature. It seems that every organ system and tissues have their intrinsic individuality to withstand these changes. Also, it varies from one individual to the other. Therefore, in most subjects the maternal systems are able to withstand this increasing conflict as the rise in BP occurs. However, once their threshold is finally reached, the protective systems crash. On this occurring, the clinical manifestations of complications like eclampsia or renal failure get precipitated.

With the rise in BP maternal protective systems become increasingly active and changes in BP are handled subclinically. However, as soon as the threshold is reached the maternal systems give way and clinical manifestations of complications become obvious. Nevertheless in some subjects thus breakdowns occur much earlier independent of the rising BP. This can be compared (albeit simplistically) to individuals who can get angry at much lower annoyance as compared to some individuals who get angry, rarely inspite of grave provocation

Also, each organ system has its own individual threshold. In some subjects, the threshold of renal system to withstand the stress is higher as compared to her brain. As a result, she may register a renal compromise much more readily and still may not register any eclampsia. These differential thresholds can easily explain the entire gamut of inconsistencies in clinical manifestations and complications of obstetric vasculopathies.

In clinical practice, numerous subjects develop abruptio placenta. However, very few of these develop a renal failure. By and large this is dependent on the amount of blood loss. But a clinician knows that some unfortunate subjects may develop a renal shutdown at much less amount of blood lost. This is due to intrinsic difference in the renal system to withstand the deprivation of blood supply.

Having had understood the concept of intrinsic tissue difference in withstanding the stress of hypertension one can now go still deeper to understand what decides this threshold. This threshold is by and large decided by the amount and competence of maternal reducing systems in response to the oxidative process which generates the vasospasm and subsequent hypertension. The maternal system generates abundant reducing systems. These increase in amount and competence as the stress rises. But a stage finally arrives when the maternal reducing systems are unable to cope up with this stress and the protective reducing systems prove insufficient and incompetent. Result—complications!

In some subjects, these protective systems might crash much earlier compared to most other females. In them, complications become manifested much earlier though on most occasions the maternal reducing systems are graded in response to the stress. Thus, more the stress more the reducing systems! But this may not hold true in all subjects. This explains the threshold difference from one subject to the other.

Concept of Competence of Reducing Systems

Modern medicine has always gone with an understanding that any protective or destructive system can be considered more active if it numerically registers a rise in its markers. To explain this with examples: more the concentration of malarial parasites in blood, more severe the malaria. Similarly increase in transaminase, in circulation, more the liver function derangement. This is a universal thinking. However, this may only be one half of the story. One very important aspect that we as students of modern medicine tend to overlook is the concept of *competence*. At all times body systems may not register a numerical rise in the pathogens or markers of protective responses. The protective systems may become more competent with the same amount of numerical values.

Thus the maternal system may clinically not show a rise in circulating reducing system still the pathological insult can get blunted. This is because the existing reducing systems may just become more competent. As a result without the need to increase the amount in circulation, these protective systems can deliver the goods by increasing their competence. This is a very important concept which can help many disease processes or the absence of these. This can help answer the argument that can come up, that in women with hypertension who may show a spate of complications much earlier, the circulating markers of reducing systems may not register a proportionate rise. Blame it or appreciate it on the "competence" of these protective systems.

Current assessment systems by and large tend to evaluate the numerical rise of any indicator or marker of health or disease. For this an example of malaria parasite concentration and circulating levels of certain enzymes has been given. We are not in a position to evaluate the competence of these enzymes or any protective system like the reducing system that is operational here. This holds a promise for the future. Science will devise ways and means by which competence of the body protective system will be evaluated. This will help in understanding of disease processes much better and devise treatment modalities more accurately.

Having had seen hypertension and its behavior in the clinical spectrum of obstetric vasculopathies other features off clinical profile will now be examined.

PROTEINURIA

Presence of protein (albumin) in urine has been known to be one of the most consistent features of obstetric vasculopathies. By and large it reflects upon the renal involvement in the process. Its popularity can be assessed from the fact that some workers have suggested that there can be a delay in diagnosis of preeclampsia as its proteinuria is mistaken for cystitis.[2] As postgraduate resident doctors in challenged settings there used to be a common teaching: if a pregnant woman is brought unconscious and has no papers to show what has produced this state of hers one should perform a heat coagulation test on her urine. If this bedside test is positive it clinches the diagnosis of eclampsia. This may in such a circumstance become even more important than hypertension. Multiplicity of reasons may cause BP to be variable. In a state of posteclamptic fit her BP may not be accurate and may be even falsely normal. In such a situation proteinuria becomes the most reliable indicator for clinching the diagnosis of eclampsia. It may be of an interest to know that when the concept of "eclampsia rooms" was prevalent, many a time there used to be a corner earmarked for performing the urine heat test in the room itself.

Proteinuria is always indicative of albuminuria in communications related to obstetric vasculopathies till and until otherwise specified. It usually develops late in the course of the disease. Fascinatingly, absence of proteinuria in presence of severe preeclampsia was considered as indicating bad prognosis.

Conventionally proteinuria is calibrated as presence of 100 mg/dL of albumin in spot urine samples taken at least six hours apart. Alternatively, it is quantified as presence of 300 mg/dL of albumin in 24 hours urine of the pregnant subject. For reasons of practical convenience the first method is more popular. The rider of using two samples at least six hours apart is added because the degree of proteinuria may vary from time to time in the same subject.

For reasons of undergraduate and postgraduate teaching calibration of the degree of proteinuria has also been done in old literature. This was by and large confined to the heat test. It varied from trace, slight turbidity to most severe form of proteinuria where the urine boils solid on heating. Though such a system of calibration appears crude on the face of it but it had a very good correlation with laboratory quantification of urinary protein.

Presence of proteinuria in whatever degree and proportion is used for both diagnosis as well as prognostication. This is more so for preeclampsia other than obstetric vasculopathies. Estimates have been done where the chances of favorable obstetric outcome has been estimated after appearance and persistent presence of proteinuria. Some estimates have predicted that persistence of proteinuria in a subject with preeclampsia indicates poor prognosis. Though these results seem to be accurate, they have a limited popularity in clinical practice.

Admittedly, there are clinical settings where decision to induce labor in a pregnant subject with preeclampsia is being taken on appearance, persistence and worsening of proteinuria. With the advent of color Doppler in the armamentarium of preeclampsia management investigative parameters like proteinuria lost their importance in day to day practice for critical interventional decision making. Presence of protein in urine is indicative of the extent of renal involvement in the disease process. Renal involvement indicates the extent of systemic involvement in the disease process. This explains the importance of proteinuria.

EDEMA

Surprisingly, very popular but one of the most unreliable clinical features of preeclampsia is edema. This feature has indeed lost its popularity due to the same and is now no more considered amongst the major features of preeclampsia. It did however occupy this exalted position for many decades in the features of preeclampsia. However, edema has not been able to retain its popularity as a reliable feature of preeclampsia because of its lack of consistency in appearance. Also, edema does not indicate the severity of the underlying pathology in any way. A subject may be having very mild form of the disease and still have a severe degree of edema. At the same time, a subject may be having severe preeclampsia or may even throw an eclamptic convulsion and she may have mild edema. In absence of reliability therefore many a times edema is mentioned as a feature of preeclampsia only to complete the list.

Weight gain is another unreliable feature linked with edema. A pregnant subject is expected to gain about 10 kg of weight by the time she reaches term. To make it simple, she gains weight at the rate of 0, –1 +1, +4, +5, +3, +3 lbs per month of her nine months of pregnancy sequentially. Excessive weight gain was considered as an indicator of a developing preeclampsia.

Similarly weight gain in pregnancy too has been found to be a very poorly reliable feature of preeclampsia and other obstetric vasculopathies. It is conventionally stated that too rapid a weight gain may be indicative of a developing preeclampsia or if preeclampsia is already present it indicates worsening of the condition. However, large studies have shown that this too is an extremely unreliable feature of preeclampsia. A subject may register preeclampsia in absence of abnormal weight gain. Similarly, she may have an excessive and at times even a rapid weight gain in absence of any features of preeclampsia or to that matter any other obstetric vasculopathy.

The reason for edema in preeclampsia is far from settled. It is believed to be due to the vasospasm and subsequent reperfusion damage that occur to the vessel wall at the level of the capillaries which prevents the fluid to be held competently within the vessel wall leading to leakage of fluid into the tissues producing edema (See Chapter 4).

One very interesting aspect of edema is worth nothing at this stage. In a given clinical situation if a pregnant subject registers a presence of edema, in absence of any other feature of preeclampsia including hypertension, the obstetric outcome especially the birth weight of the baby is likely to be much better and favorable. Thus, a subject with edema will have heavier babies in absence of any features of preeclampsia. This further adds to the lack of reliability of edema as a reliable feature of preeclampsia in the clinical spectrum.

Presence of such edema in absence of preeclampsia is attributed simplistically to heavier uterus with larger baby pressing on the large vessels in the abdomen. Conventionally, therefore, obstetrician's advice these subjects to lie down in lateral positions while resting so as to throw the heavy uterus off the large abdominal vessels. However to what extent this is helpful is a matter of conjecture.

When edema was very popular as a clinical feature of preeclampsia, even grading of edema was done thus one + edema was that on the leg upto the knee. Two plus edema was upto the lower abdomen involving the entire lower extremities. Anasarca was considered as three + edema.

Looking at the lack of reliability of weight gain some clinicians have stopped weighing mothers in pregnancy much to the intrigue of the mothers or mothers-in-law who usually accompany pregnant subjects who come for antenatal care, in socially intimately knit societies like India and the Indian subcontinent. First question that is usually asked to a clinician after he/she emerges from the examination room by the accompanying elder is "Is the weight gain adequate?" Alternatively these elders meticulously remember the weight of the gravida on last visit so the pointed question that follows is "What is her weight today?" If the answer that follows indicates that there was some weight gain, the elder is happy. She presumes that all is going well. However students, research scientists and clinical practitioners of the subject know it fully well how trivial and unreliable this feature is.

OTHER LABORATORY PARAMETERS

A series of exhaustive list of parameters are included and even recommended at sometimes or the other in management of subjects with obstetric vasculopathies. It is a very wide spectrum commencing from peripheral smear to 24 hours tests like 24 hours urine albumin and creatinine. At some instance they become popular and subsequently lose their popularity due to many reasons. Ultimately, those that have consistently remained in clinical practice includes proteinuria, serum creatinine or creatinine clearance, plasma urea and bleeding profile in terms of prothrombin time (PT) and activated partial thromboplastin time (APTT). On the other hand, these laboratory investigations have remained more as broad guiding signals to reach decisions about interventions. They in themselves are not used to clinch the decision. A clinician uses a comprehensive overview of the results of these investigations and gets a fair idea of the worsening of the picture. Also one can reasonably accurately group the disease stage into mild and severe from the results of laboratory tests.

Mild preeclampsia is termed when the systolic BP is less than 160 mm Hg, diastolic BP is less than 100 mm Hg, urinary proteins are more than 300 mg/dL in 24 hours urinary sample, and other clinical features like blurring of vision, headache, epigastric pain and convulsions are absent. Liver enzymes may be mildly elevated and fetal growth restriction may or may not be present.

Severe preeclampsia when BP shoots up systolic being more that 160 and diastolic being 110 or more mm Hg. Urine if tested on heat-test for proteinuria boils solid and forms a "coagulum". Other clinical features like headache, visual disturbances, epigastric pain are present. Plasma urea is elevated and there can be features of renal compromise like altered creatinine clearance. Such women can throw convulsions.

Grouping a subject into one of the two groups does not mean that obstetric vasculopathies especially preeclampsia is a static state. Preeclampsia is dynamic process and a subject may also be in an intermediate state neither mild nor severe. However, these groupings give a broad idea to the attending medical help as o whether the parent condition is worsening. Accordingly decisions are taken for obstetric interventions.

Plasma Urea

A word about plasma urea estimation will be worthwhile at this stage. In clinical practice, practitioners request plasma urea estimation as a basic test to assess kidney functions of patients. Rise in plasma urea has for long been relied upon in clinical practice. On the other hand in a pregnant subject this becomes an unreliable test for many reasons. In pregnancy there is a general rise in GFR. Also the renal function becomes very competent in normal pregnancy. As a result the normal non-pregnant plasma urea is pegged between 20 to 40 mg/dL. In normal uncomplicated pregnancy the plasma urea is always equal to or less than 20 mg/dL. Any rise above 20 should be considered as abnormal. This picture gets completely altered in pregnancy.

Another interesting aspect of plasma urea is its lack of reliability. It has been estimated that plasma urea may not rise till 50% of renal function is compromised. Thus, a clinician may feel that there is no problem with renal function on finding a normal plasma urea report. But in reality a significant amount of renal function may have been compromised. Therefore, renal function estimates are not done through plasma urea estimates any more, more so during pregnancy. For estimating renal function in pregnancy creatinine clearance seems to be a more reliable option.

REFERENCES

1. Desai P, Patel P, Ravat C, Desai M. Analysis of obstetric outcome in subjects having bleeding P/V in I trimester. *Jr O & G of India.* 2001;51(3):63-6.
2. Luitjes S, Franx A, van Rijn B, Bolte A. Hypertensive disorders in pregnancy: vigilance on the part of general practitioners. *Ned Tijdschr Geneeskd.* 2011;155(18):A2936.

CHAPTER

16

Differential Diagnosis of Obstetric Vasculopathies

CHAPTER OUTLINE

- Preeclampsia and Chronic Hypertension
- Transient Hypertension
- Renal Diseases
- Hepato-Hematological Involvements

INTRODUCTION

When one tries to differentiate hypertensive disorders in pregnancy from other conditions, the situation becomes challenging both for the clinician as well as the research scientists and academicians of the subject. This is because of a vast overlap of its features with other obstetric vasculopathies. Therefore, there are a series of conditions that need to be differentiated. To make this a little more clear low platelet count may be found in many obstetric conditions. This may also be found in many non-obstetric conditions where the woman may be incidentally pregnant. All these obstetric and non-obstetric conditions can come as differential diagnosis of obstetric vasculopathies in general and preeclampsia in particular. This becomes further confusing with conditions like HELP syndrome. These clinical conditions become apparent in presence of preeclampsia. However there are reports where HELLP syndrome can occur even without preeclampsia. Thus even within the domain of obstetric conditions, there can be situations where the picture may get confusing. Once the picture of any clinical condition becomes differing, delineating and then after accurately enumerating differential diagnoses becomes difficult. This is the precise reason why clear cut differential diagnoses become difficult to define in obstetric vasculopathies.

PREECLAMPSIA AND CHRONIC HYPERTENSION

This differentiation becomes critical because chronic hypertension in its nascent form may not be as devastating as preeclampsia. Chronic hypertension may or may not have a preeclampsia superimposed on it. However, the situation can become tricky if a subject with chronic hypertension become pregnant and has preeclampsia. If a subject is a known case of chronic hypertension the differentiation is by and large easy. However, if the subject had never got herself examined for hypertension prior to pregnancy and it is for the first time that a recording was done, differentiation becomes tricky. In such situations the standard order is to use fundoscopy for differentiation. If the classical features appear on fundoscopy like silver-wire appearance of vessels then it could be labeled as chronic hypertension.

Is it Terribly Important to Differentiate the Two?

The answer is both yes and no. If chronic hypertension is complicated by a superimposition of preeclampsia, the outcome can be worse compared to other subjects with preeclampsia. However, if the hypertension remains as chronic hypertension without getting complicated, it does not make it terribly important to differentiate it from preeclampsia. This is because the disease runs a relatively benign course.

One more reason to differentiate chronic hypertension from preeclampsia is the need to change the antihypertensive. If a subject is already on antihypertensives and gets pregnant, the obstetrician needs to review the antihypertensive that she is taking. Agents like ACE-inhibitors can be teratogenic and so need to be changed.

It is recommended that in women with chronic hypertension changes in blood pressure and proteinuria, rather than absolute measurements, must be used for diagnosis. Also, proteinuria can occur in a subject with chronic hypertension, it is recommended that a baseline 24 hours urine collection along with baseline serum creatinine and uric acid should be obtained for future comparison.[1]

Some tests have been credited with a capacity to differentiate preeclampsia from chronic hypertension. Presence of low platelets, elevated serum transaminases and elevated LDH has been attributed to preeclampsia. However, the catch lies in the fact that these may not be consistently found. Also, some of these tests remain system specific. This means that if that particular system is not affected in the process the test may not be altered. Hyperuricemia needs a small but separate mention. It has been said that in a given subject hyperuricemia clinches diagnosis in favor of preeclampsia. This may have some basis. This is because of the fact that there is a profound oxidative insult taking place in preeclampsia. Therefore, uric acid a potent reducing system that it is may rise. This has been referred to in detail elsewhere (See Chapter 5). However the situation become tricky again if the subject has a superimposed preeclampsia over an under running hypertension. In this situation too uric acid may rise. Experimental markers like a thrombin III and renal biopsies have been suggested. But this clinical use is limited.

For a clinician, therefore, it is important to differentiate if a preeclampsia is imposed on an under running chronic hypertension. This is because, as mentioned, the chances of complications are higher. But differentiating this superimposition from occurrence of preeclampsia de novo may not always be possible a handicap the clinician has to live within present times.

TRANSIENT HYPERTENSION

One more entity which at times needs to be differentiated from preeclampsia is transient hypertension. However this is a benign condition without remarkable complications so never became of great clinical importance. Hypocalciurea has been found to have some role in differentiating this condition. Calcium has always been in focus in some way or the other in preeclampsia. Its role in prediction of preeclampsia has been discussed elsewhere (See Chapter 5). Role of calcium supplementation in prevention of preeclampsia has also been discussed elsewhere (See Chapter 18). Hypocalciurea for diagnosing transient hypertension has been studied by Taufield et al. They have found that hypocalciuria is distinct only of transient hypertension and should suffice as the single test to differentiate it from preeclampsia.[2] Gasnier R et al have used hypocalciuria to differentiate different subtypes of hypertensive disorders. They conducted a case-controlled study of mild and severe preeclampsia, chronic hypertension, and normal pregnancy and found that measurement of calciuria can differentiate between severe preeclampsia and chronic hypertension, and hypocalciuria is also a marker for disease severity.[3] Nevertheless, the entity of transient hypertension itself did not find much bearing in clinical practice. Therefore, its importance to a clinician remains by and large limited.

RENAL DISEASES

Kidneys and its functioning have been extensively studied in preeclampsia. It is possible that some of the renal disorders may mimic preeclampsia. It, therefore becomes a clinical necessity to differentiate them from preeclampsia.

Chronic renal disease can present with hypertension, proteinuria and/or edema. It should therefore, be separated from preeclampsia. Also, they when pregnant have a higher chance of developing preeclampsia. It is understandable that most of the subjects with a chronic renal disease may find it difficult to conceive. Also if pregnant, in most of them the diagnosis is made well before the pregnancy begins. However, if one has to take a theoretical possibility of these subjects having remained undiagnosed, the clinician will indeed find it challenging to differentiate them from preeclampsia. In such a need renal function test like creatinine clearance and serum creatinine may be of value in differentiation.

Presence of persistent hematuria suggests acute nephritis. It may be present in preeclampsia as well but is rarely persistent. Specific causes of glomerulonephritis can sometimes be identified with some blood tests such as antistreptolysin O, streptozyme panel and compliment profile in poststreptococcal glomerulonephritis or screening test for collagen vascular disorders.[1] Renal biopsy any day will clinch the diagnosis and should therefore be the gold standard. However, renal biopsies never became popular pregnancy. Also the strong possibility of hemorrhage in the kidneys during pregnancy if renal biopsy is performed, deters if form being a popular tool in clinical practice.

HEPATO-HEMATOLOGICAL INVOLVEMENTS

Some hepato-hematological conditions have strong affinity and therefore association with preeclampsia. They occur independent of preeclampsia, but are usually associated with the latter. This includes conditions like HELLP syndrome, thrombotic thrombocytopenic purpura, fatty liver of pregnancy and hemolytic uremic syndrome. All of these can occur with preeclampsia, can run a furious course and can even prove fatal. Rather than differentiating them from preeclampsia (*Differential Diagnosis*) they are more like associates of preeclampsia. They are therefore, discussed in larger details in the relevant chapters (See Chapters 9, 11 and 12).

REFERENCES

1. Friedman S, Lindheimer S. Prediction and differential diagnosis. In: Lindheimer M, Roberts J, Cunningham F (eds). Chesley's Hypertensive disorders of pregnancy. 2nd edn Stamford, Appleton and Lange. 1998, Page 201-28.
2. Taufield P, Nes K, Resnick L. Hypocalciuria in preeclampsia. *N Eng J of Med.* 1987;316:715-18.
3. Gasnier R, Valério E, Vettorazzi J, Barros E, Martins-Costa S, Ramos J. Calciuria and preeclampsia: a case-control study. *J Obstet Gynaecol Res.* 2012;38(4):674-80.

CHAPTER

17

Predicting Obstetric Vasculopathies

CHAPTER OUTLINE

- Overview of Available Predicting Measures
- Application of Predicting Systems for other Uses
- The Amorphous Characterizations of Pathogenesis and Clinical Features
- Overview of the Types of Tests
- Negative to Positive Predictive Value
- Conditions Based Tests
- An Ideal Test
- Clinical Tests
- Urinary Tests
- Hematological Cellular and Non-cellular Indices
- Epidemiological Indices
- Color Doppler in Obstetric Vasculopathies: The Game Changer

INTRODUCTION

A detailed understanding of the etiopathology of obstetric vasculopathies has made one fundamental fact clear. Because of an important though amorphous genetic influence and the complex and multiplicity of factors influencing the causation of these conditions, as of now the treatment is of effects and not treatment of cause. Also, it is possible that the etiopathology described in the preceding sections (See Chapters 2–5, 14) will pave the way for devising accurate treatment mechanisms of these conditions in future. A classic example of this is devising systems which can generate substances like lysophosphotidyl choline. How and why such substances can treat obstetric vasculopathies at early stages has been described in preceding pages (See Chapter 5). In the absence of any available treatment of cause, it is understandable that science tries to predict these conditions. Their prediction can help clinicians institute measures that can prevent or ameliorate these conditions early.

OVERVIEW OF AVAILABLE PREDICTING MEASURES

Predicting measures of obstetric vasculopathies are diverse and at times complicated. This is a direct reflection of its complex etiopathology. Measures could be in the form of clinical tests at one side of the spectrum like roll-over tests; at mid-segment are biochemical tests like levels of hormones and other chemical substances and on the other extreme are tests based on complex imaging techniques like color Doppler and advanced imaging technology. All these tests have one aspect in common. They are to be performed in asymptomatic subjects before the clinical spectrum of obstetric vasculopathies becomes obvious. Some of them may require to be repeated longitudinally, whilst others may be a single-time or one-time performance.

APPLICATION OF PREDICTING SYSTEMS FOR OTHER USES

There are some tests which are reasonably accurate in predicting an impending vasculopathy. At the same time these tests can also be used to decide discontinuation of some treatment measures. They are so versatile that these tests of prediction can also be used for prognostication and even decide regarding when to deliver the baby and through which route (abdominal or vaginal route) will the delivery be safe. The versatility of some of these tests is so much that they do not stop at the mother. Tests like color Doppler can also predict the possible neonatal outcome and behavior in years to follow.

However two dichotomous or seemingly contradictory questions can then be asked. If the tests are so versatile why the treatments do still eludes medical science. Also, such versatile tests also reflect upon the fact that modern science has understood the etiopathology of obstetric vasculopathies very deeply. Even the most complicated and intricate aspects are known. That be so, the dichotomous and contradictory question, therefore is, why we not have the treatment which is accurately the treatment of the effects. This situation is comparable to many malignancies that occur in human body. Reasonably accurate predicting tests are available for malignancies. Classical examples are Pap smear test for cervical malignancies and mammography for prediction and early diagnosis of breast malignancies. While these are reasonably accurate at their job, the precise treatment still eludes medical science. Current treatments by and large are taking preventive measures so that these malignancies do not occur or if they do then the tissues or organs in which they occur are surgically removed. This prevents the invasive spread. Entire science of modern oncology revolves around this approach.

THE AMORPHOUS CHARACTERIZATIONS OF PATHOGENESIS AND CLINICAL FEATURES

It must be granted that a big challenge to the predicting tests is the fact that many variable and inconsistent features are clubbed into one bunch—preeclampsia. What BP is hypertension of preeclampsia is all guidelines based and is therefore amorphous. Also a subject can be preeclamptic and have proteinuria or can be preeclamptic without proteinuria. A subject may or may not have edema and still be preeclamptic. Similarly, in other obstetric vasculopathies, a baby may have features of IUGR but its weight may fall within the range of standard deviation. On the other hand the pregnant mother can have severe or fulminant preeclampsia or even a full blown eclampsia but the baby may still be thriving. This leaves a big challenge to the entire spectrum of tests for predicting obstetric vasculopathies.

OVERVIEW OF THE TYPES OF TESTS

On the face of it the tests for predicting preeclampsia in particular and obstetric vasculopathies in general appear very different from one another. They seem to have no connection and appear totally delinked from one another. Still most of them appear to be working and contributing to their role in some little way. A small but noteworthy group of these tests are clinical. Amongst the clinical tests, the roll-over test became very popular. This was due to the ease with which it could be performed. Also, it was amongst the earliest tests described historically to predict preeclampsia. Understandably therefore it remained in circulation for a very long time.

Amongst the clinical tests, very complicated tests have also been researched. This included tests like light stimulation tests. In this, difference in blood pressure was to be noted at midtrimester in presence of light and in darkness. Each test could never become popular due to complexity of performance and inconsistency of results.

The biggest and most researched group of these tests is the group of biochemical markers. The behaviors of different markers have been studied in preeclampsia and on the basis of the results so obtained attempts have been made to predict preeclampsia. Besides markers that needed to be serially followed, there are tests described where single estimation of a particular marker has been used to predict preeclampsia and IUGR. This includes estimation of ß-HCG, calcium: creatinine ratio, SHBG levels and the like.

There have been certain biochemical markers used initially to predict preeclampsia. However with the advances in understanding of etiopathology of these conditions their function changed from predicting the condition to prognosticator of condition. Classic example of this group is estimation of uric acid in predicting obstetric vasculopathy. It is now well understood that for reasons described elsewhere, uric acid is a competent prognosticator rather than a predictor of preeclampsia (See Chapter 5). Complex biochemical markers also need a mention. These are difficult to perform and therefore confined themselves to experimental domain. They failed to get wide entry in clinical domain. Classical example in this is renin angiotensin sensitivity tests.

The most promising of all these groups is the group of tests based on imaging technology like all fields of obstetrics and gynecology practice in particular and nearly the entire medical field in general, ultrasonography and color Doppler have proved to be the most promising of all amongst this heterogeneous body of tests to predict preeclampsia and other obstetric vasculopathies. If properly done, these tests could be very reliable. They are also very versatile in the fact that they are useful for other purposes also besides simply predicting an obstetric vasculopathy. They can be used for critical decision making in preeclampsia. They can also be used for prognostication as well as altering treatment modalities. Amazingly these tests can also be used to decide the route of delivery in the gravida.

Thus the large body of tests to predict obstetric vasculopathies singly or in combination is heterogeneous, reasonably reliable and interesting. Their heterogeneity reflects on the multiple organs and systems that this decease the absence of knowledge regarding the exact cause of this condition.

NEGATIVE TO POSITIVE PREDICTIVE VALUE

One more aspect of these tests that require a mention is the fact that most of these tests have excellent negative predictive value. By negative predictive value it means they can say that a particular pregnant subject in question is not likely or less likely to develop an obstetric vasculopathy. For a clinician, however, they need tests that are more with positive predictive value. In clinical practice obstetricians need tests that can identify subjects who may develop preeclampsia or IUGR rather than those subjects who will not develop these conditions.

CONDITIONS BASED TESTS

To add to the complexity of these tests and interpretation of their results, is the fact that some tests are more accurate with preeclampsia and others with IUGR. Those tests that reflect pathology at fetomaternal interface are good at predicting IUGR and preeclampsia both. On the other hand, tests that reflect the status of the entire maternal vasculature would predict only preeclampsia.

AN IDEAL TEST

Ideals elude reality. Probably that is the reason they remain Ideal. This is more so because the tenets of anything ideal are decided on the basis of constituting features. A summation of such features decides ideal and so ideal remains elusive. Thus an ideal test for prediction should have some features which are not found universally. These include:

- The test should be easily doable.
- It should be safe and practical.
- It should be reproducible in clinical settings. This means it should not be confined to experimental and research environment.
- It should have an excellent safety profile.
- It should be a sensitive and specific test.
- It should be noninvasive test (preferably).
- It should conform to the needs of the population.
- As none of the tests for screening for obstetric vasculopathies are "Ideal" there is a vast battery of tests available.

CLINICAL TESTS

Midtrimester BP

One of the easiest amongst all tests that predict preeclampsia is midtrimester blood pressure. It is a well-known fact that midtrimester BP in normal pregnancies tends to fall. This fall can be seen in subjects who were longitudinally followed up. This fall could be upto 20 mm of Hg systolic and upto 10 mm of Hg diastolic. It was found that those women who did not register a fall in BP in midtrimester have a higher chance of developing preeclampsia. It was further extended to predict that those subjects in whom instead of a fall if there is a rise in midtrimester BP, there is a high chance of developing preeclampsia. To make this more precise and inclusive of both the systolic and diastolic pressure, mean arterial pressure (MAP) was considered in some studies. In this regard 90 mm of Hg was taken as an arbitrary cutout figure. On serial estimation is the MAP at midtrimester fell below 90 mm of Hg the subject had a lower chance of developing preeclampsia. It was also found that when compared with other clinical markers the highest prediction for all types of hypertensive disorders was achieved by mean arterial pressure.[1]

However serial follow up is any day more cumbersome. It was, therefore, desirable to have a single estimation of BP. In this Ales et al used single midtrimester MAP evaluation of BP. It was found that midtrimester BP estimation had 23% to 47% sensitivity, poor positive predictive value of 3 to 23% and a likelihood ratio of 2 to 3.[2] (A likelihood ratio of 10 and above makes the test most conclusive). However when systolic BP is combined with chemical parameters like urinary creatinine and urinary inorganic phosphorus, the efficiency increases.[3]

Low positive predictive value is a handicap which appeared consistently in many tests used to predict preeclampsia. In the entire body of tests to predict tests with a good positive predictive value are few and far between. While still on BP in large multicenter trial simply systolic BP was used and studied for its efficacy to predict preeclampsia[4,5] 120 mm of Hg was the value used in these tests values higher or equal to these were considered as positive in predicting preeclampsia. Overall this had a low sensitive (18%), low specificity (18%) and likelihood ratio as low as 1.9 such a low likelihood ration indicated the poor reliability of this test.

Other combinations have also been tried to use BP measurements to predict preeclampsia. This included tests using only diastolic BP or 24 hours ambulatory BP for predicting preeclampsia. While some of these tests gained on likelihood ratio they got beaten up in sensitivity and positive predictive value. Therefore the ease of doing these tests explains its popularity. Also the ease of their applicability practice is well understandable. But BP proved to be incompetent in predicting preeclampsia.

One fact, however, emerges strongly. All markers based on sphygmomanometric assessment for prediction of preeclampsia had a restricted predictive efficacy.[6]

The Roll-Over Test

The popularity of this test is phenomenal. It is probably the ease with which it can be performed that explains it. Even in busy outdoors in medical college hospital settings in India, it has been performed, studied and extensively documented. It is considered as positive if the subject at midtrimester is rolled from lateral to supine position, the BP (diastolic) shows a rise of more than or equal to 20 mm of Hg. This test has both its good points and not so good points. Its estimated specificity (90) and negative predictive value are very high. However, its sensitivity (just above 30), positive predictive value (just above 30) and a likelihood ratio of a poor 3.4 makes the test of limited value. The roll-over test, therefore, can be well used for predicting that a particular pregnant subject will not develop preeclampsia. However this test is not very efficient in predicting if a particular pregnant subject will develop preeclampsia.

Hand-Grip Test

This is one more clinical test that became popular and has been quite extensively researched and studied.[7] The test is said to be positive when diastolic BP shows a rise of at least 20 mm of Hg after performing a hand-grip exercise for a time period of about 30 minutes. This test takes 30 minutes to perform which makes it time-consuming for a clinical setting especially in busy outdoor. Besides this handicap, this test also like the roll-over test was incompetent for its positive prediction value. This again means that it is good to screen subjects who will not develop preeclampsia. But this is not a good test to predict if this test will develop preeclampsia. These limitations of hand-grip test made its use in clinical practice restricted. However this test is now relegated to confines of history of the subject.

Weight Gain

This clinical parameter has a very queer popularity. In any given outdoor clinical setting, this parameter is very popular amongst lay people. A rise in weight irrespective of whether it is excessive or optimal invariably brings a smile on the face of a pregnant subject. This holds true for her husband as well as her accompanying relatives as well. It conveys a feeling of "all well" to them. It has also been studied and documented extensively for predicting preeclampsia and its other friends of obstetric vasculopathies. Many have published data on weight gain to predict preeclampsia.[8,9] However it is one of the most incompetent parameter to screen for obstetric vasculopathies in general and preeclampsia in particular. Its sensitivity is between 80 to 90 and a negative predictive value of about 95. But its specificity (< 25), positive predictive value (< 10) and a very poor likelihood ratio of just above 1 speaks volumes of its incompetence. This test has therefore, long been given up in clinical practice and confined to the realms of history.

URINARY TESTS

Microalbuminuria

Amongst tests to predict preeclampsia, microalbuminuria became very popular in studies. It occupied a prominent place in literature and journals. Somehow it also caught fancy of the clinicians thereby leading to laboratories offering these tests to predict preeclampsia in clinical practice. However, this feature was not found to be reliable in predicting preeclampsia and therefore lost popularity. Even the pathology labs that offered to do these tests in clinical practice stopped doing these in absence of large volume of referrals. It seems in using microalbuminuria to predict preeclampsia, clinicians were more skeptic than research teams. This is an example of the disjoint between research studies and luck of popularity in clinical practice. From the ease with which this assessment could be done, the clinicians should have lapped it up. But it was never to be.

Besides microalbuminuria, urinary calcium, urinary kallikrein and urinary calcium creatinine ratio have been found to be researched at sometimes or the other to predict obstetric vasculopathies.

Urinary Calcium

As regards urinary calcium excretion, reduced urinary calcium is said to have some association with preeclampsia. Besides using it for prediction of preeclampsia, hypocalciurea can be used to differentiate between severe preeclampsia and chronic hypertension, and hypocalciurea is also a marker for disease severity.[10] On the other hand Szmidt-Adjidé V et al studied 24 hours urinary calcium excretion.[11] They found that in their population, preeclamptic women had a calciuria significantly lower than controls. These are two of the many who researched on this parameter to predict preeclampsia. On basis of the statistical indices when applied to the results of this test, it has been found that the test is average at best. It has a sensitivity and specificity of 85 to 90. It has a very high negative predictive value. But when likelihood ratio is applied, urinary hypocalcium levels (hypocalciurea) remains at best average.[5] Thus this test in absence of hypocalcemia can suggest that one will not develop preeclampsia at the most, nothing beyond.

Kallikrein

Another biochemical marker that has been studied extensively is excretion of urinary kallikrein. It is believed to reflect the status of renal excretory function. Renal functions have been shown to be significantly affected in obstetric vasculopathies. Renal failure is one of the most dreaded complications of abruptio placenta. Therefore, a parameter of renal functioning capacity must be helpful in predicting obstetric vasculopathies in general and preeclampsia in particular. This is the rationale for using urinary kallikrein levels for predicting preeclampsia.

It has been hypothesized that reduced urinary excretion of kallikrein reflects reduced renal function. Reduced renal function precedes obstetric vasculopathies.[12] Initial studies by this group produced a whopping result of 83% sensitivity 91% positivity predictive value and a very high likelihood ratio. In this, they measured urinary kallikrein calcium ratio, in spot urine sample. However, in subsequent studies by others these results could not be reproduced. The sensitivity and negative predictive value remained high. But the positive predictive value and specificity were markedly low. Even the likelihood ratio reported in subsequent studies was as low as 3 or even less.[13] As this chapter is devoted to prediction of preeclampsia, tissue kallikrein activity in preeclampsia is not elaborated though it is found to be reduced in hypertensive disorders of pregnancy.[14]

These results while disproving the hypothesis of renal function compromise preceding the onset of clinical preeclampsia also showed a very important dissociation. It shows that preeclampsia can occur in absence of compromised renal function. Also, it confirms the thinking that renal involvement is just like much other systemic involvement in obstetric vasculopathies. It is more an effect of the pathophysiology rather than a part of etiopathology of obstetric vasculopathies.

HEMATOLOGICAL CELLULAR AND NON-CELLULAR INDICES

Hematological indices are probably the most studied and therefore constitutes the largest body of prediction tests of PIH in particular. The bunch of these tests and indices include very diverse components. They vary from cellular components of blood like platelets on one end to hormones like SHBG on the other end of the spectrum. Though these are apparently very diverse in appearance and function, they are indeed linked with a common chain of etiopathology running through them.

Platelets and Platelet Activation

Amongst all cellular components, the most conspicuously studied are the platelets. They have been found to have a vital role in sustaining the process of obstetric vasculopathies in the body of a pregnant human female. It is true that neutrophils (inflammatory reaction to preeclampsia) and monocytes (enhancing the process of immunological reaction) are also playing a significant role. But a change in the number or configuration of these cells has not been extensively studied. Therefore platelets remain maximally in focus.

Platelet Count and CD63

The quickest response of all scientists in medical world is to presume that there is a linear relation between any component of the body and its linked disease process. This means that the cell or biochemical molecule in question rises in a linear fashion as the disease gets activated and/or progresses. Classical example of this is in measuring the platelets. In this linear relationship, it is presumed that with the pathophysiology of obstetric vasculopathies becoming active, platelets rise proportionately. However, it was well known that though the platelets did not consistently alter in their population, their functioning gets altered. This is, what is described elsewhere as platelet activation (See Chapter 4).

For this markers of platelets activation are to be studied. Several techniques have been used to assess platelet activation in P-EC. Detection of aberrations of platelet function and activation appeared to have predictive value for its diagnosis.[15] One such parameter or marker studied was surface CD63 expression in activated platelets. Konijnenberg A et al studied CD63 expression to predict preeclampsia.[16] They found results inconsistent to what was expected. Also when the statistical indices were applied platelet activation marker CD63 in first trimester had poor sensitivity (< 50%) and a dismal predictive value of less than 15%. The likelihood ratio did not even touch 2. These results were still worse when studied for second trimester. But when CD63 was studied in combination with in subjects with first visit diastolic BP of 75 mm of Hg or more, the sensitivity remained low but the positive predictive value and likelihood ratio improved. The likelihood ratio rose to nearly 9.5, best being 10. This hinted at a strong possibility of platelet activation when BP changes have already begun. But the test has never become popular for mass screening. It seems Yi ZS et al, therefore, used wisdom when on basis of their results on assessment of CD62p and CD63 expressions stopped short of recommending the use for predicting preeclampsia. Instead they just stated that high levels of platelet glycoprotein CD62p and CD63 expressions are present in patients with preeclampsia, suggesting the presence of platelet activation in these patients.[17]

Uric Acid

If one follows the importance of uric acid estimation in preeclampsia it is a very fascinating story. Uric acid was initially thought to have a very good role in predicting preeclampsia. There were two reasons for this—first, scientific and the other probably rates to English language!

Uric acid is said to be excreted through kidneys and so a high level of uric acid meant impaired renal efficiency. This was thought to be preceding preeclampsia. Delić R and Stefanović M showed that when parameters such as uric acid (and urea) were included into to predict the occurrence of preeclampsia based on multivariate logistic regression model, they could correctly predict in 79.6% patients.[18] In a bivariate meta-analysis and decision analysis to assess the accuracy of serum uric acid as a predictive test for maternal complications in preeclampsia, it was found that in the strategy where women with an increased serum uric acid were supposed to have labor induced, whereas women with serum uric acid levels below the threshold were managed expectantly, based on the decision analysis, serum uric acid seems to be a useful test in the management of preeclampsia under realistic assumptions.[19] While on uric acid levels plasma uric acid levels more than 350 μmol/L is thought to be predictive of preeclampsia in high-risk subjects.

Besides the scientific reason of impedance of renal function, another amusing possibility of it finding a place in predicting preeclampsia seems to be the English language itself. Urea rhymes with urine which rhymes with uric acid. Therefore, it was probably presumed that uric acid should have some role in screening for preeclampsia. This assumption got a scientific backing in the fact that renal function compromise has some association with preeclampsia and other vasculopathies.

The popularity of uric acid in preeclampsia did not confine to the realms of prediction. It is also a regular entry on the list of "essential" investigations to be carried out in subjects being managed for preeclampsia, in many big and small hospitals. It is further amusing that an undergraduate and postgraduate examinee is expected to mention uric acid estimation as an essential investigation when asked to enumerate the list of investigations in a case of preeclampsia. All these become a little comical with the advent of science indicating that alterations in uric acid levels if any are not for diagnosing renal function impairment in preeclampsia. Uric acid level estimation is more sensitive for prognosis of preeclampsia. This is interesting.

As indicated elsewhere, uric acid is one of the most sensitive reducing systems in the body (See Chapter 5). Therefore, estimating uric acid is not renal function assessment but more for assessments of oxidative stress that is prevalent. When oxidative stress has become so important in the etiopathology of obstetric vasculopathy reducing systems like uric acid will have a significant role to study the process. It is now well known that the reducing systems have a great protective role in the body against oxidative insult. Before oxidative reactive substances reacts with a body tissues and substances, the reducing substances react with them and prevent injury.

The Police-riot Model to Understand the Role of Uric Acid in Obstetric Vasculopathies

One can compare the role of uric acid as that of a policeman in preventing riots or mischief in the society. During riots if someone finds that the posse of policemen has remarkably increased over a period of time, it indicates that the situation is grave. It indicates that the riots are not coming under control. It can also mean that there is a great possibility of one fresh wave of rioting. So as to combat the rioters before the latter can cause havoc on this society, the policemen are increased. Thus more policemen or an increased movement of policemen indicates an increased violence or rioting. Applying this to uric acid, serial estimation of uric acid can show a rise in levels or levels by and large same. Rising levels of uric acid indicates that the riots of oxidative stress have still not been effectively quelled. This means that the process is not coming under effective control. In that case the prognosis is not good. A rising level of uric acid indicates poor prognosis. Levels of uric acid expectedly and understandably do not fall till the placenta is out of the body. Till the process and its nidus is not out of the body (fetomaternal interface) the policeman (uric acid) stays put though not lessening.

In clinical practice, if one finds that the uric acid levels are same and have not increased remarkably it means the prognosis is not bad or the situation is not worsening. The maternal reducing systems have been able to effectively stem the mischief. Thus the reducing systems are not produced increasingly more. The prognosis is not bad. Hence estimation of uric acid in a given case of preeclampsia should be done for prognostication of the disease forces and not for diagnosing of screening of the condition.

Fibronectin

Fibronectin is a glycoprotein that has been much referred to in etiopathology of obstetric vasculopathies. It is involved in many fundamental cellular functions. Therefore it is not surprising to find its role being investigated in prediction of preeclampsia. Many studies are in circulation in this regard. Besides prediction of preeclampsia, fibronectin has been studied extensively in predicting preterm labor. However there are very few good quality tests to help deduce the efficiency of fibronectin in predicting preeclampsia. Aydin T et al showed that elevated maternal plasma fibronectin level over 40 mg/dL is capable of predicting preeclampsia with a sensitivity of 73% and a specificity of 92% suggesting that serial plasma fibronectin measurements before 24 weeks' of gestation may be helpful in the early detection of preeclampsia in normotensive gravid women who are destined to become clinically preeclamptic.[20] However Paarlberg et al[21] studied about 350 (347 to be precise) subjects. This group calculated a cut out value of 230 mg/L. Values higher than this were considered to be predictive of preeclampsia. It was found that fibronectin was found to be incompetent in PIH prediction. It had a low sensitivity and specificity at around 69% and 59% in that order. The likelihood ratio worked out to be less than 2. This made the assessment of fibronectin not a very good test for predicting preeclampsia. Also, a technicality of assessment renders the testing of fibronectin impractical for mass screening.

β-HCG

β-HCG has also been used to predict preeclampsia. Trophoblastic activity is reflected in circulating levels of β-HCG. Levels more than 2 MOM at midtrimester were found to be useful in predicting preeclampsia and allied adverse obstetric outcomes.[22] In one of our studies we found that when low-dose aspirin was given to subjects with raised ß-HCG at midtrimester adverse obstetric outcomes like miscarriages were reduced and favorable outcomes like full-term deliveries increased.[23]

EPIDEMIOLOGICAL INDICES

One of the easier options to predict any medical condition is to identify its epidemiological indices. Once identified, they are bunched together and then singly or collectively used to predict that condition. Many scoring systems also get developed based on the factorization of these individual indices. On the basis of scores so evolved attempts to predict the condition are evolved. However using epidemiological indices to predict preeclampsia has not proved to be very useful.[24] The factors that were associated with increased risk of preeclampsia were as follows:

1. First pregnancy
2. Preeclampsia in previous pregnancy
3. > 10 years since previous pregnancy
4. > 40 years of maternal age
5. BMI of > 35 at booking
6. Family history of preeclampsia
7. Diastolic BP of > 80 mm of Hg at booking
8. Proteinuria at booking
9. Multiple pregnancy and
10. Underlying medical conditions including:
    - Chronic hypertension
    - Renal disease
    - Diabetes
    - Presence of antiphospholipid antibodies.

When these were applied individually or in different combinations or as an entire bunch, epidemiological parameters have found to be poor and incompetent predictors of preeclampsia in particular and obstetric vasculopathies in general.

While on predicting preeclampsia and obstetric vasculopathies many clinical and epidemiological factors came into focus at some time or the other. However, they are listed here only to be stated. They have never become popular or valid for mass screening or prediction. These can be tabulated as in Table 17.1.

It, therefore, appears that amongst the clinical and hematological tests to predict preeclampsia none of the tests alone or in combination are complete and competent. If some appeared promising on predictive values they lacked a good specificity and/or sensitivity. The important standard of likelihood ratio was also very poor in most of these tests. It, therefore, becomes imperative to examine new frontiers in science. In this regard imaging technology needs to be closely

TABLE 17.1: Risk factors evaluated at sometime or the other to predict obstetric vasculopathies[25]
• Limited sperm exposure
• Primi paternity
• Pregnancy after donor insemination
• Oocytes donation
• Embryo donation
• Extremes of maternal age
• Rheumatic disease
• Maternal low birth weight
• Obesity and insulin resistance
• Maternal infections
• Preexisting thrombophilia
• Maternal susceptibility genes
• Hydropic degeneration of placenta

evaluated for this purpose color Doppler seem to be one such investigative parameter which needs to be thoroughly analyzed for its function in predicting preeclampsia. However, when one actually goes deep in this technology it is found that color Doppler goes well beyond the mere prediction of obstetric vasculopathies.

COLOR DOPPLER IN OBSTETRIC VASCULOPATHIES: THE GAME CHANGER

Ultrasonography is one development in science which changed the face of how obstetrics is practiced. Gone are the days when so much was left to imagination. X-rays were the only principle imaging modality for medical science till as late as the early 80s. Students of the subject who have been a witness to the introduction of ultrasonography for widespread use in clinical practice have experienced the joy and ease of diagnosing and managing obstetric situations hitherto left to imagination. Ultrasonography, therefore, is the game changer for obstetric practice.

The advent of color Doppler as an extension tool to ultrasonography has been proving to be a similar game changer in managing obstetric vasculopathies. What began as a non-invasive imaging technique to study the blood supply and its complexities, has become a potent weapon for effective prognostication and decision maker in different stages of obstetric vasculopathies.

The Diastolic Notch

As a part of routine second trimester obstetric scan, a good imaging spectrum always includes a mention of the presence of diastolic notch in the uterine artery. Some reports include the imaging of uterine artery. Bilaterally, this feature is imaged along with the scan of 12 weeks and then about.

What is the Diastolic Notch?

Diastolic notch is the marker of incomplete second wave of trophoblastic invasion. Extensive mention of this has been done elsewhere (See Chapter 19). It is a critical phenomenon in the advent of obstetric vasculopathies. It has been proved conclusively that subjects in whom the second wave of obstetric vasculopathy fails or is incomplete obstetric vasculopathies result. The second wave of trophoblastic invasion is expected to get complete at or around 20 weeks of pregnancy. At 12 weeks scan the second wave is not expected to be complete so, in a scan at this duration of pregnancy, one should expect the presence of diastolic notch, in uterine artery.

As the pregnancy advances the second wave of trophoblastic invasion goes on to complete itself. This event is documentable on color Doppler. The diastolic notch in uterine vessels that is usually evident in 12 weeks scans or there about now disappears at 20 to 22 weeks scan. This is a very good predictor of obstetric vasculopathies. Disappearance of the diastolic notch in the uterine artery at 20 to 22 weeks scan indicates that the second wave of trophoblastic invasion is complete in a given subject. Clinically this reflects as a low risk for development of clinical manifestations of obstetric vasculopathies including preeclampsia.

Persistence of diastolic notch at 20 to 22 weeks and there after indicates a strong possibility of the second wave of trophoblastic invasion proving to be incomplete and incompetent. This means that the subject has either already developed obstetric vasculopathy or has a strong possibility of developing it clinically. This has been conclusively proved in many studies.[26,27]

It is strange but true that in most reporting's of colour Doppler, the indices are relied upon for drawing fair conclusions. These include the resistance index (RI), the pulsatility index (PI) and the systolic to diastolic (SD) ratio). However, in prediction of obstetric vasculopathies, there is no consensus for the change of these values. In this only, the presence or disappearance (absence) of diastolic notch is all that has been agreed upon for prediction of obstetric vasculopathies. Infact when workers have relied on these indices they have concluded that color Doppler is not a good method to predict vasculopathy. This is because of the inconsistency in these indices.

Review of Indices

In the earlier days of application of color Doppler in obstetric world, there was no agreement on the index or a combination of indices to be used for predicting adverse to be used for predicting adverse situations of obstetric vasculopathies. Jacobson et al used RI for predicting preeclampsia. They scanned both uterine arteries at around 20 to 24 weeks in high-risk subjects for preeclampsia. Based on standard deviation they chose an RI of 5.8 as a cutout. An RI of more than 5.7 was examined for eventual development of preeclampsia. They did not find this index to be reliable enough for predicting preeclampsia.[28] Similar results on single measurements of RI at or around midtrimester were also reported by Steel et al.[29] With such dismal results appearing in scientific journal color Doppler was nearly given up by the medical world for prediction of obstetric vasculopathy. However, another study by Bower et al revived the interest.[30] This group used the disappearance of diastolic notch to predict obstetric vasculopathy. They found a higher sensitivity and a higher positive predictive value for this index for predicting obstetric vasculopathies. Besides introducing the diastolic notch for prediction of preeclampsia and other obstetric vasculopathies, this study used a two-stage test. They studied the subjects first at 18 to 22 weeks of pregnancy. Then they studied them again at 24 weeks and found disappearance of diastolic notch to be a good predictor of obstetric vasculopathy.

Florio P et al used a combination of Doppler alteration with serum markers like Activin A and Inhibin A. They found that the measurement of serum Activin A and Inhibin A levels may add significant prognostic information for predicting preeclampsia in pregnant women showing specific Doppler alterations in the late second trimester.[31]

It seems the out-of-the-box thinking of Bower et al[30] of using the diastolic notch was a game changer in the field of prediction of obstetric vasculopathies. However, in the mid 1990s and early 2000 studies continued to appear in literature which gave conflicting results. Thus color Doppler failed to gain its rightful place in prediction obstetric vasculopathies. This led Friedman S.A. and Lindheimer S.A. to state that Doppler does not appear to be useful in screening low-risk patients but may have a role in research protocols seeking to define a high-risk population.[32] However, they did leave a window open stating that the presence of diastolic notch seems to be very promising in prediction of obstetric vasculopathies. Around a decade or more down the line, these early results proved to be the most important early results on which the subsequent edifice of using color Doppler in prediction of obstetric vasculopathies was built.

It was very interesting to study the diastolic notch and the behavior of indices at around 12 weeks and then again at or around midtrimester. Basically the indices PI, RI and SD ratio help us in identifying the quantum of diastolic flow in the uterine vascular system. This can be better understood if correlated with the pathophysiology occurring at or around this time. The process of second wave of trophoblastic invasion is expected to get competently completed at or around midtrimester. In this process, the moulding of spiral arterioles in the maternal vasculature gets done. With this moulding the maternal vascular bed becomes a low resistance—high flow pool of blood. It becomes nearly shielded off from the other changes that are taking place in the maternal systems. It also gets shielded off from the pressor substances that may be in circulation in the maternal system at some time or the other. The sum total effect of all these changes is an increase in blood flow to the pregnant uterus. That apart, this increase in blood flow is continuous and guarded by blunting the effects of sympathetic and parasympathetic systems on spiral arterioles.

The uterine arteries can be readily accessed to color Doppler as it crosses the iliac vessels just before entering the uterine musculature and just after giving the cervical (descending) branch. In old literature, uterine artery is also referred to as ascending uterine artery. This is more so as a corollary to descending cervical. However the adjective ascending was subsequently dropped. As a result the hitherto ascending uterine is referred to as uterine artery plain and simple. A substantial risk of complications is associated with impedance to maternal changes at the level of uterine circulation has been demonstrated.[33,34] Therefore persistence of diastolic notch has been agreed upon by and large to be a good predictor of obstetric vasculopathies.

It is, therefore, wise to believe that uterine artery Doppler is a path breaking and game changer in the amorphous world prediction of obstetric vasculopathies.

REFERENCES

1. Abdelaziz Nassar A, Maaher Hussein M, Sayyed T, Bazeed M, Hassanien N. Early pregnancy screening for hypertensive disorders in pregnant women without a-priori high risk. *Ultrasound Obstet Gynecol.* 2012.
2. Ales K, Norton M, Druzin M. Early prediction of antepartum hypertension. *Obstet Gynecol.* 1989;73:928-33.
3. Kuromoto K, Watanabe M, Adachi K, Ohashi K, Iwatani Y. Increases in urinary creatinine and blood pressure during early pregnancy in preeclampsia. *Ann Clin Biochem.* 2010;47(4):336-42.
4. Sibai B, Gordon T, Thom E. Risk factors for preeclampsia in healthy multiparous women: A prospective multicenter study. *Am J Obstet Gynecol.* 1995;172:642-48.
5. Sibai B, Ewell M, Levine R. Risk factors for preeclampsia in healthy nulliparous women. *Am J Obstet Gynecol.* 1997;177:1003-10.
6. Vollebregt K, Gisolf J, Guelen I, Boer K, van Montfrans G, Wolf H. Limited accuracy of the hyperbaric index, ambulatory blood pressure and sphygmomanometry measurements in predicting gestational hypertension and preeclampsia. *J Hypertens.* 2010;28(1):127-34.
7. Baker P, Johnson I. The use of the hand-grip test for predicting pregnancy-induced hypertension. *Eur J Obstet Gynecol Reprod Biol.* 1994;56(3):169-72.
8. Shi J, Yang Z, Chen L, Wang J. Early warning signs of severe preeclampsia, *Zhonghua Fu Chan Ke Za Zhi.* 2009;44(5):337-40.
9. Thomson A, Billewicz W. Clinical significance of weight trends during pregnancy. *Br Med J.* 1957;1:243-7.
10. Gasnier R, Valério E, Vettorazzi J, Barros E, Martins-Costa S, Ramos J. Calciuria and preeclampsia: a case-control study. *J Obstet Gynecol Res.* 2012;38(4):674-80.
11. Szmidt-Adjidé V, Vendittelli F, David S, Brédent-Bangou J, Janky E. Calciuria and preeclampsia: a case-control study. *Eur J Obstet Gynecol Reprod Biol.* 2006;1;125(2):193-8.
12. Millar J, Campbell S, Albano J, Higgins B, Clark A. Early prediction of preeclampsia by measurement of kallikrein and creatinine on a random urine sample. *Br J Obstet Gynecol.* 1996;103(5):421-6.
13. Kyle P, Campbell S, Buckley D, Kissane J, de Swiet M, Albano J, et al. A comparison of the inactive urinary kallikrein: Creatinine ratio and the angiotensin sensitivity test for the prediction of preeclampsia. *Br J Obstet Gynecol.* 1996;103(10):981-7.
14. Khedun S, Naicker T, Moodley J. Tissue kallikrein activity in pregnancy. *Aust N Z J Obstet Gynaecol.* 2000;40(4):451-4.
15. Kazmi R, Cooper A, Lwaleed B. Platelet function in preeclampsia. *Semin Thromb Hemost.* 2011;37(2):131-6.
16. Konijnenberg A, Stokkers E, van der Post J, Schaap M, Boer K, Bleker O, et al. Extensive platelet activation in preeclampsia compared with normal pregnancy: Enhanced expression of cell adhesion molecules. *Am J Obstet Gynecol.* 1997;176(2):461-9.
17. Yi Z, Zhou S, Meng F, Feng R, Liu Q, Lin R. Detection of platelet activation by flow cytometry in patients with preeclampsia. *Di Yi Jun Yi Da Xue Xue Bao.* 2003;23(10):1095-6.

18. Delić R, Stefanović M. Optimal laboratory panel for predicting preeclampsia. *J Matern Fetal Neonatal Med.* 2010;23(1):96-102.
19. Koopmans C, van Pampus M, Groen H, Aarnoudse J, van den Berg P, Mol BW. Accuracy of serum uric acid as a predictive test for maternal complications in preeclampsia: bivariate meta-analysis and decision analysis. *Eur J Obstet Gynecol Reprod Biol* 1. 2009;46(1):8-14.
20. Aydin T, Varol F, Sayin N. Third trimester maternal plasma total fibronectin levels in pregnancy-induced hypertension: Results of a tertiary center. *Clin Appl Thromb Hemost.* 2006;12(1):33-9.
21. Paarlberg K, de Jong C, van Geijn H, van Kamp G, Heinen A, Dekker G. Total plasma fibronectin as a marker of pregnancy-induced hypertensive disorders: A longitudinal study. *Obstet Gynecol.* 1998;91(3):383-8.
22. Desai P, Rao S. Predictive value of raised midtrimester HCG in PIH. *Jr O and G India.* 2002;52(1):68-70.
23. Desai P, Rao S. Role of low dose aspirin in mothers registering high serum HCG levels at midtrimester. *Jr O and G of India.* 2002;52(5):30-2.
24. Duckitt K, Harrington D. Risk factors for preeclampsia at antenatal booking systematic review of controlled studies. *Br Med J.* 2005;330,565-71.
25. Mukherjee J, Seal S, Banerjee G. Current concepts in pregnancy induced hypertension. In: Gita Ganguly Mukherjee (Ed). Current Obstetrics and Gynecology. (Ist edn). Jaypee Publishers: Delhi. 2007;93-100.
26. Phupong V, Dejthevaporn T. Predicting risks of preeclampsia and small for gestational age infant by uterine artery Doppler. *Hypertens Pregnancy.* 2008;27(4):387-95.
27. Hafner E, Metzenbauer M, Höfinger D, Stonek F, Schuchter K, Waldhör T, et al. Comparison between three-dimensional placental volume at 12 weeks and uterine artery impedance/notching at 22 weeks in screening for pregnancy-induced hypertension, preeclampsia and fetal growth restriction in a low-risk population. *Ultrasound Obstet Gynecol.* 2006;27(6):652-7.
28. Jacobson S, Inhofe R, Manning N. The value of Doppler assessment at the uteroplacental circulation in predicting preeclampsia and IUGR. *Am J Obstet Gynecol.* 1990;162,110-4.
29. Steel S, Pearce J, Mc Par land P, Chamberlain G. Early Doppler ultrasound screening in prediction of hypertensive disorders of pregnancy. *Lancet.* 1990;335:1548-51.
30. Bower S, Bewley S, Campbell S. Improved prediction of preeclampsia by two-stage screening of uterine arteries using the early diastolic notch and colour Doppler imaging. *Obstetric Gynecology.* 1994;82:78-83.
31. Florio P, Reis F, Pezzani I, Luisi S, Severi F, Petraglia F. The addition of Activin A and inhibin A measurement to uterine artery Doppler velocimetry to improve the early prediction of preeclampsia. *Ultrasound Obstet Gynecol.* 2003;21(2):165-9.
32. Friedman S, Lindheimer S. Prediction and differential diagnosis. In: Lindheimer M, Roberts J, Cunningham F, (Eds). Chesley's Hypertensive disorders of pregnancy. (2nd edn). Stamford, Appleton and Lange. 1998. pp. 201-28.
33. Hernandez–Andrade E, Brodzki J, Lingman G. Uterine artery score and perinatal outcome. *Ultrasound Obstet Gynecol.* 2002;19:438.
34. Lees C, Para M, Missfelder Lobos H. Individualized risk assessment for adverse pregnancy outcome by uterine artery Doppler at 23 weeks. *Obstet Gynecol.* 2001;98:369.

CHAPTER

18

Prevention of Preeclampsia and other Obstetric Vasculopathies

CHAPTER OUTLINE

- What is the Difference between Disease and Derangement?
- Preventing Obstetric Vasculopathy is a Challenge
- Which Subjects may Benefit out of Preventive Measures
- Measures Prevent Occurrence or Prevent Worsening
- Preventive Measures of Obstetric Vasculopathies
- Prevention of Eclampsia

INTRODUCTION

Once the etiopathology involved in causing a disease is understood, science always tries to attack this area to prevent the disease states. However due to multiplicity of reasons, obstetric vasculopathy becomes difficult to prevent by measures influencing the etiopathology. In such a situation the effects of the disease are attempted to be prevented. This can be compared to flood prevention measures in some community. The basic cause of floods is excessive rainfall in that area. This is beyond the control of human beings. In such a situation resilient human minds try to find out measures by which flood waters get diverted in such a way that floods do not cause devastation. Thus measures like dams, check dams, ground water harvesting and the like come into effect. The aim therefore is: till the time that the cause cannot be controlled, try controlling the effects. This is the approach in clinical practice for management of obstetric vasculopathies including pre-eclampsia. Another area in which preventive measures have had a reasonable success is through early detection.

However when one is studying preventive measures it is wise to know that human body doest perceive obstetric vasculopathies as a disease process but as processes of derangement. This difference is very important because a disease can be cured but a derangement can be prevented or detected in time and controlled.

WHAT IS THE DIFFERENCE BETWEEN DISEASE AND DERANGEMENT?

The basic difference between the two is in the body response. The body response to a disease state is furious and having a tendency to stem the rot. In derangements body response is muted and becomes furious only when the condition heavily worsens. As a result protective or treatment measures in derangements give inconsistent response. On the other hand body response to diseases is consistent. This seems to result from the perception of derangement by the body as its own innate process but the disease as an attack on itself.

Before making the matter more complex it would be easier to understand this through examples. Malignances can be called derangements and malaria is a disease. Malignances anywhere in the body do not incite an immediate response on occurrence. They tend to run an insidious course with the body protective mechanisms themselves trying to handle and suppress the condition. It therefore grows slowly and produces hardly any clinical features. It is therefore said in euphemism that malignancies usually do not pain and therefore a mass that pains is not malignant usually. On the other hand, the body responds very torridly to malaria. Fever with rigor, headache, generalized body ache and similar series of clinical features develop. It is produced by an exogenous element the malarial parasite and therefore perceived as alien by the human body. Malignancies, atherosclerosis and on similar lines obstetric vasculopathies are not perceived as aliens by human body. They are a part of its own for the body. Therefore the response of the body to these is muted and insidious. The features that occur are only of the complications and systemic effects of these derangements.

There is still more to this. By understanding the difference between derangement and disease, one can predict if these conditions will be cured or will be controlled. Diseases get cured derangements get controlled. Thus anemia in pregnancy is a disease. In most cases nutritional anemia are found. These are diseases. They can be cured by administering the nutritional hemopoietic substance. On the other hand non-nutritional anemia due to sickle cell disease or thalassemia is a derangement. The genetic abnormality results from derangement of the system that produces normal disease. Therefore those conditions cannot be cured. They can either be controlled or if the entire marrow is replaced, they can be changed. But they cannot be cured. Diabetes too is a derangement. It is a derangement of the insulin production, activity and metabolism. The basic cause is insulin deficiency which may be genetic or age acquired. Therefore diabetes can be controlled it cannot be cured. Diabetes is therefore not a disease it is a derangement.

One more illustration to this differentiation will not be out of place. The condition in focus is myocardial infarction. When angioplasty or bypass vascular surgeries are done, does myocardial infarction get cured? Not at all! The dead myocardium or the infracted myocardium remains as such. The blood supply which was proving deficient gets restored. The patient gets relieved but is never cured of myocardial infarction.

On the other hand viral hepatitis though has seemingly no cure. But from medical science, it is a known viral disease. Once the viral load is overwhelmed by the body resistance mechanisms, the disease gets cured. Like anemia, jaundice can also be a derangement. Types of liver derangements which result from factors that produce a permanent dysfunction of liver function as in Hepatitis C are derangements. They elude a cure. Liver transplant replaces the dead liver tissue by a healthy and functioning new hepatic tissue. But that is not a cure of the original disease. It is only a circumvention of the diseased system.

Why is this differentiation so terribly important? This differentiation is very important from the cure point of view. Scientists in search of immortality continue to find cures for derangements. Cures which never exist and will never be created. Derangements are incurable. They can be controlled, their complications prevented, their progress thwarted but they cannot be cured. Disease get cured not derangements. Atherosclerosis causing the disease like myocardial infarction may be preventable but the derangement atherosclerosis cannot be cured.

This does not mean that the difference between the disease and a derangement gets blurred. In the initial stages derangements can be transiently reversed or their progress slowed and worsening postponed. But the process continues to lurk at the cellular level. It can strike again. This is because there is no cure for a derangement. There is only follow-up and surveillance to keep a watch on deterioration. One very interesting point comes up here regarding progress of Cervical Intraepithelial Neoplasia (CIN). CIN-I can progress to CIN-II and get reversed. But once CIN-III occurs, it becomes irreversible. Gynecologists may then use fanciful names of removing the lesion by cone biopsy or loop excision or even hysterectomy. But they can not cure or reverse it. In very early stages therefore the condition gets cured. As soon as the cervical junction gets deranged permanently it starts producing cells that are malignant or potentially malignant. Now these cann not be cured. This is no more a disease.

Can stem cells cure a derangement? The answer technically is no. Stem cells act by marrow replacement in leukemia or thalassemia. It replaces the deranged manufacturing line. It generates a totally different and new line that is healthy and competent. Clinically the patient will be free of the condition but technically he/she was not "cured". The dysfunctional system was not restored to regain its function. Therefore even stem cells will not be able to "treat" a derangement. They will only replace the derangement by healthy systems.

Having had known and understood this difference well, it can now be understood why treatment of obstetric vasculopathies in general and preeclampsia in particular is not found. Obstetric vasculopathies in general and preeclampsia in particular are derangements. They cannot be cured. They can be controlled. They can be prevented from worsening. Their complications can be prevented. But the parent condition cannot be cured.

In a greatly dramatized mention Lindheimer M et al have photographed and inserted it in their book Chesley's hypertensive disorders of pregnancy a picture of placards honoring famous physicians who have made major contributions to the field of obstetrics. This placard holder stands at Chicago Lying-In Hospital. They point at an empty plaque which they say is reserved for a person who discovers the cause and cure for pre-eclampsia. This plaque is reportedly still empty.[1] This plaque is empty for decades. If the custodians of this plaque holder are and shall remain honest to the causes and purpose of erecting this plaque holder, the plaque for person finding the cause and cure of preeclampsia will remain vacant till eternity. This is because there is no cure or cause of pre-eclampsia. Preeclampsia is not a disease. Preeclampsia is a derangement. It will never open its cause. It will never get cured. It can be controlled. It can be prevented from worsening its complications can be prevented or kept to bare minimum. But cure does not exist. Derangements do not get cured. Once humanity accepts this limitation of its existence, the struggle and needless useless attempts shall become relegated to history. It is possible that staring at this empty plaque for decades, its custodians may finally compromise and insert the name of the person who described the etiopathology of this condition. But if they are wanting the name of the person who cures it or tells us what causes it in all honesty: the plaque is destined to remain empty.

PREVENTING OBSTETRIC VASCULOPATHY IS A CHALLENGE

Having had clearly understood that preventing preeclampsia in particular and obstetric vasculopathies in general is very challenging as these are derangements and not diseases, it is now timely to explore the different options available for this.

WHICH SUBJECTS MAY BENEFIT OUT OF PREVENTIVE MEASURES

This is a very important and at the same times a very tricky question. The answer to the question at the first step seems very easy. Those subjects that are at a high-risk of developing obstetric vasculopathy are the ones that should benefit out of preventive measures. But the bigger question is which of these subjects are at a high-risk. A series of studies and experiences from clinical practice can identify most of these subjects. Past history of adverse outcome can give vital clues of a subject at-risk of obstetric vasculopathy. Any one or more than one manifestations of obstetric vasculopathy like preeclampsia remote from term or recurrent missed abortion in late first trimester early second trimester IUGR, accidental hemorrhage and the like are some of the conditions which can make a subject vulnerable to recurrence of obstetric vasculopathy. It is not necessary that the same vasculopathy will occur again. It may be preeclampsia remote from term in one pregnancy and the other time she can have an IUGR. This can agreeably take an ill-informed obstetrician off guard. But any of these conations singly or in combination indicate the process. There are the subjects at a higher-risk for recurrence. Therefore preventive measures may help in them.

Nullipara

It is well know that nulliparous subjects are at a higher risk of developing pre-eclampsia. This therefore brings out a very pertinent question should all nulliparous subjects be provided with the umbrella of prevention. This can be compared to iron and calcium supplementation being routinely provided to all pregnant subjects in countries like India. Should this basket of antenatal prescriptions also include preventive substances for pre-eclampsia? The answer is a big No! Not routinely. The increase propensity of nulliparous subject to development of preeclampsia is a statistical result. It does not need a clinical intervention of such a large scale. It is a statistical figure and the clinician is just expected to bear it in mind. If there are some other associated features like H/O lupus, then a nulligravida gets a card for inclusion in the list of preventing measures.

Abnormal Uterine Artery Doppler

Color Doppler reflecting the flow of blood, the resistance to it if any and the pulsatility of the vessel with which the vessel successfully propels the blood ahead is a very valuable tool for gaining insight into what is happening inside. The uterine artery Doppler is a valuable tool for predicting preeclampsia as has been discussed in the chapter on Prediction of Obstetric Vasculopathies (See Chapter 17). However it has got an important role in identifying a subject at risk for preeclampsia in particular and other obstetric vasculopathies in general. At around late first trimester the uterine artery shows a presence of diastolic notch. It is reflecting that the second wave of trophoblastic invasion is not complete. At or around midtrimester this diastolic notch should disappear. Persistence of diastolic notch is an indicator of the second wave of trophoblastic invasion still not complete. These subjects are at a high risk for developing all obstetric vasculopathies single or multiple in different combinations. This feature of uterine artery color Doppler puts it one step ahead of the other methods and parameters to identify "at risk" subjects.

By and large most studies have concentrated on the persistence and disappearance of the diastolic notch in the uterine arteries. It is however a known fact that Doppler flow velocimetry also calculates certain critical indices from the blood flow. These indices seemingly have not found favor with the scientists as regards their utility in identifying subjects at a risk for developing obstetric vasculopathies. Indices like Pulsatility Index, Resistance Index and S:D ratio as it is called popularly seems not to be very helpful. Yet a clinician who backs up his practice by doing color Doppler's of his patients himself, will definitely be a witness to one very important observation. Irrespective of the presence of absence of diastolic notch, there is a wide variation in values of PI, RI and S:D ratio in subjects in whom uterine artery color Doppler is done at late first trimester (about 12 to 14 weeks.) How these variations translate into identifying subjects at risk for obstetric vasculopathies is a matter unanswered.

Inconsistent Presence of Diastolic Notch: Any Significance?

One more aspect needs to be covered here. It is the matter related to the consistency of diastolic notch. While diastolic notch is expected to be consistently present in all subjects in all waves at first trimester (12 to 14 weeks scan) there are subjects in whom some peculiar inconsistency is observed. There are at least three if not more wave forms in every ten waves in which one may not find diastolic notch. As of now this is reported as diastolic notch to be present. But three, four or even five waves irregularly regularly showing an absence of diastolic notch is an intriguing phenomenon. Do these subjects have a low-risk for developing obstetric vasculopathies? What is the significance of this inconsistent presence of diastolic notch? These questions have either remained unexplored or an answered.

If some answer is found to the two points raised viz; value of color Doppler indices and inconsistency of diastolic notch presence these can have a huge bearing on identifying high-risk subjects. As of now only disappearance of an already present diastolic notch at midtrimester identifies low-risk for obstetric vasculopathies. For this the clinician has to wait upto midtrimester. Through them high-risk subjects can be identified as early as 12 to 14 weeks. In studies currently available by and large abnormal uterine artery Doppler studies use RI of more than 0.58 at 18 to 24 weeks. This can potentially change in times to come.

This is in no way an attempt to run down the currently used parameter the diastolic notch. It is very effective and very reliable but it tends to get a little late. By the time a clinician comes to know that his subject is at a high-risk of developing severe PIH, preventive measures may be a little late to institute. Any day, sooner the better!

Subjects with Obstetric Challenges

This includes subjects with obstetric conditions like multifetal pregnancy, past history of adverse outcome due to obstetric vasculopathies, diabetic subjects, subjects with obesity, subjects with renal disease and those with chronic hypertension. All of these are more susceptible to development of obstetric vasculopathies. Nevertheless the question that arises in them is: should preventive measures be started universally? The answer is: Yes! If there is a past history of obstetric vasculopathy, it is advisable to start preventive measures universally in such subjects. But for others it would depend on findings of color Doppler and individualization of the case.

One more group of subjects is of those in whom screening tests for obstetric vasculopathies are positive, should preventive measures be started? Screening tests for obstetric vasculopathies have been extensively discussed in the chapter on Prediction of Obstetric Vasculopathies (See Chapter 17). The answer to this question therefore is: if the method to predict these conditions definitively identifies a subject, then preventive measures should be started across the board.

But most of these tests like the Roll-Over Test and The Handgrip Test are more efficient in ruling out the possibility of developing obstetric vasculopathy in a given subject rather than committing the possibility. Thus, they have a more efficient negative predictive value. Such tests are a little handicapped. To pontify on whether preventive measures should be started on basis of these tests if they are positive may be risky. Thus it needs to be clarified that decision to start preventive measures should be individualized and left on the clinician to decide.

MEASURES PREVENT OCCURRENCE OR PREVENT WORSENING

This is a very important question. Many preventive measures are initiated in subject in whom milder forms of these conditions have already developed. On the other hand there are clinical situations where the preventive measures are initiated to prevent the occurrence of these conditions altogether. There is a considerable overlap. Measures used to prevent worsening are also being used to prevent the occurrence of these conditions all together.

Salt Restriction

In society like ours where food and rest are given undue importance in day-to-day life for well being and health, low salt diet or even salt free diet is suggested more often than not by the pregnant subject and her family for preventing preeclampsia rather than the attending obstetrician. When the doctor announces that the pregnant subject has a tendency to develop a rise in blood pressure, the first response of the pregnant subject and her family is "shall we give her salt free diet?" Worst still is a situation when the doctor is informed on subsequent visits that the family has stopped serving her food containing salt. All this is when the medical staff has never advised ever.

It seems that the concept of salt free diet is deeply ingrained in the society for prevention of hypertension. This thinking comes from experiences of elderly subjects in the family who are having an age-related hypertension and have been advised a low salt or salt free diet, by their attending physician. A quick and hasty extrapolation is done. Little do they realize that both are absolutely different conditions and hypertension is the only external manifestation common to both. While it is well known that salt free or low salt diets do not in any way help in managing or preventing hypertensive disorders of pregnancy, infact the results might be actually reverse. It is well possible that in an overzealous attempt to restrict salt in the mother the fetus suffers from vital electrolyte deprivation. There is some fear that maternal salt restriction may actually produce a stunting of fetal growth.

A popular advice given by obstetricians of Indian subcontinent is to avoid consuming salt rich foods. This includes pickles for example. However this has not been scientifically validated and therefore seems to be an advice given by convention or by the word-of-mouth. It has not been proved to give any great advantage to the hypertensive or potentially hypertensive subject.

Diuretics

Use of diuretics for preventing obstetric vasculopathies especially those complicated by preeclampsia is a habit that obstetricians seem to have borrowed from their physician counterparts. This habit seems to be more confined to the senior generation of obstetric practitioners probably the youngest of the lot seem to be aware of the fact that these not only do not help in preventing preeclampsia but may in fact cause complications. The use of these agents is also instituted in subjects with edema in pre-eclampsia.

If one knows the pathophysiology of edema in preeclampsia well, it is not difficult to guess the error in this decision of prescribing a diuretic for treating edema of pre-eclampsia. Edema in preeclampsia is not due to increase in the circulating fluid load as the kidneys are unable to excrete the fluid. In preeclampsia edema occurs due to altered albumin distribution as well as loosening of the vascular wall cellular arrangements. Therefore using diuretics to treat edema of preeclampsia or prevent preeclampsia occurrence is both irrational and even harmful. It is feared that long-term use of diuretics in pregnant subjects can in-fact lead to worsening of IUGR. This seems to be due to the drastic electrolyte loss that occurs in the process of diuresis. Therefore the use of diuretics in prevention of preeclampsia or treatment of edema in pre-eclamptic subjects only mentioned to be condemned.

Antihypertensives

Uses of antihypertensives have been proposed by some for subjects of chronic hypertension. In these subjects continuing use of antihypertensives on which she has been stabilized is in order. However expecting this antihypertensive to prevent the superimposition of preeclampsia over the under running chronic hypertension may not work. The chronic hypertension may me controlled but in no way is the occurrence of preeclampsia prevented. Two critical analyses have also corroborated this contention.[2]

It should however be noted that if a subject is stabilized on a particular antihypertensive for treating her chronic hypertension. It may be necessary to change this agent if it is found to be teratogenic or having some adverse fetal effect. In such a situation the clinician may be warranted to changes the antihypertensive, preferably when she is planning a pregnancy. However if the subject is already pregnant when she reports to the obstetrician and is on such an antihypertensive the drug be changed immediately in joint consultation with her attending physician. The most frequent drug that warrants such a change is the group of ACE inhibitors which are contraindicated in pregnancy. Thus use of antihypertensives in prevention of preeclampsia and other obstetric vasculopathies is not recommended.

Calcium Supplementation

Dietary calcium and extraneous calcium supplementation to prevent specifically preeclampsia caught the attention of obstetric scientists. Fodor A et al reviewed this matter in details. They felt that calcium supplementation seems to be a good opportunity to prevent pre-eclampsia.[3] One more study that initiated the thought process in this regard was performed by Belizean et al. In this study an inverse association was found between dietary calcium intake and development of pre-eclampsia. It therefore meant that if the calcium content of diet was low there was a higher chance of the subject to develop pre-eclampsia.[4] These two studies invited a series of activities for calcium supplement for reducing the incidence of pre-eclampsia.

Though most of the world started agreeing to this concept, all of them missed one very vital concept. In countries like India calcium supplementation to pregnant women has been a routine for decades. It would have been pertinent to study the behavior of preeclampsia in these societies. However based on these type of publications cited above a series of studies got published in many journals. Most of these studies extolled the virtue of calcium supplementation during pregnancy for preventing pre-eclampsia. However as usually happens in modern medicines all studies were not so positive about this. This initiated an undertaking of a large review of all such published data at Cochrane data base. It was attempting to find some answers to the questions: Does calcium supplementation really prevent pre-eclampsia. If the answer to the first was yes than in what dose? A meta-analysis of large number of studies on this matter showed calcium supplementation appears to almost halve the risk of pre-eclampsia, and to reduce the rare occurrence of the composite outcome 'death or serious morbidity'. There were no other clear benefits, or harms.[5] But this had a rider attached to it: Calcium supplementation would help only those subjects in whom dietary intake of calcium was already low. In these subjects supplementation of calcium to reduce preeclampsia would be effective.

However it seems that this review of calcium by Cochrane data base is more a research analysis of published data. It seems to be more of statistical exercise than of clinical ground reality. There are reasons to believe so: As has been hinted in a couple of preceding paragraphs, in the body of pregnant subjects seeking antenatal care in public hospitals in countries like India calcium content of their diet is expectedly low. These subjects are by and large nutritionally challenged. Iron deficiency anemia in particular and other nutritional anemia in general is rampant in these pregnant subjects. Calcium content also is expectedly low. Now if one is in the know how, supplementing calcium to these subjects free of cost or at a highly subsidized rate is a routine. This practice is prevalent for more than half a century. If the results of the study reviewed at Cochrane data base was clinically relevant, the incidence of preeclampsia in these subjects should have been either negligible or low. In clinical practice in these countries, incidence of preeclampsia remains fairly constant and therefore by and large unchanged. This seriously challenges the validity of the review of Cochrane data base. In conclusion at this stage one can only say that calcium supplementation in pregnancy even in those subjects in whom dietary intake of calcium is low, has limited role for prevention of pre-eclampsia.

Other Trace Elements Like Magnesium and Zinc

The possibility of magnesium in preventing preeclampsia got examined on a simplistic background that magnesium sulphate is used successfully in eclampsia and severe preeclampsia to prevent a convulsion. Obstetric scientists wanted to explore if it was effective in preventing preeclampsia all together. Magnesium supplementation through diet or tablets containing magnesium failed to produce any significant change in causation of pre-eclampsia.[6,7]

Similarly zinc supplementation in pregnancy does not influence the course of preeclampsia or to that matter any other obstetric vasculopathies in any way worth mentioning. Though levels of zinc in plasma and in the leucocytes may be reduced n pre-eclampsia, counteracting this by extraneous zinc supplementation is too simplistic and irrational.

Immunoglobulins

Literature references confine the use of immunoglobulins for treating subjects with recurrent pregnancy loss of immunological basis. Prevention of this obstetric vasculopathy would have an indirect bearing on prevention of other obstetric vasculopathies like pre-eclampsia. This is because preeclampsia is known to be more frequent in subjects with obstetric vasculopathy producing recurrent pregnancy loss.

Even we were using immunoglobulins for some years in late last century and the early part of 2000 for prevention of recurrent pregnancy loss. This immunoglobulin was administered as a 16.5% in a 2 mL dose every three weeks. In the initial years we felt this was indeed effective. We did not have an explanation for this. We therefore attributed it to a possible immune-potentiation of the maternal system that it may be bringing about. However, over a period of years we have found that this administration is not useful or give any advantage in preventing immunological recurrent pregnancy los. We have given up this practice altogether for nearly a decade now.

It is also noteworthy that during the late 1990s considerable interest had developed in administration of intravenous immunoglobulins for prevention of recurrent pregnancy loss. This practice too was subsequently abandoned due to its limited utility and high cost involved.

PREVENTIVE MEASURES OF OBSTETRIC VASCULOPATHIES

If we carefully go through the basics of obstetric vasculopathies we know that all these seemingly diverse conditions on clinical presentation are actually diverse manifestation of the same etiopathology and pathogenesis. However, when one evaluates their preventive measures one cannot miss the fact that most of these preventive measures are mentioned, evaluated and used for pre-eclampsia. There are very few measures for preventing other obstetric vasculopathies. Also, one cannot but note the fact that these preventive measures are most of the times for one single obstetric vasculopathy. For example antihypertensives or calcium supplementation is used for prevention of pre-eclampsia. Immunoglobulins or progesterone is used for prevention of recurrent miscarriages. DHA and nitric oxide donors like L-Arginine are evaluated and used if found useful for prevention of IUGR. Literature and clinical practice therefore remains diverse and apparently amorphous on this aspect.

This has to be understood in the light of historical timeline in the events that led to the understanding of the disease process. For upto the turn of this century it was perceived that these were all diverse conditions without any credible link with each other. Therefore scientists and clinicians tried to tackle them independently separately. The overlaps were confined to the prevention of preeclampsia what was perceived then as its complications like accidental hemorrhage of IUGR. The measures should have been focused on prevention of preeclampsia or IUGR or immunological causes of miscarriage all together through prevention of the basic pathology of obstetric vasculopathy.

There are only two credible methods in this regard: (A) Aspirin and (B) Heparin. These can be grouped as antithrombotic agents. Another potential group of pharmacological agents that may also be able to attack obstetric vasculopathies at its basics is the group of antioxidants. However as of now antioxidants have not become so popular with obstetric scientists. The reasons why antioxidants though promising but not effective enough in clinical practice for prevention of obstetric vasculopathies, has been extensively discussed elsewhere (See Chapter 5). Here it can only be repeated that what is needed is an antioxidant which can specifically prevent the disease processes resulting from oxidative stress.

However nowhere should their effect bear influence on the physiological or health promoting processes based on oxidative process. Till that time that such an "ideal" antioxidant is found, the use of currently available antioxidants for preventing obstetric vasculopathies will remain limited.

Progesterone in Prevention of Obstetric Vasculopathies

Progesterone as a hormone seems to be a misfit in the basket of preventive measures examined in reference to obstetric vasculopathies. This is because most obstetric vasculopathies like preeclampsia and IUGR are events of later half of pregnancy. However amongst obstetric vasculopathies recurrent missed abortions is a very important component. Here the role of progesterones in prevention of miscarriages arising out of obstetric vasculopathies is being examined.

Progesterones interestingly are most controversial and also most studied components of obstetric vasculopathies. There have been phases in time where progesterones have been found to be the only helpful agent in prevention of miscarriages. This belief changed quickly to the other extreme wherein progesterones were outright rejected as being completely useless in prevention of miscarriages. The progesterone pendulum has swung again to became one of the most used hormone now not only for prevention of miscarriages but even preterm labors. We too had moved with this pendulum. In our early days of working in the field of obstetric vasculopathies, we were prescribing progesterone for prevention of miscarriages. We too perceived its limited utility in the matter and therefore stopped using it for many years. Following the publication of a meta-analysis by Cochrane data base we have restarted using progesterones for prevention of miscarriages of late 1 trimester and II trimester. This too has a rider that these should essentially be abortions due to fetal demise and are recurrent.

Which Progesterone

Many forms of progesterone entered the market. Most of these have fallen by the wayside over a period of time. However progesterones that have stuck on either due to merit or due to aggressive pharma companies or both are now very few. One clear fact emerges from this and that is which progesterone does not matter! All progesterones are equally efficient (or inefficient—either way) in preventing miscarriages due to obstetric vasculopathies. Progesterones if they are to be used, they should be prescribed from the luteal phase of the menstrual cycle. This is to take advantage of the influence that progesterones have on the implantation window. This aspect has been discussed in greater details elsewhere (P···). We have been using natural micronized progesterone. This preference is more out of habit and not showing any special privilege to this form of progesterone. It is neither superior nor inferior to any other progesterone.

How Do Progesterones Possibly Act

Many theories exist to explain the action of progesterone in prevention of miscarriages. These ranges from placentotrophic action to keeping the implantation window open for a longer time to immune modulation have all been proposed to be acting singly or in combination.

What Dose Progesterone

As has been stated in the previous pages (P···), we have been using natural micronized progesterone for this purpose. The dosage that we are using is of 200 mgm twice a day vaginally. We do not use 100 mgm or 400 mgm preparation for this purpose.

Progesterone administration route is usually decided on patient compliance. As has been stated there is nothing much to select between different types of progesterone. In the same way there is very little to choose between the vaginal route of administration and intramuscular route of progesterone administration. Both are equally effective.

In this situation patient's preference and compliance is the only factor considered. All those subjects who do not mind vaginal administration are prescribed those formulations. However those subjects who prefer a less frequent administration or who find vaginal route to be cumbersome or sentimentally unfavorable, in them we prescribe intramuscular preparation of progesterone. For the purpose intra-muscular progesterone a depot preparation of 200 mgm is administrated once every week.

We start administering progesterone as early as possible. Those subjects who are with us even before they conceive in them progesterone administration is begun early in luteal phase itself. However the bigger majority report to us early in pregnancy but not before they have missed the period. In such cases we administer progesterone as soon as they register with us.

Decision making regarding discontinuation of progesterone is based on the age-old concept that human pregnancy is a two phase pregnancy. By this it is meant that in the first phase the corpus luteum supports the pregnancy. In the second phase the efficient placenta takes over the function of the corpus luteum. Corpus luteum seems to be acting upto 12 weeks of pregnancy at a minimum. Therefore we administer progesterones upto 12 weeks of a viable pregnancy.

We do not discontinue progesterone even if the subject develops spotting per vaginum or reports bleeding per vaginum during these 12 weeks. The important prerequisite here is the pregnancy should be a viable pregnancy as confirmed on an ultrasound scan. Present of fetal heart activity is enough to continue progesterone administration even if the subject is spotting. If the fetus is viable this bleeding is usually never excessive. It soon stops on its own.

It is irrational to use locally acting hemostatics in subjects with early pregnancy bleeding and we do not use them.

Side Effects of Progesterone

There is a large list of possible Adverse Drug Reactions (ADRs) with progesterone. Most of these are mild, transient and self limiting. The list includes allergic reactions, excessive sleeping to some theoretical effects on the fetus. But these fetal effects are not found with progesterones used for prevention of miscarriages.

HCG in Prevention of Obstetric Vasculopathies

One more hormone that requires to be touched here is hCG or Human Chorionic Gonadotropin. In these pages its role in preventing obstetric vasculopathies is being examined.

Hormonal Basis of hCG Administration

The rationale proposed for administering hCG is that endogenous hCG released through the zygote and then the chorionic tissue, stimulates the production of progesterone through the corpus luteum in pregnancy. This progesterone then acts to support a successful and healthy nidation and growth of the conceptus. On the other hand there are some objections raised to this rationale: The dosage required to stimulate corpus luteum by exogenous hCG will be massive as pregnancy is a state of hormonal boom. Massive amounts of hormones are produced and utilized in the body for a successful non-vasculopathic obstetric outcome. In that case will administering 5000 IU of hCG weekly suffice? Also, the dosage of hCG used by our group previously was 5000 IU intramuscularly every week. The half life of hCG is at best 72 hours. Thus administering hCG at the duration of once a week may be a low dose. This brings out one very important question: Is there something beyond the simple endocrinal action of hCG?

Immunological Basis of Using hCG

Due to the above reasons one low dose of hCG administration and weekly administration it was perceived that hCG should technically if administered in this way should not produce any results. But inspite of this “low dose”, there were studies and experiences in which hCG did produce results even at these schedules and dosages. This led to exploring of the possibility of hCG having effects beyond its biological half-life. The endocrinal (biological) half life of hCG is indeed 72 hours. Why it is that there are experiences which showed a successful prevention of obstetric vasculopathy even on administration at a weekly duration? The answer lies in the immunological face of hCG.

Every hormone has an endocrinal face and an immunological face. This immunological face is what seems to be acting if at all, in prevention of late I trimester and II trimester fetal demise leading to missed abortions. hCG is a master conductor of the immunological orchestra that brings about the immune tolerance in the mother. This aspect of immune tolerance has been extensively touched in other chapter (See Chapter 3).

The hCG oversees and even induces distinct changes in the maternal milieu in such a way that the mother learns to tolerate the alien immunological protein the fetus. It either generates changes in the trophoblasts to make them resist the immunological rejection of the mother. Alternatively it may be subduing the immune rejection process. It is also possible that exogenous and endogenous hCG may be doing both.

This brings one closer to the understanding of why lower doses of hCG are effective. Any immunological substance generates its effects much beyond the pharmacological dosage of its administration. The classical example of this is vaccine inoculums. Miniscule doses of vaccine antigens are able to generate a massive antibody response saving from specific diseases for years. Vaccine inoculums continue to have protective affect much beyond its presence in the body of the host. Decades after an immunologically active vaccine has been administered, the host gets protected from diseases for which the vaccine was administered. On the same basis low dose immunologically active substances can produce effects much more and totally disproportionate to the amount injected.

This is not to say that hCG is a vaccine. It indeed is not one. But this rationale helps understanding how its low doses can produce effective results much beyond the pharmacological half-life of the hormone administered. Therefore the immunological half-life of hCG seems to far outstrip the endocrinal half life. It is for this immunological face that hCG is effective at lower doses and that too well beyond the duration of its endocrinal activity.

We use hCG only in very few subjects for prevention of obstetric vasculopathies. These are essentially refractory subjects in whom fetal demise have occurred inspite of progesterone administration in the past. We also feel that till the time as hCG efficacy is completely ruled out or committed in science, it should be left to the discretion of the attending clinician if and when he/she wants to administer hCG in clinical practice. As mentioned we administer hCG only in refractory subjects in a dose of 5000 IU every weekly. This is commenced from the diagnosis of pregnancy as early as possible in 1-trimester. We continue hCG till 12 weeks of pregnancy. This is with a rationale that placenta takes over the function of corpus luteum. Also by this duration the immunological tolerance in whatever form is nearly set in the maternal system.

Antithrombotic Agents (Aspirin with or without Heparin) for Prevention of Obstetric Vasculopathies

Antithrombotic agents are as a group maximally researched and used in obstetric vasculopathy. What is all the more interesting is that the final answer to the efficacy of aspirin in prevention of obstetric vasculopathies still eludes us. Nonetheless the combination of aspirin and heparin has been found to be indeed effective in prevention of obstetric vasculopathy. Antithrombotic agents (aspirin and heparin) are efficient in small or large extent in preventing all obstetric vasculopathies. It is also to the credit of these two agents that they have remained popular with clinicians for more than two decades now and still continued to be used extensively. In this section it is planned to examine their possible mechanism of action, their activity singly and in combination and all allied aspects of these agents.

Possible Mechanims of Action of Antithrombotic Agents

The mechanism of action of both these antithrombotic agents is basically the same. However the details their action singly and in combination is reviewed here. Obstetric vasculopathies have vasospasm as its basic pathology. It is during this vasospasm that slowing down of blood circulation takes place. During this sluggish phase of blood circulation the lipids LDL and VLDL have a tendency to go closer to the activated endothelial lining. Some actually sink into the intercellular spaces. This space is between two endothelial cells.

In the intercellular space the free radicals are on the prowl. They quickly denature the lipids (VLDL and LDL) molecules that have sunk within. These free radicals have been generated by the activated endothelial lining at the fetomaternal interface. This activation has the failure of trophoblastic invasion and inefficient spiral arteriolar moulding at its root. This matter has been extensively discussed in chapters related to etiopathology of obstetric vasculopathies (See Chapters 3-5, 11).

Once denatured by the free radicals, these lipid molecules get flushed into the system when vasospasm locally is reduced. In this phase of reperfusion the denatured lipids go into the circulation. Wherever they go these denatured lipid molecules produce a vasospasm. This generates a vicious cycle of vasospasm - reperfusion—vasospasm. If confined to the fetomaternal interface it produces IUGR, still births and such fetal complications, when it is involving the entire maternal vasculature it results in pre-eclampsia.

Antithrombotic agents do not release the vasospasm. They act by preventing the sluggishness of blood stream while facing the obstruction of reduced vessel caliber in vasospasm. They tend to act by keeping the blood 'more liquid'. As a result blood continues to flow as a result of which the VLDLs and LDLs find it extremely difficult to come close to the endothelial lining. Resultantly these lipids do not get enough time to sink into the intercellular spaces. This prevents a denaturation and subsequent reperfusion damage. A sluggish blood stream is a strong prerequisite for the entire pathophysiology of obstetric vasculopathies to get triggered.

Antithrombotic agents predominantly combat this sluggishness. It therefore becomes clear by now that antithrombotic agents are not combating the cause of the vasospasm or the effects of decidual and other endothelial activation. This activation generates the free radicals which are all out to denature the lipid molecules that come in their close proximity. Antithrombotic agents therefore treat the effect of sluggishness and not the cause (vasospasm and reperfusion damages).

Studies that have concentrated on the dominant effect of antithrombotic agents on thromboxane prostacyclin imbalance have therefore produced inconsistent results thereby disillusioning the investigation. Those that concentrate on the balance expect antithrombotic agents to combat the cause of obstetric vasculopathies. Antithrombotic agents, on the contrary are preventing the effects and not the cause. They prevent the sluggishness of blood stream.

If the cause is intact and the effect is only combated the results are bound to be inconsistent. When the cause is neutralized the efficacy would be most conspicuous. Antithrombotic agents therefore have disillusioned those who concentrated on the treatment of cause and getting the preventive effects. On the other hand those who have grasped the entire pathophysiology in greater depth of both the disease as well as treating agents expect the results of their agents to be a shade lower as they are known to prevent the effects.

Bearings of Low Dose Aspirin

Traditionally aspirin is used in a dose of 300 to 500 mgm /day. But for prevention of obstetric vasculopathies this dose is not found to be necessary and can be downright harmful. The recommended dose of aspirin for this indication therefore is 1.2 mgm/kgs/day. This will come to 60 to 75 mgm of aspirin per day in an average sized woman.

Another important bearing that low dose aspirin has is on is adverse drug reactions. While aspirin makes the blood less hypercoagulable it does not paralyze the coagulation system significantly. The action of low-dose aspirin is predominantly on the platelets. Therefore if in a given clinical situation, a clinician needs to perform a cesarean section on a subject in whom aspirin could not be timely stopped, there would not be much serious Intraoperative difficulty. At the most there will be some increase in minor bleeds making the operative field a little more sanguine than normal. This can be easily handled by taking the stitches tightly it being a platelet based bleeding it is easily stopped by a tight pressure generated by tight stitches.

One more fear that aspirin use had was premature closure of Ductus Arteriosus in the fetus of pregnant subjects in whom it is antenatally given. As is well known prostaglandins have a very important role in maintaining the patency of Ductus Arteriosus during intrauterine life of the unborn fetus. Aspirin is also as antiprostaglandin NSAID. There were fears in the initial days of aspirin administration of this possible adverse drug reaction leading to intrauterine fetal death.

The Early Days

We remember a subject in whom we had stated aspirin in very early days of our using this agent. The subject indeed had an unexplained intrauterine fetal death. At that time we did try to attribute it to the aspirin that we had given. It was not until later in late 1990s and early 2000 AD that we realized that the dosage in which we gave aspirin the chances of premature closure of Ductus Arteriosus was nil. Those were the days of clinical monitoring of the fetal conditions. We did not have an access to CTG and color Doppler technology was still settling.

This case did not leave our mind till the detailed analysis that we did for years solved our dilemma. This subject was given aspirin after her preeclampsia had become clinically manifested. Therefore if at all aspirin can prevent, the prevention is more or less confined to prevention of worsening of obstetric vasculopathy. Also in absence of an access to CTG or color Doppler it was not possible to accurately know much about the fetal well being. Therefore what seemed to be sudden unexplained fetal death could actually be a slow, steady and progressive deterioration in the condition of the fetal condition. Finally post mortem of the fetus could not be done as the parents refused consent. As a result years later we analyzed to find that it may not have been the premature closure of ductus at all that killed this fetus.

However this one event made us refine, review and re-review our administration of aspirin very watchfully. As a result after more than two decades of its use we are now much better equipped and much more confident in handling antithrombotic agents in prevention of obstetric vasculopathies.

While still on early days it is timely to record one more challenge that we faced in administering aspirin. It was related to the availability of low dose aspirin. Aspirin that was then available to us was in the more popular 300 mgm tablets. To convert this to 75 mgm we had to use nutcrackers and divide each tablet into four seemingly equal parts. Thereby we could get our first access to 75 mgm of aspirin what subsequently became popular as low dose aspirin. It was nearly five years of our administering in this way that one pharmaceutical manufacturer locally agreed to use the wastage generated from making a round tablet of aspirin of 300 mgm to produce 75 mgm aspirin formulation for us.

We transmitted this good news of getting a well made scientific formulation of low dose aspirin available to our colleagues that the non-skeptics amongst us also started using this formulation. Soon international early literature also started flowing in on this matter. Once the pharmaceutical manufactures realized the potential of this formulation many other companies also started manufacturing this 75 mgm and even 60 mgm formulations solving our problem completely.

As pioneers in this aspect of the subject there were many questions on all possible aspects of this agent. I vividly remember an episode that happened when I had delivered an oration on the subject decades ago. One cardiologist also attended the oration. He pointedly asked about what I meant by "low-dose aspirin". This I could very well reply as we were already working in this field for nearly a decade by then. As if by miracle even in cardiology this dose soon got accepted and rest as they say is history.

In one of our studies on allied aspects of these conditions, we found that when low-dose aspirin was given to subjects with raised β-hCG at midtrimester adverse obstetric outcomes like miscarriages were reduced and favorable outcomes like full term deliveries increased.[8] This has already been referred to in the chapter on Prediction of Obstetric Vasculopathies (See Chapter 17).

Low-Dose Heparin

The other most popular and rational use for prevention of obstetric vasculopathy is heparin. Heparin is being used by us for nearly two decades now. It has met with a reasonable success. Heparin is usually used in combination with low dose aspirin.

Rationale: The rationale for use of heparin in obstetric vasculopathies is similar to aspirin. It permanently paralyses the platelets by its action on cyclooxygenase enzyme. Thus rendered incompetent the blood continues to flow with relative ease through the reduced caliber of blood vessels thereby preventing the denaturation process of lipids. Another possible rationale that acts concurrently is the possibility that platelet activation a very important component of etiopathology of obstetric vasculopathies gets blunted. Thereby the perpetuation of the entire chain of event that activates the process of obstetric vasculopathies is broken. Thus heparin acts by preventing the causation and sustenance of the process of obstetric vasculopathies.

Which heparin: A very consistently asked question is which heparin should be given? Two types of heparin are available in the market. One is the regular heparin as it is called and the other is the low molecular weight heparin. The answer to this question is critical as price factor is involved. The low molecular weight heparin is much more costly than regular heparin. The answer to this question is: does not matter. Both these formulations are equally effective. There is no significant difference in the ADRs of both these formulations of heparin. In late 1990s and early 2000 there was a belief that regular heparin needed much more monitoring for alteration in coagulation profile when administered for a long period of time. Therefore it was recommended that the two platelet dependant parameter prothrombin time (PT) and activated partial thromboplastin time (APTT) should be performed every two to three weeks in subjects on regular heparin. No such monitoring was required for low molecular weight heparin.

However over a period of time it has been found that none of the two need any such monitoring in the dosage in which they are given. Therefore if cost is an important factor, regular heparin can be safely given for prevention of obstetric vasculopathies.

Dose of heparin: We use regular heparin as cost is a factor in our practice. The dose of heparin that we use is 5000 IU subcutaneously (SC) daily. This heparin is started as soon as pregnancy is diagnosed and is continued till 36 weeks of pregnancy. It is discontinued thenafter and labor induced at 37 weeks. There are many aspects involved in reaching this recommendation of heparin dosage and schedule. It is necessary to examine each of these.

About 5000 IU of heparin is the prophylactic dose of heparin. The therapeutic dose of heparin is upto 10,000 IU given SC daily. However in prevention of obstetric vasculopathies we are not using its therapeutic action but prophylactic action. so it is not necessary to administer 10,000 IU of heparin SC daily.

The rationale of discontinuing heparin at 36 weeks and then allowing a gap of seven days for any obstetric intervention is also warranting an explanation. As has been clarified in the mechanism of action, heparin acts by rendering the platelets incompetent and suboptimal in activity. This change is mediated through the cyclooxygenase pathway. This change is permanent. The average life span of platelets is 72 hours. By 72 to 96 hours the entire crop of platelets in the body is replaced. As a result of this if any operative obstetric performance is to be performed, it will be under a fresh crop of platelets. Thus there will not be any excess oozing in the operative field even if cesarean section is performed.

While still on the dosage, it is worth mentioning that since last five years we have been using a higher dose of heparin in some specific indications. This dosage is 5000 IU given SC twice a day (instead of once a day). This dosage schedule is used for refractory subjects of obstetric vasculopathies. By refractory subjects it is meant as those subjects who do not respond to the usual 5000 IU given SC every day. They develop obstetric vasculopathy and also have pregnancy wastage like a severe IUGR or a still birth. Subjects who develop a severe preeclampsia or a full blown eclampsia are also considered as refractory obstetric vasculopathy. Basically these are subjects who had an obstetric vasculopathy in the past. They were once managed with 5000 IU of SC heparin. But they failed to register a favorable outcome in the next pregnancy. These subjects are managed with 5000 IU of heparin administered SC twice a day every 12 hourly.

The basis of this alteration in dosage schedule of heparin is the fact that obstetric vasculopathy seems to be furious in these subjects. While striking a balance between therapeutic dose of 10,000 IU given SC twice a day and 5000 IU given SC once a day, 5000 IU given SC twice a day is the mean that is worked out. This is between the full therapeutic dose and the low prophylactic dose.

Monitoring subjects on heparin: One cumbersome aspect of heparin that clinicians find difficult to follow is the possible need to monitor subjects on heparin. However it is being restated that there is no need to specially monitor subjects of low dose heparin for any adverse side effects. This is applicable to both types of heparin the regular heparin and low molecular weight heparin. This is in relation to the alteration in coagulation profile that may occur due to heparin administration.

One more fear that is occasionally expressed regarding such relative long-term use of heparin is the possibility of osteopenia. It has not been found in subjects on heparin use for prevention of obstetric vasculopathies.

When to stop heparin? (compliance issues): The recommendation of stopping heparin at 36 weeks one week before a planned intervention is a general recommendation that is being followed for years now. However in science, any fact or policy remains settled only till someone else unsettles it. Such an unsettling seems to be on the horizon for discontinuation of heparin. Long-term use of heparin is a big challenge to the compliance of the subjects who are placed on it. Apparently clinicians have been able to achieve this compliance due to the fact that the subjects have undergone unnerving adverse obstetric outcomes due to obstetric vasculopathies. As a result they are understandably ready to undertake this cumbersome dosage routine of subcutaneous heparin administration daily.

Most of these subjects or their partners learn how to administer heparin eliminating the need to go to a clinic or a hospital daily. Their morale is further boosted by counseling them to the fact that subjects with insulin-dependent diabetes have to take insulin in the same way once or twice a day for years together. All these efforts and understandings together have been able to achieve a near complete compliance for heparin use in subjects for preventing obstetric vasculopathies.

When to stop heparin (different perspective): Modern technology and understanding of the etiopathology in better details seem to open up new possibilities regarding discontinuation of heparin. This needs to be understood in details before reaching clinical conclusions. Going back to the etiopathology of obstetric vasculopathies, it is now settled and well understood that the critical phenomenon of second wave of trophoblastic invasion moulds the spiral arterioles at the fetomaternal interface to get a healthy and thriving pregnancy going. Defective, suboptimal or failure of this phenomenon is the basis of obstetric vasculopathies.

Color Doppler documents the successful completion of second wave of trophoblastic invasion or failure of the same. The most well documented sign is the disappearance of the diastolic notch at midtrimester. Persistence of diastolic notch in uterine artery color Doppler is a sign of suboptimal or failed trophoblastic invasion in its second wave. This imaging sign can be used to discontinue heparin in clinical practice.

Heparin is started in any given subject of obstetric vasculopathy for prevention, as soon as the diagnosis mentioned this heparin is continued till 36 weeks or if a rare adverse obstetric outcome warranting an obstetric intervention whichever occurs earlier. However we have been discontinuing heparin in subjects in whom the diastolic notch disappears at midtrimester about 20 to 24 weeks of pregnancy. The rationale for thus early discontinuation is the fact that once the second wave of trophoblastic invasion has been complete there is no need to continue heparin. In these subjects heparin can be discontinued much earlier. As and when a subject and heparin shows a disappearance of diastolic notch, there is no reason to continue with heparin. The oxidative stress which if at all it occurs is at a very low intensity. This can be easily combated by the maternal reducing systems. In other words these subjects will not develop severe and stormy forms of obstetric vasculopathies. Therefore they can be put off heparin now.

Indications of heparin: By and large, heparin is not started as a first-line defense against obstetric vasculopathies. This is principally because of the need to administer it in the form of injectable preparations. There are some subjects however in whom heparin needs to be started as first-line defense. This includes.

- Subjects in whom aspirin has failed in the past
- Subjects who test positive for LAC as well as anticardiolipin antibodies
- Subjects in whom life threatening complications of obstetric vasculopathies like renal or coagulation failure or term fetal demise have occurred.

In these subjects aspirin plus heparin combination is started at the first instance. In other subjects however only aspirin is administered as anti-vasculopathy agent. It is also relevant at this stage to note that aspirin plus heparin in combination always gives better results than aspirin alone. Had it not been for the route of administration of heparin, this combination would have easily become the first line management against obstetric vasculopathies.

Practical clinical challenges with heparin use: Besides the route of daily administration of heparin there are certain challenges in heparin administration, which tends to make an average clinician a little fearful of this drug. These are never major challenges and therefore when a need to administer heparin arises, a clinician should not hesitate to do so. By deciding against administering just because of our fear, the subject of vasculopathy is deprived of a very nice agent to prevent her from getting stormy adverse obstetric outcome.

The biggest fear is the fear of a need to carry out any operative intervention in subjects on heparin. It is not relevant here as to which indications of surgery may be required but more important is the fact that heparin acts on platelets. It permanently paralyzes their activity. In such an event if any surgical intervention is undertaken the subject can have some amount of diffuse and minor oozing from the tissue which is more than normal. However this bleeding is never life threatening. Also, this bleeding can be easily handled by applying local pressure as this is platelet related bleeding. The operating doctor has to suture the tissues a little more tightly than is being normally done. Therefore this bleeding should never be a fear to postpone a surgery or not starting heparin in subject with history of vasculopathy.

It goes without saying that if it is a planned surgery it would be advisable to postpone the surgery by a week during which heparin is discontinued after which the surgery is undertaken. The rationale for this has already been discussed.

One more point that clinicians consider and ask opinion about is regarding administering oral anticoagulants. Through oral anticoagulants have been tried in pregnancy, they were thought to be teratogenic and therefore having a limited use in pregnancy. Over a period of time however Warfarin has been used and tried in pregnancy. The fear of teratogenicity seems to have been overhyped. In spite of this the use and popularity of oral anticoagulants in general and Warfarin in particular has remained limited.

Another practical question that is asked by clinicians relates to the use of antidotes to heparin in subjects warranting emergency surgery while still on heparin. Antidotes like protamine sulphate have been found to be very effective in preventing and neutralizing the actions of heparin. But in clinical practice the situation is never so severe enough to warrant Protamine Sulphate administration. It is important to note that heparin is administered in dosages of 5000 IU subcutaneously. In such a dose, protamine administration may not be necessary at all.

Another point that is raised is related to the fear of stopping heparin for a week before an elective surgery is planned. The fear is will it worsen the under running obstetric vasculopathy. The answer to this is no. In the entire plan of things, obstetric vasculopathy prevention is a long drawn process. Thus suspending the prevention method by a week or maximum ten days will not make any significant difference.

Antithrombotic Agents: Review of Literature

Having had examined and discussed the intricacies of antithrombotic agents in the prevention of obstetric vasculopathies, it will be worthwhile to review the literature available and published on this matter. One study performed a meta-analysis to assess the influence of gestational age at the time of introduction of ASA on the incidence of preeclampsia in women at increased risk, on the basis of abnormal uterine artery Doppler. It was found that ASA treatment initiated early in pregnancy is an efficient method of reducing the incidence of preeclampsia and its consequences in women with ultrasonographic evidence of abnormal placentation diagnosed by uterine artery Doppler studies.[9] A series of studies on this matter were subjected to a meta-analysis that concluded that aspirin in low-dose is highly effective in preventing obstetric vasculopathies especially preeclampsia and IUGR.[10]

Two large multicentric trials were undertaken amidst, popularly known as CLASP and ECPPA trials. They showed limited utility of low-dose aspirin in prevention of preeclampsia CLASP study in fact did show a reduction in the incidence of proteinuric hypertension and IUGR.[11,12] However these and other large trials were roundly criticized for poor compliance, gestational age at randomization and heterogeneity of dosage of the drug, etc. inspite of all these, doubts were raised on the efficacy of aspirin in consistently reducing the incidence of pre-eclampsia. Similar studies have also been under way as regards aspirin and low-dose heparin combination.

PREVENTION OF ECLAMPSIA

Another area which has evinced keen interest in obstetric vasculopathy is prevention of eclampsia. One of the most furious and potentially lethal forms of obstetric vasculopathies is eclampsia. Maternal mortality and morbidity climbs up steeply as soon as the subject throws an eclamptic fit. Measures to prevent eclampsia have been more intensely studied than other obstetric vasculopathies.

Thankfully in this matter quite clear and convincing messages emerge from the results and experiences available. Prevention of eclampsia is based or three pronged approaches:

1. Prevention of eclampsia by preventing the worsening of pre-eclampsia.
2. Prevention of preeclampsia itself and
3. Prevention of subsequent attack of convulsion in a subject who has already thrown a convulsive episode.

For the prevention of developing eclampsia in a subject with severe preeclampsia is now well established. Also preventing subsequent convulsion in a subject with eclampsia is now a settled issue. For both these magnesium sulphate is universally established as the agent of choice.

While focusing on measures to prevent eclampsia, magnesium sulphate has been found to be singularly effective globally. The scientific world continues to tinker with the dosage schedule of the drug. The original dosage schedule proposed as the so called "Parkland Memorial Regime" was administration of 5 gms. of magnesium sulphate every four hourly in subjects of reverse preeclampsia (or imminent eclampsia as they have described). This administration was recommended for upto 24 hours post-delivery.

For a subject who already has at the least one convulsive episode, the dosage schedule that was recommended was 14 gms bolus dose initially followed by 5 gms intramuscularly every four hourly. This was to be continued till 24 hours of delivery or 24 hours of the last convulsive episode whichever was earlier. 14gms. bolus was recommended to be administered as 5 gms on each buttock and 4gms of magnesium sulphate administered slowly intravenously, over a period of twenty minutes. This was very promising and was giving best results.

The earliest change in the dosage schedule came from developing countries including our group. This was found to be necessary due to low weight and body mass of mothers in our part of the world. 5 gms of the drug administered was found to have a higher chance of development of toxicity of magnesium sulphate. As a result the dosage was changed from 5gms 4 hourly to 5 gms 6 hourly. All other aspects like the bolus dose for prevention of subsequent convulsion and continuation of the drug till 24 hours after delivery/last convulsion whichever was earlier remained unchanged.

Another change that was followed by some groups was a complete shift to intravenous magnesium sulfate. This schedule of administration included intravenous continuous administration of magnesium sulfate at the rate of 1gm. of magnesium sulfate per hour. This is continued till 24 hours of last convulsion whichever was earlier.

Another dosage schedule that was recommended was the so called low-dose magnesium sulfate. In this the dose of drug administered was reduced. There were two principle fears with magnesium sulfate that led to this myriad of different dosage schedules. One was the fear of magnesium sulfate toxicity. This toxicity could be potentially lethal and therefore scary. The other fear was the reduced requirement of the drug in the tropics. It was perceived that these petite women in the tropics especially the Indian subcontinent needed less drug for achieving results of preventing eclampsia.

There is a small group of subjects who present as recalcitrant eclampsia. In these subjects it is recommended to give a top-up dose of magnesium sulfate early. Thenafter the subsequent doses are calculated as per the time duration of six hours from this top-up dose.

While still on prevention of eclampsia, it will be worthwhile to mention prevention of fits in status eclampticus the dreaded form of eclampsia. In these subjects Pentothal sodium remains the agents of choice.

Besides magnesium sulfate many other agents were used to prevent eclampsia. It is beyond the scope of the current discussion to review them. They are mentioned only as a passing reference. It included agents like diazepam, pethidine, Phenargan and a tizzy combination of these in the form of lytic cocktail. All these were basically sedatives more than anticonvulsives. Their results therefore were suboptimal and so they lost their popularity over a period of time.

REFERENCES

1. Lindheimer M, Roberts J, Cunningham F, Chesley L. In: Lindheimer M, Roberts J, Cunningham F, editors: Chesley, Hypertensive disorders of pregnancy. Stamford, Appleton and Lange. 2nd edn. 1998, Page 36
2. Sibai B. Treatment of hypertension in pregnancy women. *N Engl J Med.* 1996;335:257-65.
3. Fodor A, Gyorffy A, Váradi M, Fülesdi B, Major T. The possible options for the prevention of preeclampsia. *Orv Hetil.* 2012;153(4):144-51.
4. Belizean J, Villar J, Repke J. The relationship between calcium intake and pregnancy induced hypertension: Upto date evidence. *Am J Obstet Gynecol.* 1988;158:898-902.
5. Hofmeyr G, Lawrie T, Atallah A, Duley L. Calcium supplementation during pregnancy for preventing hypertensive disorders and related problems. *Cochrane Database Syst Rev.* 2010;4(8):CD001059.
6. Briceño-Pérez C, Briceño-Sanabria L, Vigil-De Gracia P. Prediction and prevention of preeclampsia. *Hypertens Pregnancy.* 2009;28(2):138-55.
7. Oken E, Ning Y, Rifas-Shiman S, Rich-Edwards J, Olsen S, Gillman M. Diet during pregnancy and risk of preeclampsia or gestational hypertension. *Ann Epidemiol.* 2007;17(9):663-8.
8. Desai P, Rao S. Role of low dose aspirin in mothers registering high serum hCG levels at mid trimester. *Jr O and G of India.* 2002;52(5):30-2.
9. Bujold E, Morency A, Roberge S, Lacasse Y, Forest J, Giguère Y. Acetylsalicylic acid for the prevention of preeclampsia and intra-uterine growth restriction in women with abnormal uterine artery Doppler: a systematic review and meta-analysis. *J Obstet Gynaecol Can.* 2009;31(9):818-26.
10. Bujold E, Roberge S, Lacasse Y, Bureau M, Audibert F, Marcoux S, Forest J, Giguère Y. Prevention of preeclampsia and intrauterine growth restriction with aspirin started in early pregnancy: a meta-analysis. *Obstet Gynecol.* 2010;116(2 Pt 1):402-14.
11. CLASP: A randomized trial of low dose aspirin in prevention and treatment of preeclampsia among 9364 pregnant women. *Lancet.* 1994;343:619-29.
12. ECPPA: Randomized trial of low dose aspirin for the prevention of maternal and fetal complications' in high-risk pregnant women. *Br J Obstet and Gynecol.* 1996;103:39-47.

CHAPTER

19

Color Doppler in Obstetric Vasculopathies

CHAPTER OUTLINE

- Color Doppler in Early Pregnancy
- Third Trimester Color Doppler in Obstetric Vasculopathies
- Color Doppler for Discontinuation of Antithrombotic Agents
- Fetal Aortic Doppler Studies

INTRODUCTION

It has been previously mentioned that color Doppler is the "game-changer" in the entire approach and understanding of obstetric vasculopathies in relevance to different points in this monogram. Though it may sound repetitive, this matter is being covered separately as a complete chapter to give one-stop information on color Doppler in obstetric vasculopathies comprehensively. It is not envisaged to cover the basic physics and similar aspects of the technology involved but only the clinical applications of this technology is covered.

In recent years, the characterizations of Doppler ultrasound patterns and fetal surveillance have contributed significantly to decrease the adverse perinatal outcome in obstetric vasculopathies. In this regard, there is one study that needs to be mentioned here. Imdad A et al performed a systematic review with a focus on reduction of obstetric vasculopathy (IUGR) related stillbirths. They found that Doppler velocimetry of umbilical and fetal arteries and appropriate intervention is associated with 29% reduction in perinatal mortality.[1] This is important also from the negative aspect of the fact that it does not have much role in monitoring low-risk subjects for obstetric vasculopathies. This makes it result-competent.

COLOR DOPPLER IN EARLY PREGNANCY

In early pregnancy, color Doppler use step in at around 12 to 14 weeks. This is the time when and USG becomes a very vital contributor to management of subjects with history of obstetric vasculopathies. Latest by 13 to 14 weeks, if not earlier pregnant subjects are subjected to soft tissue screening for chromosomal anomalies like T21, T18, etc. This is done by achieving scan markers like nuchal translucency (NT), presence of nasal bone (NB), tricuspid incompetence and study of blood flow through ductus venosus. Although none of these markers are in a position to predict any of the obstetric vasculopathies singly or together, uterine artery Doppler at this stage may be able to have some importance.

In normal pregnancy, almost always at this duration, the uterine artery will show a presence of diastolic notch. This is the small dip in the wave found just before the diastolic wave begins (Fig. 19.1). Presence of a diastolic notch at this stage of pregnancy is usual and normal. However, there will be some subjects in whom even as early as 12 to 14 weeks of pregnancy, the diastolic notch is absent. These are subjects of interest. Presence of diastolic notch suggests that the second wave of trophoblastic invasion is still not complete. It also suggests that the process may be ongoing but still not over. Presence of diastolic notch in these subjects has got no much significance except indicating that the process is ongoing.

Nevertheless, those small percentage of subjects in whom the diastolic notch is absent as early as late 1 trimester, the second wave of trophoblastic invasion can complete so early. There is no rule that trophoblastic invasion can never occur so early. In some subjects it does and one can predict the chances of developing obstetric vasculopathies so early. They will be low in these subjects.

What is Diastolic Notch?

In normal pregnancy almost always at 12 to 14 weeks of duration, the uterine artery shows presence of a diastolic notch (Fig. 19.1). This is the small dip found just before the diastolic wave begins as mentioned in the preceding paragraph. Presence of diastolic notch suggests that the second wave of trophoblastic invasion is still not complete. It suggests that the process may be ongoing but still not over. Presence of diastolic notch in these subjects at 12–14 weeks may not have much significance except indicating that the process is ongoing. Disappearance of the diastolic notch seems to be a very reliable predictor of obstetric vasculopathy. This occurs at around mid-trimester or thereafter anytime.

Over a period of time disappearance of diastolic notch seems to be a popular predictor of obstetric vasculopathies especially of preeclampsia and IUGR.

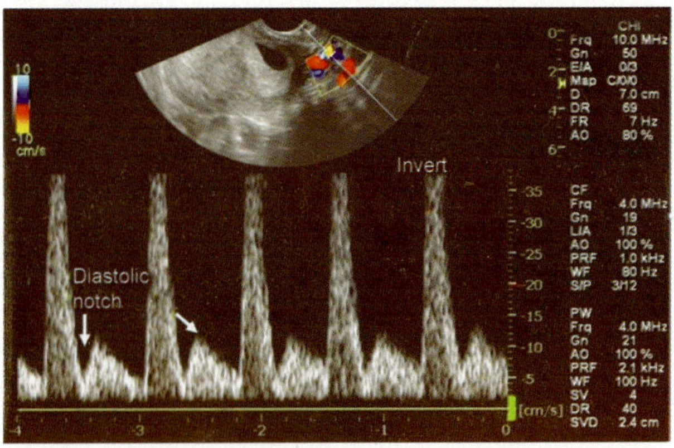

Fig.19.1: Uterine artery diastolic notch

Chan and coworkers showed that the combination of a diastolic notch and an abnormal resistance index in both uterine arteries at 20 weeks gestation is the most accurate indicator in predicting severe pregnancy complications. These subjects are almost eight times more likely to develop either clinically significant hypertension and/or deliver prior to 32 weeks and/or have a perinatal demise or have an infant with a birth weight of less than 1500 grams.[2]

Disappearance of diastolic notch at mid-trimester (Fig. 19.2) alone has also been studied for this purpose. However, one study has shown that in high-risk subjects, disappearance of diastolic notch at mid trimester in uterine artery Doppler waveform analysis if used alone, may not be a good screening method for obstetric vasculopathies.[3]

Inconsistent Notch

One more point needs to be reviewed here. There is always a distinct group of subjects who show "inconsistent" presence of diastolic notch. By this, it is meant that in at least four (arbitrarily decided figure) out of ten waves examined the diastolic notch is absent. It is present in other waves but not all. What is the significance of such inconsistent notch is a matter of further study.

Inconsistent presence of diastolic notch has been found even in subjects at mid-trimester (to be covered in details later). Do these have any meaning? Does it indicate that some amount of trophoblastic invasion is complete? Does it mean that these subjects may not require any preventive measures? Does it mean that preventive measure can be discontinued? These entire set of questions remain to be answered.

Notch Index and Notch Depth Index

Quantitative index: The Notch Depth Index (NDI) has been developed and evaluated for its association with the risk of obstetric vasculopathies like preeclampsia and a small-for-gestational-age (SGA) infant. It is calculated as the depth of the diastolic notch divided by the maximal diastolic velocity (Fig. 19.3).

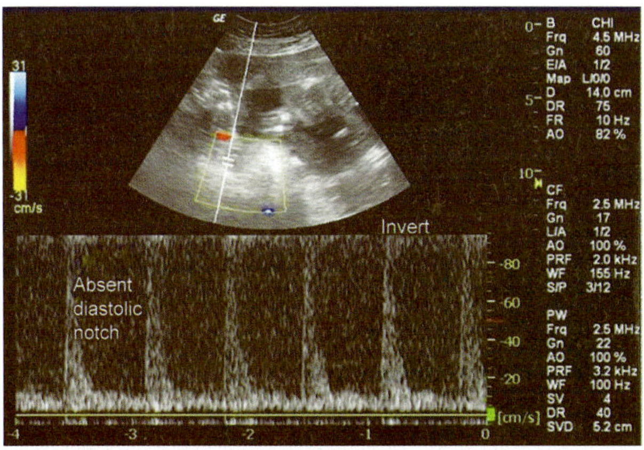

Fig. 19.2: Disappeared diastolic notch in II trimester

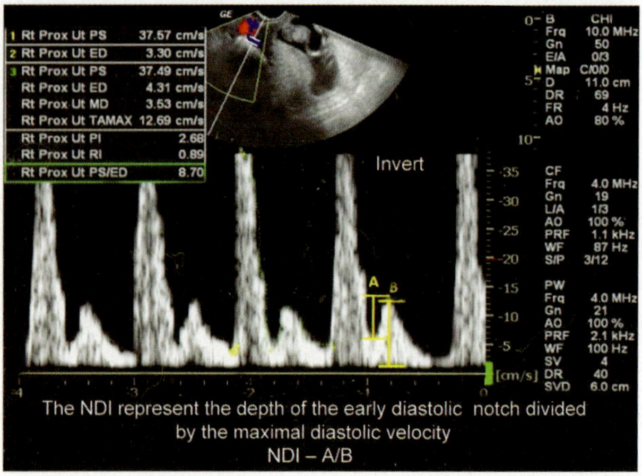

Fig.19.3: NDI: Notch depth index

Ohkuchi A et al evaluated association of the NDI with the risk of pre-eclampsia and a small-for-gestational-age (SGA) infant and to compare its clinical usefulness with that of the uterine artery resistance index (RI) and the peak systolic to early diastolic velocity (S/D) ratio. They studied in 288 consecutive healthy pregnant subjects at 20.2 ± 2.0 (range 16.0–23.9) weeks of gestation and found that the NDI value in the second trimester is associated with the later onset of pre-eclampsia, and is clinically more useful in predicting pre-eclampsia than the two conventional indices.[4]

Color Doppler Indices in Early Pregnancy: Any Role in Prediction?

There are very few signs based on technology whose presence or absence has a great value indicating some clinical event. Technology right from the time thermometers were introduced to measure fever, have calibrated values. So the values range or ratios are expressed to indicate and measure different aspects of human body. The diastolic notch seems to be an exception to this rule. Apparently simplistically, disappearance of the diastolic notch seems to be a very reliable predictor of obstetric vasculopathy. However, as is well known, color Doppler also calculates blood flow and this is expressed as different indices. The most useful and popular among these are the Pulsatility Index (PI), Resistance Index (RI), and Systolic to Diastolic ratio (S:D ratio). These values are calculated by the machine itself.

The majority of blood flow to the uterus is supplied by the uterine arteries. Blood flow through these vessels can increase up to ten to twelve fold by the time term is reached. Besides the second wave of trophoblastic invasion, the massive increase in blood volume also adds to the increase in blood flow through uterine arteries. The shape of blood flow through uterine arteries is unique and changes its configuration as pregnancy advances. These changes are a valuable tool for the clinician in many decision makings in obstetric vasculopathies.

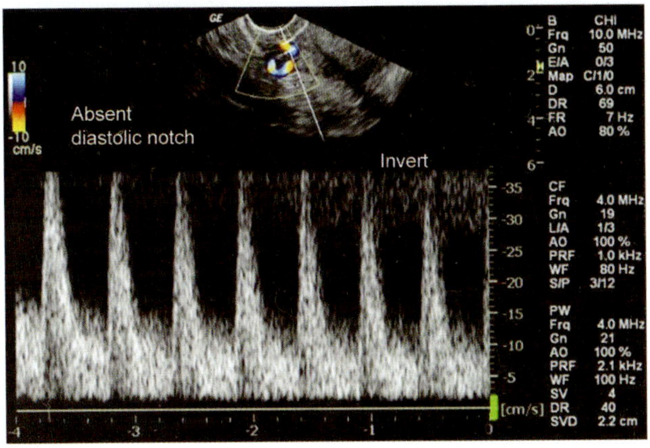

Fig. 19.4: Diastolic notch disappeared in first trimester itself

Although most of the scientific world involved in uterine artery Doppler study for prediction of obstetric vasculopathy concentrated on disappearance of diastolic notch there were some who considered the indices also. It was found that a change of uterine artery PI between the first and second trimesters is the best index in predicting early preeclampsia and preeclampsia of early onset.[5] Interestingly, Belfort M et al have used Middle Cerebral Artery (MCA) Doppler resistance indices to predict development of preeclampsia. They found that low MCA resistance values in the second trimester are predictive of the subsequent development of preeclampsia in a low risk, ethnically homogenous population.[6]

There are also some studies that have studied the role of these indices in I trimester between 11 to 13 weeks. In clinical practice, one sees many occasions when the diastolic notch may disappear in I trimester itself (Fig. 19.4). How accurate was I Trimester assessment of this finding singly or in combination with other indices of uterine artery blood flow for early prediction of obstetric vasculopathies warranted a review. Rattanapuntamanee and Uerpairojkit determined uterine artery pulsatility index (PI) to describe the characteristic of uterine artery Doppler velocimetry in pregnant Thai subjects at 11–13 (+6) gestational weeks. They found that when segregated for gestation age, uterine artery PI was 1.78 ± 0.41 at 11 weeks, 1.72 ± 0.41 at 12 weeks, and 1.66 ± 0.43 at 13 weeks' gestation. The uterine artery Pl was 1.84 ± 0.37 with presence of notching and was 1.59 ± 0.43 without notching. The uterine artery notching was present in 19.3%, 16% and 18% of the patients at 11, 12, and 13 weeks respectively. The uterine artery notching was absent in 18%, 15.3% and 13.3% of patients at 11, 12, and 13 weeks respectively.[7] This group found that even in I trimester uterine artery diastolic notch in combination with other parameters seems to be a good test for prediction of obstetric vasculopathies particularly PIH and IUGR.

Another study assessed the role of uterine artery Doppler studies at 11–14 weeks in screening for pre-eclampsia (PET), small for gestational age (SGA) fetuses, and placental abruption—all major constitutes of obstetric vasculopathies. It is a prospective study on 1,123 subjects presenting for routine ultrasound examination at 11–14 weeks for nuchal translucency measurement. Uterine artery blood flow (Fig. 19.5) was studied by transvaginal color Doppler, the mean pulsatility index (PI) was calculated, and the presence of a diastolic notch was recorded. It was found that abnormal uterine Dopplers at 11–14 weeks identified one-third of subjects with severe early onset pre-eclampsia, all fetuses with SGA ≤ 5th centile that were delivered at ≤ 34 weeks, and 40% of cases with placental abruption. Uterine artery Doppler examination at the 11–14 weeks scan can identify a high-risk population in which preventive or therapeutic interventions might be effective.[8]

Another study undertaken to evaluate the association between uterine artery Doppler velocimetry performed between 10 and 14 weeks gestation and intrauterine growth restriction. The uterine artery mean resistance index (RI) for the entire cohort was equal on the right and left sides (0.59 ± 0.14). Of the 1067 subjects, 34.2% had unilateral or bilateral diastolic notches, 1 notch was observed in 23.8%, and bilateral notches in 10.4%. It was found that subjects with a high uterine artery mean RI (≥ 75th percentile) were 5.5 times more likely to have IUGR (95% CI 1.6–18.7). There was no significant relationship between notching and IUGR. It concluded that elevated first trimester uterine artery mean RI is significantly associated with IUGR.[9] This study further confirmed the efficacy of uterine artery diastolic notch in combination with other parameters in prediction of obstetric vasculopathies even in I trimester.

It therefore seems clear that even I trimester screening of uterine artery blood flow is reasonably competent in identifying high-risk subjects for developing conditions of obstetric vasculopathies. The advantage of such an early screening is obvious. It will allow an early instituting of preventive measures. These results are still very early and so as of now the presence or absence of diastolic notch at mid trimester remains the only established indicator of an impending obstetric vasculopathy.

THIRD TRIMESTER COLOR DOPPLER IN OBSTETRIC VASCULOPATHIES

In advanced pregnancy the role of color Doppler becomes more extensive and versatile. There is no need of its predictive role. At this stage the vessels under study completely change. Also, at this stage venous Doppler also steps in and

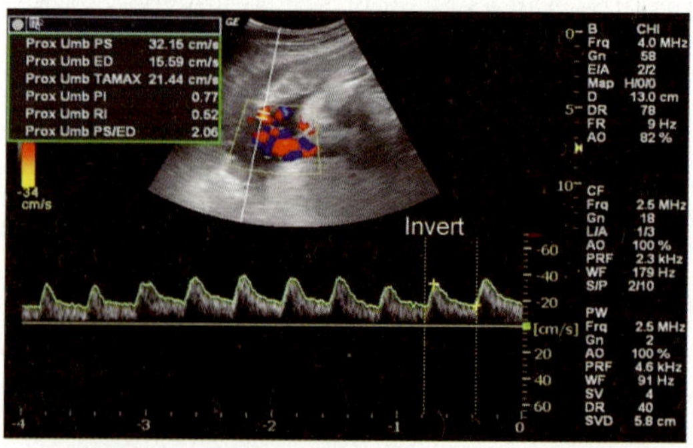

Fig.19.5: Normal uterine artery flow at 39 weeks

has an important role to play. The main arteries that are imaged for obstetric vasculopathies are umbilical artery (UA) and middle cerebral artery (MCA). The venous flow that is most commonly imaged is the flow in ductus venosus (DV), IVC and sometimes in the umbilical vein. It should however, be noted that if the flow through the arteries is good and is maintained so in spite of the obstetric vasculopathy, there is no need of venous flow imaging.

Umbilical Artery Flow

It is well known that blood flow faces very little resistance while flowing through the umbilical arteries. As pregnancy advances this low impedance or low resistance flow is also characterized by a good diastolic flow. Technically this is expressed as a umbilical flow being a low impedance flow with the end diastolic flow increasing progressively as pregnancy approaches term. This is a direct reflection of the increase in requirement of well-oxygenated blood by the developing fetus. The fetus not only grows in size but requires well-oxygenated blood. This supply is seen through the umbilical arteries. It is true that umbilical arterial flow reflects the status of placental circulation. Also the increase in end-diastolic flow reflects an increase in the number of tertiary stem villi that takes place with placental maturation.

In the two most prevalent obstetric vasculopathies preeclampsia and IUGR, there occur profound changes in vascular caliber and blood flow. As a result, the umbilical artery flow accurately reflects the happening at the fetomaternal interface. Obliteration of these vessels leads to a progressive decline in the end diastolic flow (Fig. 19.6) showing absent end-diastolic flow followed terminally by reversal of flow is seen.

Reversal of diastolic flow is a grave sign. It is estimated that more than 70% of vascular channels get obliterated to register this sign. Reversal of diastolic flow in umbilical artery is of grave connotation and warrants an immediate decision-making for intervention leading to delivery. Interestingly it is consistently associated with oligohydramnios.

For reasons of making things complex, different studies have compared the standard three color Doppler indices (PI, RI, and S:D ratio) in different segments of the umbilical cord. Through there may be some minor differences, these are

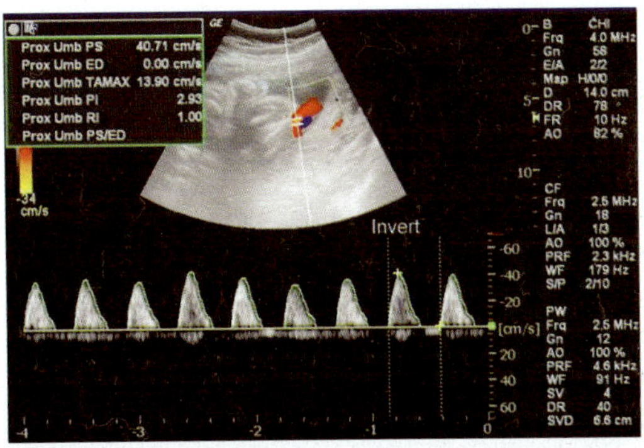

Fig.19.6: Absent end-diastolic flow in umbilical artery

never so profound to make much differenc in clinical practice. Technically, therefore, we do not bother much on this aspect in our practicee.

Because of its easy accessibility to examination and sensitivity in reflecting the status of fetal circulation, umbilical artery imaging is the most popularly studied of all vessels in the fetus. It is interesting that alterations in umbilical artery indices are consistent and show a distinct stability in all the three indices (PI, RI and S:D ratio). They all show a decline progressively with advancing pregnancy. All these indices do show a distinct fall early in pregnancy. This is usually attributes to the fall in fetal heart rate. But color Doppler studies of early pregnancy umbilical artery is not of much clinical significance.

Middle Cerebral Artery Flow

Among all the central vessels, middle cerebral artery (MCA) is most accessible to Doppler imaging. Also this vascular channel carries most of the cerebral blood and has a great importance in diagnosis and decision making in obstetric vasculopathies. It is estimated that it carries upto 80% of cerebral blood.

In normal circumstances middle cerebral artery flow is a high-impedance flow. It is also a continuous forward flow all throughout the cardiac cycle in both its phases, systolic and diastolic. It is very interesting to note that the body tends to give a priority to cerebral circulation. By this priority it is meant that even when the other body organs and tissues are facing a dearth of oxygen supply, body makes all attempts to see that the brain gets oxygenated blood even in most stressful and critical times. For this, the cerebral vessels bring about many changes as compensation. These changes can be misleading for the clinician as it may still reflect a picture of all being well. However, any further decompensation can crash the entire system and cause a fetal demise.

Although imaging these vessels the landmark that is considered is the Circle of Willis. The right and the left middle cerebral arteries represent the major branches of Circle of Willis. On the other hand the circle receives it blood supply from the internal carotids and vertebral arteries. It is a well-accepted fact that the imaging of middle cerebral artery is obtained from the proximal portion of the vessel immediately after it's branching from the Circle of Willis has best reproducibility. This is the accepted point of reference for all imaging of MCA (Figs 19.7 and 19.8).

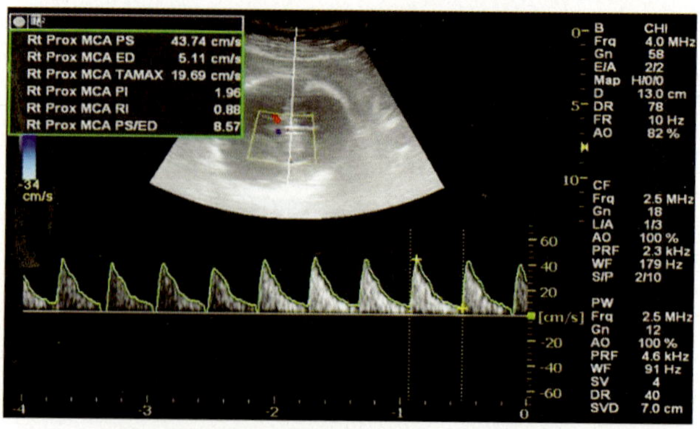

Fig.19.7: Normal middle cerebral artery flow

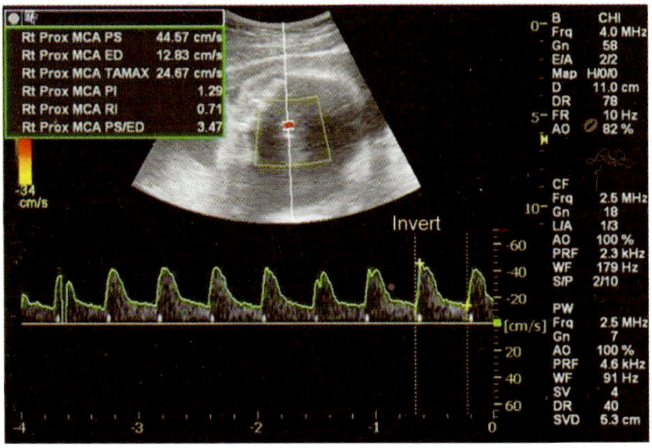

Fig.19.8: Abnormal flow through middle cerebral artery

Initially the body of the pregnant fetus that gets chronically challenged by asphyxia increases its flow to the MCA. This is reflected by a high S: D ratio. The PI also rises correspondingly. However, as time passes and hypoxia continues or worsens, the S:D ratio starts getting low. Now with continuance of asphyxia, the systolic flow may remain the same but as compensation the diastolic flow raises. Ultimately this leads to a fall in S: D ratio again. This redistribution of blood is a warning sign for the clinician to intervene. If steps are not taken the fetus gets acidosis and subsequently there occurs a fetal demise.

Venous Doppler

At the stage when fetal decompensation steps in, fetal venous Doppler imaging becomes important. It will help reaching two critical decisions:

1. How quickly should one intervene and
2. What route of delivery of the fetus is used for safe delivery.

A Doppler waveform from the central circulation of the venous segment reflects the status of the right ventricle. It is now well known that specific and reasonably accurate information with regards to the right ventricle preload, myocardial compliance and right ventricular end-diastolic pressure can be derived from Doppler flow studies of inferior vena cava and ductus venosus. The technique of imaging for any vessel arterial or venous is not being described here as it is not within the scope of this discussion.

Arterial Doppler abnormalities are first to appear in fetal compromise because of chronic hypoxia. Once these appear and the stage appears for planning a delivery, arterial flows are not of much use. This is a critical phase in IUGR pregnancies as the clinician needs a clear message and guidance. He needs to decide if the intrauterine environment is hostile enough for the fetus to bring about a delivery. For this purpose, the venous Doppler becomes important. This is because venous Doppler abnormalities found in the ductus venous and inferior vena cava are associated with advanced and even terminal stages of fetal compromise.

It is also interesting to note that progressive deterioration of fetal arterial flow and a subsequent venous flow (Fig. 19.9) by and large precedes the fetal cardiotocograph abnormalities. It is also believed that CTG abnormalities show the state of fetal compromise over a period of time, on the other hand fetal arterial and venous Doppler imaging indicate the status of fetal oxygenation at that particular moment of time when the examination was actually performed.

This can be compared to blood sugar estimation in diabetic patients. Assessment of blood sugar levels (e.g. FBS—Fasting blood sugar and PG2BS—Post-glucose blood sugar after 2 hours of consumption) indicate the sugar levels at that material moment of time. However, estimation of glycosylated hemoglobin or Hb1AC indicates blood sugar level status over a period of time. This example is given for better understanding of Doppler and CTG assessments.

Coming back to Doppler, the limitation of arterial Doppler was succinctly put by Bacchant AA et al. Once arterial centralization occurs, however, no clear trend is noted in the observational period, and thus, arterial redistribution may not be helpful for timing of delivery.[6] However, if reversal appears in the end diastolic flow in the umbilical artery it is a norm to consider immediate delivery of the fetus. Continuing such a pregnancy exposes the fetus to a dangerous and grave possibility of intrauterine fetal demise.

At this stage fetal venous Doppler steps in to decide how quickly (matter of hours if not days) and the route of delivery. It goes without saying that such babies have a very high chance of needing on NICU admission. It also depends on the maturity and birth weight of the fetus. Currently in a setup like that of ours, a fetus with 30 to 32 weeks of pregnancy and a birth weight of greater than 1000 grams has a reasonable chance of survival. Needless to say, these improved chances are positively consolidated if the mother has been given steroids antenatally for enhancing the fetal systemic maturity especially the fetal lung maturity.

It is interesting to note that about one-third of fetuses show early signs of circulatory deregulation, a week before the biophysical profile deteriorates and in most cases Doppler deterioration precedes biophysical profile deterioration at least by one day.[10]

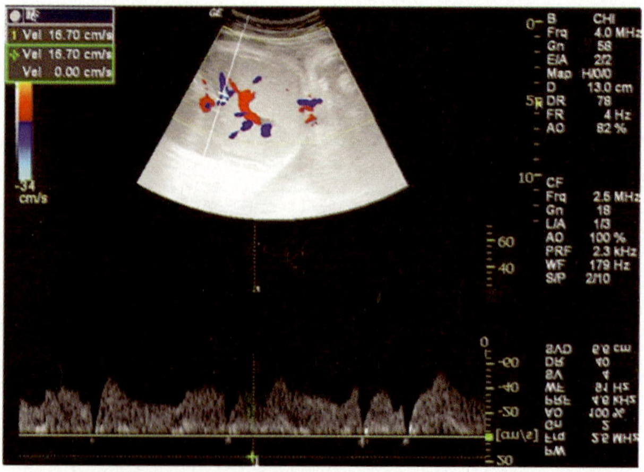

Fig.19.9: Normal flow through ductus venous

It is also pertinent to understand the limitation of color Doppler studies after 34 weeks of gestation. It has been found that deterioration of fetal Doppler values do not prognosticate the fetal outcome very efficiently after 34 weeks. It is possible that in such gestations the umbilical flow may still be normal and the fetal middle cerebral artery flow may show deterioration. This disjoint can be misleading and even dangerous. Therefore the word used for applying color Doppler studies in clinical management of IUGR after 34 weeks is *caution*.

Limitations of Venous Doppler

On the positive side of limitations it has already been stated that if the fetal arterial Doppler studies are normal, there is no need to do venous Doppler. On similar lines the universal application of venous Doppler may not be very much necessary. The pattern of consequential and progressive deterioration decides when to do venous Doppler.

The arterial Doppler deterioration is followed by:

A. Venous Doppler abnormalities in turn followed by
B. Fetal heart rate abnormalities in turn followed by
C. Deterioration in fetal biophysical profile.

Therefore, if the fetal arterial Doppler is not good and is coupled by heart rate or CTG abnormalities, it implies that the venous Doppler must also not be good. Sequential event A and C indicate that B also must have occurred.

Statistically too some interesting values have been found. About 70% of fetuses with IUGR show significant deterioration of all vascular beds by the time they are delivered and about 10% showed no change in circulation at the time of delivery in a study.[10] While the sequential model of event A to B to C has been suggested there is also a flip side to it. In a prospective study, 505 of fetuses with IUGR who were delivered because of abnormal CTG tracings actually had a normal venous Doppler. Thus the event C can sometimes occur without event A.[11]

The progressive fall in all the three indices as pregnancy advances in the III trimester is attributable to declining peripheral resistance. A variation in these indices in pregnancies complicated by obstetric vasculopathies is attributable to increase peripheral resistance especially at the fetoplacental interface. Absent end-diastolic flow that is also expressed as loss of end diastolic flow is a reflection of a severe state of peripheral resistance. This resistance being high the forward flow in the umbilical vessels toward the placenta could not be sustained. In absence of such peripheral resistance, the blood pushed out by the cardiac systole is able to keep flowing all throughout the cycle in the umbilical artery. This merges with another peak systolic push wave. But in deteriorating cases of fetomaternal vascular resistance a distinct gap occurs toward the end of the flow wave. This is expressed as absent diastolic flow.

As an extension to the same, fetal cerebral-umbilical Doppler ratio has also been used in prediction of fetal distress in patients with preeclampsia. By measurement of pulsatility indices in medial cerebral and umbilical arteries Cerebral-umbilical (C/U) ratio can be calculated. The C/U ratio values obtained from in fetal vessels showed a highly significant correlation with fetal pH at birth in the patients with preeclampsia. It indicates the reliability of C/U ratio in estimation of fetal condition in preeclamptic patients. Very low C/U ratio values in patients with preeclampsia indicate that in these fetuses fetal acidosis and fetal distress may be expected.[12]

Further increase in resistance at the fetoplacental interface leads to the blood actually being thrown back from the placenta because of intense resistance (or opposition to flow). As a result there occurs a reversal of flow. This is a very dangerous sign and can indicate an impending perinatal death. These fetuses are most consistently suffering consequences of obstetric vasculopathies (usually IUGR and preeclampsia). It is therefore wise to plan a delivery in such subjects within days if not hours. However the fact remains that umbilical artery parameter singly is not to be considered for decision-making. It is the comprehensive picture that emerges from other Doppler vascular studies coupled with CTG tracings and result of the fetal biophysical profile that will decide the ultimate decision making in intervention.

It is obvious that each fetus even if sick due to IUGR it has its own responsive system. Like any adult the fetus too maintains its individuality in its response. While many of the IUGR fetuses will have a sequential pattern of deterioration in circulation, there will be about half of the fetuses who will not follow this pattern. They will therefore maintain the individuality of their response. This makes the consistency of venous Doppler and its reliability vulnerable. It is for that reason wisdom to do venous color Doppler but use the results for ancillary assistance in decision making. They will not be the only findings but in combination with other findings.

Umbilical Venous Flow

With progressive hypoxia, there is an increase in the right ventricular after load. This leads to a reversal of flow in the vena cava during the contraction of right atrium. With the pathology further worsening the fetomaternal interface becomes an intensely high impedance wall. In such a critical situation, the entire vascular system gets involved. In this process, therefore, the inferior venacava and umbilical vein starts developing pulsatility. Thus, a constantly forward moving non-pulsatile bloodstream through the umbilical vein can get converted into a pulsatile blood flow. If and when this happens is a very ominous sign. Such a subject needs an immediate delivery. This baby is likely to be acidotic at birth. The delivery has to be accomplished within hours if not minutes. If not, this can lead to an intrapartum fetal demise.

Venous Doppler for Deciding the Route of Delivery

Although accepting that venous color Doppler individually will not necessitate a clinician to decide the need for delivery, it has some important role in deciding the route of delivery. By and large in modern obstetric practice, IUGR has become an important indication for cesarean section. This has two reasons: one a clinical reason of the baby running into an added acute distress while travelling through the maternal passages. The second reason is statistical where it has been shown that IUGR babies statistically can be more asphyxiated if delivered vaginally. Understandably, therefore, the clinician will be attracted to a softer and apparently safer option of cesarean section. Yet in medicine there is never anything that is absolute. As is euphemistically stated in medicine there is nothing like never, it is *usually never*. On these lines venous Doppler may be able to identify subjects who can be allowed a vaginal delivery, inspite of having an IUGR fetus. Those few IUGR subjects who on color Doppler are showing abnormality in arterial circulation (both in umbilical artery as well as MCA) but still do not show a venous Doppler change may be candidates for vaginal delivery. Needless to say these labors have to be very closely monitored and carefully selected. But there will be some IUGR subjects who will have enough oxygenated blood pool to withstand the stress of labour and allow a vaginal delivery.

COLOR DOPPLER FOR DISCONTINUATION OF ANTITHROMBOTIC AGENTS

This area of application of color Doppler is a very exciting area based on sound understanding of scientific events. It will need to revisit uterine artery color Doppler again. At about the end of 1-trimester or early II trimester scans color Doppler's consistently show a presence of a diastolic notch in the uterine artery tracings. This diastolic notch is expected to disappear in the mid-trimester at or about 20 to 27 weeks of gestation. The cellular event to which it is attributed to is the second wave of trophoblastic invasion. This all important event in normal pregnancy is found to be deficient or incomplete in subjects who develop clinical manifestations of obstetric vasculopathies. As a result, uterine artery continues to register a diastolic notch even beyond II–trimester.

With this background, it would be interesting to know that if antithrombotic can be continued or discontinued with the help of color Doppler. In those subjects in whom antithrombotic agents have been started currently the norm is to discontinue at 36 weeks of pregnancy or on intervention whichever is earlier. This has been extensively discussed in the chapter of prevention of obstetric vasculopathies (See Chapter 18). This norm has been established with obstetric considerations rather than cellular events and their background. It therefore seems scientific, if a clinician decides to discontinue antithrombotic agents at the stage of disappearance of the diastolic notch. Disappearance of diastolic notch will indicate that the second wave of trophoblastic invasion is over. In that case, there is no fear of generation of their process of obstetric vasculopathy now on in these subjects. This pregnancy is now behaving like any other normal pregnancy and so antithrombotic agents can be safely discontinued.

The most cumbersome antithrombotic agent is heparin. The compliance issues of heparin have been discussed elsewhere (See Chapters 18, 21). Therefore, if heparin can be discontinued earlier, it can reduce the need of the pregnant subject to take the injection daily. While disappearance of diastolic notch at any stage after mid- trimester signals a possibility of stopping heparin, if a clinician is apprehensive, aspirin may be continued and heparin can be discontinued.

Continuing aspirin is more related to apprehension of abrupt withdrawal of protective cover of antithrombotic agents. Stormy adverse obstetric outcomes in subjects under treatment in the past can further make them apprehensive. Therefore, more out of this apprehension rather than scientific rationale, aspirin is continued. But low dose heparin, the more cumbersome of the two, can at the least be discontinued on basis of color Doppler findings.

One more group requires to be mentioned here. There is a small but distinct set of subjects who have a bad obstetric history because of obstetric vasculopathy. In some of these there is an absent diastolic notch as early as the 12 weeks to 14 weeks scan. In these subjects, it seems that the second wave of trophoblastic invasion is competently completed by early second trimester. In such subjects it may be possible to recommend a discontinuation of heparin as early as 12 to 14 weeks. However, it is still early in the day to make this recommendation applicable to clinical practice.

The scientific basis for discontinuation of antithrombotic agent use using uterine color Doppler seems to be promising. However, it still needs to be supported by a large clinical experience. It is therefore necessary to strike a word of caution that it may still be very early in the day to adopt this as a policy. Thus, as of now discontinuing heparin in potential subjects of obstetric vasculopathy should be individualized and a close watch on such pregnancies continued.

It is also worth noting here that there are some causes of fetal IUGR where an association is found with maternal condition but a temporal relationship may not have been yet established. This includes causes like maternal bronchial asthma. In these subjects, if there is a concurrent possibility of IUGR because of obstetric vasculopathy it may not be advisable to discontinue using heparin. This is not to suggest that heparin prevents IUGR of non-temporal causes. But these subjects have an added high-risk factor for IUGR. In such situations on taking a holistic view, it would be advisable to continue using heparin till term. This takes care of the component of IUGR that is likely to come from obstetric vasculopathy. This makes the going a little easier for the mother as well as the clinician.

To make this simpler discontinuing use of heparin in obstetric vasculopathy by using the marker of disappearance of diastolic notch should be individualized. If any indexed pregnancy has an added factor in the mother that may also have a likelihood of producing IUGR in the fetus it would be wise not to discontinue heparin in these subjects till term.

Cardiac Doppler in Obstetric Vasculopathies

It seems that cardiac Doppler may add a dimension to the entire spectrum of imaging in the management of obstetric vasculopathies. It has been found that in IUGR specifically, there are distinct changes in the preload, ventricular compliance, and contractile power of the heart muscles as well as the afterload. Makikallio et al have shown that there is an increase in after load seen at the level of right ventricle is because of high vascular impedance in IUGR.[13] This same group has also demonstrated an increase in afterload at the level of left ventricle owing to decreased cerebral impendence, associated with brain-sparing effects in IUGR.

Myocardial contractility is also reduced severe IUGR. Rizzo G et al have shown that the ventricular ejection force is decreased at the level of right and left ventricle in fetal growth restriction. IUGR fetuses seem to be acidotic with reduced ventricular ejection force and a higher incidence of non-reassuring fetal heart tracing.[14] Currently the principal color Doppler marker used to strongly suspect an acidotic fetus is the reversal of blood flow in the ductus venous. Reduced ventricular ejection can add to this assessment parameter further alerting the clinician for an immediate need for intervention. Alternately in fetuses where the arterial color Doppler is affected and tracings are none reassuring, if the ductus flow is still inconclusive, one can use the ventricular ejection imaging for a quick decision making for early intervention in IUGR. This will also be an indication for immediate cesarean section.

Understandably, the fetal heart plays a central role in adaptive mechanisms for hypoxemia and placental insufficiency. Figueras et al have shown through a longitudinal study of the hemodynamic sequence that the umbilical artery and middle cerebral artery are the first variables to become abnormal. These are followed by the deterioration in right cardiac diastolic indices followed by the right systolic indices and finally by both the left and the right indices.[15]

The body of the fetus does most adaptive mechanisms to ensure that the brain gets well-oxygenated blood to the last. Left side systolic function becoming the last to get affected is a part of these adaptive changes of ensuring oxygenation to the fetal brain even in most trying and near terminal situations.

It seems to be promising to study and include myocardial function assessment in the functioning of IUGR. Very early attempts in these directions were done when sometimes the cardiac size was measured. This was with the rationale that in IUGR-there is a chronic deprivation of well-oxygenated blood to the fetoplacental interface. The heart as a compromise has to work more. This gets reflected in the different alterations now identified in the cardiac systolic and diastolic functioning. Such functional alterations are achieved by increased muscular activity of the heart. Any increase in muscular activity cumulatively leads to increase in the size of that organ in question, the fetal heart. However, it seems that there was not much changes in the overall size of the heart though it's muscular, functioning does get altered. While importance of all currently used vascular indices cannot be run down, inclusion of cardiac functioning indices may add to the accuracy in decision making for the clinician for IUGR management.

FETAL AORTIC DOPPLER STUDIES

In the basket of vessels examined for Doppler studies, fetal aortic studies are now not much popular. But in the late last century when this technology was evolving they seemed popular. In uncomplicated pregnancy the descending aorta shows a continuous forward flow throughout the cardiac cycle. The blood volume traversing through the fetal descending aorta progressively increases upto 37 weeks. After this, it plateaus off. In pregnancies that are complicated by fetal IUGR the absent. End diastolic flow (EDF) is predictor of a poor fetal outcome.[16] It has also been found that pregnancies with absent EDF in fetal aortic circulation are more likely to be delivered by cesarean section. These babies, besides having a lower birth weight also have a poor perinatal outcome.[17]

Reversal of EDF suggests a worst form of vascular impedance at the vascular bed that it supplies. The blood that is pushed through now is unable to flow. It therefore hits against the resisting into circulation. This produces the reversal of EDF. In subjects with a reversal of EDF in the aorta of the fetus it is recommended to deliver the baby in less than 24 hours. If not, there is a grave likelihood of an intrauterine fetal demise.

Though the aortic flow showed good correlation between the perinatal outcome and changes in its flow, over a period of time it lost its prime position to umbilical artery and MCA flow studies. This is predominantly because of more consistent results from these two studies. However, fetal aortic color Doppler studies continues to be used as a supplementary to fetal MCA and umbilical artery flow studies.

Over a period of years other vessels especially those supplying blood to the fetal brain have also been studied. This includes vessels like to internal carotid artery, the common carotid artery and the most popular middle cerebral artery. Internal carotid is the most difficult among all these to access but may be the most accurate in reflecting the fetal cerebral flow status. In normal pregnancy the internal carotid artery flow remains fairly constant forward flow with a very high PI (pulsatility index). Like the descending aorta it plateaus off around 37 weeks or may even show some downward trend.[18] In cases complicated by IUGR, this flow through the internal carotid shows a progressive increase in the diastolic component. This will get reflected in lowering of the pulsatility index—PI. Interestingly this reflects the so, called brain sparing effect where the fetal brain gets a privileged status. The fetal oxygenation is maintained by compensatory mechanisms of blood flow through foramen ovule and ductus arteriosus. In subjects with IUGR because of obstetric vasculopathy, fetal brain sparing effect is demonstrated. However, if the IUGR is because of other cause like congenital anomalies or some chromosomal problem, this type of brain sparing effect is not seen.

However, the ease of access and near equal reliability of results has made MCA to be more popular for studying the status of fetal cerebral blood flow. Other vessels are by and large given up or if at all used it is for the purpose of research studies or for supplementing results of MCA.

REFERENCES

1. Imdad A, Yakoob M, Siddiqui S, Bhutta Z. Screening and triage of intrauterine growth restriction (IUGR) in general population and high-risk pregnancies: a systematic review with a focus on reduction of IUGR related stillbirths. *BMC Public Health*. 2011;11(3):S1.
2. Chan FY, Pun TC, Lam C, et al. Pregnancy screening by uterine artery Doppler velocimetry—which criterion performs the best. *Obstet Gynecol*. 1995; 85:696-02.
3. Pongrojpaw D, Chanthasenanont A, Nanthakomon T. Second trimester uterine artery Doppler screening in prediction of adverse pregnancy outcome in high-risk subjects. *J Med Assoc Thai*. 2010;93(7):S127-30.
4. Ohkuchi A, Minakami H, Sato I, Mori H, Nakano T, Tateno M. Predicting the risk of pre-eclampsia and a small-for-gestational-age infant by quantitative assessment of the diastolic notch in uterine artery flow velocity waveforms in unselected women. *Ultrasound Obstet*. 2000;16(2):171-8.
5. Napolitano R, Melchiorre K, Arcangeli T, Dias T, Bhide A, Thilaganathan B. Screening for pre-eclampsia by using changes in uterine artery Doppler indices with advancing gestation. *Prenatal Diagn*. 2012; 32(2):180-4.
6. Belfort M, Van Veen T, White G, Kofford S, Allred J, Postma I, et al. Low maternal middle cerebral artery Doppler resistance indices can predict future development of pre-eclampsia. *Ultrasound Obstet Gynecol*. 2011.doi:10.1002/uog.11078.

7. Rattanapuntamanee O, Uerpairojkit B. Reference range and characteristic of uterine artery Doppler in pregnant Thai subjects at 11–13 (+6) gestational weeks. *J Med Assoc Thai.* 2011; 94(6):644-8.
8. Pilalis A, Souka AP, Antsaklis P, Basayiannis K, Benardis P, Haidopoulos D, et al. Screening for pre-eclampsia and small for gestational age fetuses at the 11–14 weeks scan by uterine artery Dopplers. *Acta Obstet Gynecol Scand.* 2007; 86(5):530-4.
9. Dugoff L, Lynch AM, Cioffi-Ragan D, Hobbins JC, Schultz LK, Malone FD, et al. FASTER Trial Research Consortium. First trimester uterine artery Doppler abnormalities predict subsequent intrauterine growth restriction. *Am J Obstet Gynecol.* 2005;193(3 Pt 2):1208-12.
10. Baschat AA, Gembruch U, Reiss I, Gortner L, Weiner CP, Harman C. Relationship between arterial and venous Doppler and perinatal outcome in fetal growth restriction ultrasound. *Ultrasound Obstet Gynecol.* 2000;16(5):407-13.
11. Ferrazzi E, Bozzo M, Rigano S, Bellotti M, Morabito A, Pardi G, et al. Temporal sequence of abnormal Doppler changes in peripheral and central circulatory systems of the severely growth retarded fetus. *Ultrasound Obstet Gynecol.* 2002;19(2):140-6.
12. Jurisić A, Jurisić Z, Pazin V, Vasiljević M, Janković-Raznatović S, Dragojević-Dikić S. Fetal cerebral-umbilical Doppler ratio in prediction of fetal distress in patients with pre-eclampsia. *Vojnosanit Pregl.* 2010;67(6):487-92.
13. Mäkikallio K, Vuolteenaho O, Jouppila P, Räsänen J. Ultrasonographic and biochemical marker of human fetal cardiac dysfunction in placental insufficiency. *Circulation.* 2002;30;105(17):2058-63.
14. Rizzo G, Capponi A, Rinaldo D, Arduini D, Romanini C. Ejection force in growth retarded fetuses. *Ultrasound Obstet Gynecol.* 1995; 5(4):247-55.
15. Figueras F, Puerto B, Martinez J, Cararach V, Vanrell J. Cardiac function monitoring of fetuses with growth restriction. *Eur J Obstet Gynecol Reprod Biol.* 2003;110(2):159-63.
16. Laurin J, Marsál, Persson P, Lingman G. Ultrasound measurement of fetal blood flow in predicting fetal outcome. *Br J Obstet Gynaecol.* 1987;94(10):940-8.
17. Hackett G, Campbell S, Gamsu H, Cohen-Overbeek T, Pearce J. Doppler studies in growth retarded fetus and prediction of neonatal necrotizing enterocolitis, hemorrhage and neonatal morbidity. *Br Med J* (Clin Res Ed). 1987;294(6563):13-6.
18. Wladimiroff J, Tonge H, Stewart P. Doppler ultrasound assessment of cerebral blood flow in the human fetus. *Br J Obstet Gynaecol.* 1986;93(5):471-5.

CHAPTER

20

Cardiotocography in Obstetric Vasculopathies

CHAPTER OUTLINE

- Physiology and Cardiotocography
- Hypoxia and Fetal Heart Rate
- Cardiotocographies in subjects with APA Syndrome
- Color Doppler and Cardiotocography Correlation

INTRODUCTION

Like color Doppler, cardiotocography (CTG) also has a very important contribution in modern management of obstetric vasculopathies. Not only does it warn of an impending disaster, it also reveals a hidden condition. These will be discussed in this chapter at length. It will also be necessary to understand how to correlate and use both technologies, color Doppler and CTG simultaneously to the maximum advantage of the mother and her unborn fetus. For understanding any technology and its results, it is imperative to know and understand the physiology that provides the basis. This can then be applied to the pathology involved to draw valid conclusions.

PHYSIOLOGY AND CARDIOTOCOGRAPHY

Basal Heart Rate and its Variability

Fetal heart musculature, like any smooth muscle system is autonomous in its function. It does not need external stimulus to keep it going. Nevertheless, neurological innervations can alter its function. The human fetal heart as that of its adult counterpart has innervations from the autonomic nervous system. Its efferents are originating from both the autonomic nervous systems, the sympathetic and parasympathetic. In the healthy and optimally innervated fetal heart (like the adult heart) the rate and the rhythm can be modified by these innervations.

The fetal heart has a rate and a rhythm at which it beats. The rhythm of the heart beat varies nearly at every beat. As a result of this the heart rate appears to vary at every set of beats. It is healthy to see a well oxygenated fetal heart beating at variable rates like 130-132-130-144-140-144-130-150-145-130-144-148-135-130-146-144 and on. This continuous variation in the heart rate is expressed as heart rate variability. Presence of these variations in heart rate is expressed as variable heart rate or variability. The average rate of fetal heart beating is 144 and the variability varies from 5 to 15 beats per minute.

The parasympathetic system matures later than the sympathetic nervous system. The parasympathetic system has a tendency to slower the heart rate. The sympathetic system has a tendency to accelerate the heart rate. Due to a delay in maturity of the parasympathetic nervous system in premature fetuses the heart rate tends to be faster than the term fetuses. This parasympathetic control becomes fully manifested at or around 32 weeks. Therefore at this duration the basal heart rate of a fetus completely settles with full variability.

Fetal heart beats at an average heart rate of 144 beats per minute. Much is written about the possible errors in this absolute figure. The biggest point of discussion is the fact that heart rates and usually measured for 15 seconds and then multiplied by four presuming that it will remain constant through the other three quarters also. With the introduction CTG in measuring the fetal heart activity the fetal heart rate could be measured at any given instance of time and its behavior all over the minute could be understood.

During cardiotocograph monitoring one can realize that the sympathetic nervous system continuously accelerates the heart. As a result the heart rate has a tendency to rise. To counteract this is the parasympathetic innervation. It decelerates the heart. The continuous variation that one sees on the CTG panel of heart rate is this interplay between the two nervous systems.

A poorly oxygenated heart will show that the heart rate does not vary much. The innervations of the heart tend to get temporarily dysfunctional in states of deoxygenation. As soon as the heart gets well oxygenated again, this interplay of nerves gets restored. Thus a good variability in the heart rate is a sign of a well oxygenated and healthy heart. Absence of this is ominous. It indicates a hostile intrauterine ambience for the fetus and therefore a need for the clinician to intervene.

Accelerations in Heart Rate

A healthy fetus accelerates its heart rate when it moves. This is exactly like the adult heart rate which also registers acceleration when there is physical activity. Thus an increase in heart rate in response to movement of the fetus indicates a well oxygenated heart and a healthy fetus. In chronically asphyxiated fetus if the myocardium also gets affected, the heart does not accelerate on fetal movement. Lack of heart acceleration in IUGR or PIH fetus indicates an ominous sign and therefore a need for intervention. Acceleration in a well oxygenated heart is abrupt, equal to or more than 15 bpm and is independent of uterine contractions. Any day presence of accelerations on a CTG tracing is a very reassuring feature and indicates that there is no need to hasten the intervention for affecting a delivery.

Decelerations in Heart Rate

In any CTG tracing, decelerations are not a welcome feature. But all forms of decelerations need not indicate an emergency. Decelerations should be looked at vey attentively. Principally there are three types of decelerations with clinical bearings: Early decelerations, late decelerations and atypical decelerations.

Early Decelerations

These are also known as type 1 decelerations. They occur early in reference to contractions. The hallmark of early deceleration is that the nadir of the deceleration corresponds with the maximum height of the contraction. They are believed to be physiological decelerations. They occur possibly due to the compression of the head leading to vagal stimulation. This being a physiological phenomenon need not warrant any alert or alarm.

Late Decelerations

The fall in heart rate in these types of decelerations commences after the onset of contraction. It reaches its nadir after the peak of the contraction. The heart rate returns to baseline after the contraction has ceased. The possible pathophysiology of this deceleration is totally different from early decelerations. This deceleration reflects a deoxygenated state. During contractions, the uterine blood flow is very significantly reduced. It may be completely shut off at the peak of the contraction or may be reduced to a faint trickle during the rising or falling of the contraction. This is that small period of time when the fetus has to rely on the pool of blood in the placenta that is shut off from movements due to contraction. In a well oxygenated and healthy fetus this impoverishment of oxygen supply is not of much consequence. This is because the fetus has robust mechanisms by which it can handle this short phase of oxygen deficiency. However in babies with IUGR or pre-eclampsia the entrapped blood pool is also impoverished of oxygen. As a result the fetus reacts to this added burden of low oxygenation in the form of a late deceleration.

Initially the fetus manages its heart rate by its protective mechanisms. But further deprivation of oxygen (even for a few seconds) cracks its protective mechanisms and the heart begins to decelerate. Its takes a little more time correspondingly to return to the baseline levels. This is vividly reflected in the pattern of late decelerations. The commencement and peak of acceleration does not show change in heart rate the protective mechanisms are holding. The deoxygenated state at its peak of the contraction now starts cracking the fetal protective mechanisms and soon the heart starts decelerating. By this time however the peak of the contraction has ceased and the uterus stars relaxing. But the deoxygenated heart continues to decelerate needing some time to recuperate. As a result by the time the heart rate reaches to baseline once again it is late as compared to the contraction which has long since ceased. A late deceleration is therefore an ominous sign and indicates a responsive system of the fetal body. It reflects a hypoxia fetus and alerts the clinician to a need for intervention to bring the baby out of the hostile (deoxygenated) environment.

Variable Decelerations

Their pattern and occurrence is variable in respect to the uterine contraction. They are reflective of the umbilical cord of the fetus getting compressed and temporarily shutting off the blood supply leading to a fall in heart rate. Cord compression can occur irrespective of the uterine contraction. It can occur due to a change in maternal posture or a fetal movement. It can occur due to uterine contractions. As a result the deceleration can occur at variable instances for variable period of time and for variable intensity.

Shouldering

This is the small hump that is seen in variable decelerations just before the hart rate starts sinking or just after the trough, before it restricted the baseline. The heart rate seems to overshoot at this point registering a small and transient rise. This is called shouldering. There are different explanations that are given for this. The most popular of all is that when compression occurs, first to collapse is the umbilical vein. This is because its thin wall. This leads to a sudden reduction in blood volume in circulation which stimulates the sympathetic innervations resulting in a rise in heart rate. However the process of compression is still ongoing. Now it occludes the arterial walls also which leads to vagal stimulation (parasympathetic) resulting in a sharp and sudden fall in fetal heart rate. This small interval of a rise in heart rate just preceding the deep fall is called shouldering.

When the compression is released with the uterine wall relaxing the normalcy is restored in the reverse order with the arterial flow getting released first followed by the venous flow. This leads to one more overshoot just at the end of deceleration. Shouldering disappears as cord compression becomes more and more profound and persistent. It seems all are not buying this explanation for the process of shouldering and many are of the belief that it does not have any significance and can be harmlessly ignored. One fact however always remains and that is variable deceleration occur due to cord compression and this is worsened or even precipitated by oligoamnios. Some workers have suggested that absence or disappearance of shouldering in subjects with variable decelerations suggests acidosis in the fetus and warrants immediate delivery. This seems to be overhyped.

HYPOXIA AND FETAL HEART RATE

Having had seen and understood all the three types of decelerations early, late and variable it will now be important to understand their correlation with hypoxia and its clinical applications. In subjects with obstetric vasculopathy there can be different types of hypoxia that can affect the fetus. The fetus can be affected by a gradually developing hypoxia or acute hypoxia.

Acute Hypoxia

The most notable obstetric vasculopathy that has acute hypoxia is accidental hemorrhage. Rendering the placenta detached from its attachment understandably causes a sudden hypoxic state in the fetus. As a result of this acute hypoxia parasympathetic or vagal stimulation occur leading to sudden bradycardia.

Gradual Hypoxia

This is found in subjects who develop oligohydramnios due to obstetric vasculopathies like IUGR and pre-eclampsia. Over a period of time this gradually developing hypoxia initially leads to increase in cardiac output now causes a rise in fetal heart rate. This gradually rising FHR (Fetal Heart Rate) subsequently gets associated with fetal acidosis. Once compensatory mechanisms fail acidosis sets in. This gets reflected in the fetal heart activity recordings on CTG as reduced baseline variability. Acidotic fetuses have poorly responding cardiac innervations resulting in loss of healthy variability. Persistent respiratory acidosis now leads to metabolic acidosis and subsequently resulting into direct myocardial damage both functional and structural. On CTG tracings this gets manifested as bradycardia and late decelerations.

Chronic Hypoxia

A classic example of this in obstetric vasculopathy is the phenomenon of IUGR and pre-eclampsia. This is a reflection of chronic fetomaternal interface compromise. In absence of uterine contractions, their fetuses register reduced baseline variability on CTG and absence of healthy decelerations. Once uterine contractions set in decelerations occurs. These are usually shallow decelerations but are ominous and may warrant a need for early intervention. These are situations where both CTG and color Doppler tracings are necessary for managing such pregnancies. A comprehensive picture that emerges from use of both these would guide the clinician for the need and method of intervention.

CARDIOTOCOGRAPHIES IN SUBJECTS WITH APA SYNDROME

We performed longitudinal observations of deterioration of cardiotocographic parameters in subjects with adverse outcomes of APA Syndrome. In this 84 consecutively enrolled subjects who tested positive for APA and in whom weekly CTGs could be done from 33rd. week onwards were observed for serial deterioration if any in their CTG reports. We found that a progressive deterioration in CTG reports of mothers with APA syndrome is ominous. It is an indication and has a high chance of having an asphyxiated newborn.[1]

COLOR DOPPLER AND CARDIOTOCOGRAPHY CORRELATION

Color Doppler and CTG are two relatively new technologies that have been deployed in obstetrics. The process of decision making has undergone a sea change in quality due to these. This decision making is usually related to the timing of delivery. When to deliver a pre-eclamptic mother's baby or an IUGR baby is guided by these. Also, in some situation how to deliver the baby also comes through these. Finally the two together help in diagnosing conditions of obstetric vasculopathy like accidental hemorrhage.

The Two together in Preeclampsia

In a subject with pre-eclampsia, the clinician needs to decide when to deliver the child. The balance in decision making is needed when the child is still preterm and the maternal BP starts deteriorating. A rising BP can produce scary morbidities in the mother and can even prove fatal. On the other hand if the baby is delivered unnecessarily preterm, there can be problems of iatrogenic prematurity. Also, the quality of neonatal backup may vary from set up to set up and skill of the neonatal intensivists. In an average set up a 1200 gms newborn with a maturity of 32 weeks in fairly salvageable. There are many setups where 1000 gms babies with a maturity of 30 weeks or even a shade less can be saved.

For the clinician the challenge lies in pulling the pregnancy till salvageable levels amidst rising BP and impending complications. The question is: which environment is safer the intrauterine environment or the extrauterine environment. In such a situation a combination of both these technologies is of great help to the clinician. If the CTGs show that there are no accelerations to satisfaction or variability is reduced it means that PIH has started affected oxygenation at the fetomaternal interface. In the light of the same, a colour Doppler following an alerting CTG can show a flow that is normal at umbilical artery but redistribution at MCA. In this situation the obstetrician has got some time. If the mother has not yet been given antenatal steroids, this is the time to give it.

If the variability needs is at the lower side of normal and there are no decelerations on record a critical situation for decision-making develops. These situations do not have a two plus two is equal to four like easy answer. The BP is progressively rising but the baby is still preterm. Here color Doppler helps to buy some days of time.

On the other hand if the CTG tracing show a good trace with satisfactory variability and healthy accelerations there may not be a need to do the color Doppler at all. Pregnancy can be prolonged if the BP is brought under control and there are no systemic complications developing in the mother.

Another situation arises when the BP is high but not rising any further and CTG shows alerting picture. In such a situation the color Doppler may show that both the arterial flows are affected. The venous Doppler has to be employed now. This is the situation where the clinician has only hours for decision-making. If the flow of the ductus venosus is still normal it means that the pregnancy needs an intervention but not a crisis intervention. If color Doppler and CTG can be repeated six to eight hourly such pregnancies can be prolonged for even 24 hours. This latitude of time can prove a breather and help to shift the mother to a better and more competent NICU setting.

One more picture where decision-making is helped by the two is when the CTG is ominous, the arterial flows are affected but the venous flows are still not affected. This situation though warrants an immediate intervention there may be a scope for vaginal delivery. If vaginal delivery is attempted, it should be with all arrangement of an urgent cesarean section standing by. If and whenever the baby shows evidence of distress during labor the clinicians can cesar out. If not vaginal delivery can still be tried if the venous Doppler is still unaffected.

The last scenario is when the CTG is ominous and the flow of the ductus is even affected in a subject with PIH. In such a scenario the care takers of this pregnancy are on a very tight leash. Not only have they to intervene quickly but even a cesarean section may be warranted.

From this it is evident that the CTG gives the oxygenation status over a period of time and color Doppler gives the oxygenation status of the fetus at the material moment.

The Two together in IUGR

Basically in obstetric vasculopathies that manifest late in pregnancy like pre-eclampsia and IUGR, there is a progressive deprivation of oxygen at the fetomaternal interface. In IUGR this can occur in absence of hypertensive disorders or along with. Usually IUGR is picked up on clinical examination coupled with USG scans. Cardiotocographic manifestations may occur at any stage of the ongoing pregnancy. It is therefore imperative to examine the pregnant subject for fetal wellbeing very vigilantly, more so in the last trimester. Now the fetus becomes more and more salvageable progressively. Secondly, the fetal compromise occurs rapidly in this trimester making the fetus vulnerable to demise in the uterus in this trimester.

On a routine monitoring of a CTG trace may be usually reassuring with excellent variability and healthy robust accelerations without decelerations. Till that time that such a trace continues to get recorded, the clinician can continue the pregnancy with close monitoring. There may not be any need to institute color Doppler in this management plan at this stage. Needless to say this time is to be used by the clinician for administration of antenatal steroids. Also this is the time when the neonatologist has to be alerted of such an ongoing pregnancy which may warrant labor intervention. The frequency with which the CTG recordings may be done should be decided by the clinician based on duration of pregnancy and intensity of fetal compromise. On these bases CTG monitoring may be required twice weekly and if the deterioration starts looming CTG tracings may be required more frequently twice a week, daily or even six hourly. If non-reassuring trace is recorded on any of the CTG monitoring, there would now be a need to institute color Doppler to zero down on the exact timing of intervention and type of intervention. If the baby has reached of reasonable salvagability for the neonatal backup system that is associated with the clinician, even with a good CTG, or with earliest induction changes in CTG, labor induction can be done. In such a liberal induction policy, chances of vaginal delivery are bright for IUGR can be reduced.

Once the tracings turn non-reassuring the color Doppler support becomes important. On an early non-reassuring CTG trace in the form of lack of good robust accelerations but still a reasonable variability if the arterial flows of the fetus are good, pregnancy can be continued. Alternatively if the neonatal salvagability for that duration of pregnancy is good, labor can be induced and vaginal delivery can be reasonably anticipated. But if the CTG shows non-reassuring patterns in the form of absent accelerations on non-stress test and/or reduced variability, color Doppler can still show a satisfactory arterial flow. In such a situation labor can be induced and vaginal delivery anticipated.

While anticipating a vaginal delivery a close monitoring of the fetal heart rate (if need be even a continuous CTG monitoring) may be required. At any stage if there is a further deterioration on the trace, a cesarean section needs to be done. However if the NST CTG is non-reassuring and the arterial flows register a compromise the venous flows should be studied. Very bold clinicians do tend to induce labors in anticipation of a vaginal delivery in subjects in whom the flow at the ductus venosus is still normal. However now onwards color Doppler is going to be very important. If there is any deterioration in the venous flow especially the ductus venous there is a need for cesarean section. This deterioration is usually in the form of increased frequency and amplitude of the flow through it. However if the ductus venosus registers a reversal of flow this is a very dangerous situation. If the pregnant subject is in labor her CTG will now show poor variability. These tracings can also show late decelerations and even sinusoidal pattern. Such a situation should not be allowed to occur in a closely monitoring obstetric unit. However, if this does occur, this is an indication for instant cesarean section. It indicates that the fetus is acidotic and severely distressed. In such cases the baby may be born asphyxiated and may need aggressive resustitatory measures.

Summarizing, therefore, cardiotocograph has proved to be a very valuable tool in the management of obstetric vasculopathies. When combined with color Doppler, the two together can make decision making regarding the need urgency and method of delivery accurate and scientific. While CTG gives an idea of the oxygen status and resulting asphyxia due to its deprivation over a period of time, color Doppler gives that information about the same for that material moment. Singly too CTG is capable of giving lots of information about the oxygenation status of the fetus and many decisions can be taken even from it alone. Thus these two technological advances have completely changed the picture of management of the two principles and most frequent obstetric vasculopathies, pre-eclampsia and IUGR.

REFERENCES

1. Desai P, Shah A. Longitudinal observations of deterioration of CTG parameters in subjects with adverse outcomes of APA syndrome. *Jr O & G India.* 2003;53(3):244-7.

CHAPTER

21

Treatment of Obstetric Vasculopathy: Recurrent Miscarriages

CHAPTER OUTLINE

- Corticosteroids: Not Used Any More
- Folic Acid
- Low Dose Aspirin
- Heparin
- Progesterone is Treatment of Immunological Miscarriages
- Treatment of a Subject of Miscarriage always for Prevention

INTRODUCTION

In this section treatment of recurrent miscarriages will be discussed. However there is no intention of conducting a discussion of all causes of recurrent miscarriages. There are many diverse and at times totally unrelated causes of recurrent miscarriages. Yet in the pages to follow the discussion will be confined only to recurrent miscarriages where obstetric vasculopathies are causing the same. These are recurrent miscarriages of immunological origin.

As has been extensively reviewed in sections related to immunology of obstetric vasculopathies, both autoimmune and alloimmune causes can cause obstetric vasculopathies which ultimately leads to recurrent miscarriages. These types of miscarriages are essentially characterized by those occurring as missed abortions. Also, they occur late in First-trimester or in second trimester presenting as fetal demise. In these subjects cardiac activity has usually been seen after which the fetal demise occurred.

The treatment mainstay for both types of immunological causes is antithrombotic agents: Aspirin and Heparin. The rationale for use of these agents has been extensively and scientifically discussed in other sections. Several studies have examined to use of these agents and reported an improved outcome beyond the pale of doubt.[1,2]

CORTICOSTEROIDS: NOT USED ANY MORE

In early years, prednisolone was recommended for use. It is possible that the basis of this would be those papers where inflammation has been found to have as some role to play. This aspect related to the role of inflammatory process has been covered extensively elsewhere. With the understanding of this pathophysiology going deeper it became obvious that inflammatory process is just an associated feature and does not have much role to play. As a result, we have stopped using prednisolone in subjects with history of recurrent immunological miscarriages.

Another remote possibility of why prednisolone entered the prescribing list for these subjects could be due to the possible immunomodulator role of corticosteroids. Immunomodulation is term which is used quite popularly in these discussions. However, if one is to consider this term holistically all agents and treatment modalities used for managing immunological aspect of obstetric vasculopathies can be called immunomodulators. These are principles of treatment which tend to modulate or attenuate the ill effects of immunology of pregnancy which ultimately leads to fetal rejection and or fetal demise.

Therefore, eulogizing only corticosteroids or hormones like progesterone as immunomodulators may not be very accurate. All treatment modalities cannot summarily paralyze the immunology involved. At the most they can modify the effects and therefore all of these treatments are immunomodulatory. It is also worth noting in this comprehensive discussion that studies that reviewed aspirin and prednisolone combination for recurrent immunological miscarriages suggest that the complications connected to prednisolone use outweigh the benefits. Therefore, their use is summarily discontinued.[2]

FOLIC ACID

Folic acid is popularly used for subjects of recurrent miscarriages where hyperhemocystenemia is attributable. It has been found that 5 mg/ms of folic acid started at least three months before pregnancy gives most satisfactory results. Therefore in subjects of hyperhemocystenemia folic acid is thus administered. It is relevant to note here that hyperhemocystenemia is also believed to be acting through the thrombomodulin pathway. This is has a role in the immunological causes of pregnancy failures. Folic acid remains the agent of choice in these conditions.

There are some clinical setups where investigations for hyperhemocystenemia may still not be done. In such situations too starting folic acid empirically may not be unwise. This is because as such the current norm of prescribing in pregnancy order administration of folic acid for prevention of neural tube defects and allied benefits. Therefore, even in absence of a clinical proof for hyperhemocystenemia it is wise to start folic acid 5 mg/ms in all subjects planning pregnancy.

While on folic acid supplementation, there have of late been big onslaughts of many pharmaceutical companies which have added many other compounds with folic acid. These are recommended for both treatment of hyperhemocystenemia as well as for prevention of birth defects. On this matter at this stage it would be wise to state that no compound gives results as consistent as folic acid. Therefore, folic acid alone has been found to be summarily most effective for prenatal and preconception supplementation. All other combinations still need more evaluation for inclusion on the prescription list of a rational medical practitioner.

LOW DOSE ASPIRIN

In subjects with recurrent immunological miscarriages (as has been discussed in the section related to antithrombotic agents in prevention of obstetric vasculopathies) 1.2 mg/kg of aspirin is recommended. This is to be given as soon as pregnancy diagnosis is made. However, there is a school of thought which recommends the use of low dose aspirin preconceptionally. It is recommended by these groups that aspirin should be started in the same low dose at least three months prior to conception. It should then be continued though the trimesters once pregnancy occurs. It is discontinued at 36 weeks and intervention be planned at 37 weeks. However the advantage of such an administration before conception is not well, established. Therefore, the order of the day is to individualize and leave it to the obstetrician.

FAQs on Aspirin

Though low dose aspirin is a settled issue there still remains a few doubts in the minds of some clinicians. However, we are now seeing that the fears in the minds of clinicians have been taken by and large care of. They are quite comfortable with the use of low dose aspirin. As a result the questions have become sparse.

Q. Teratogenicity of Aspirin

A. In doses of aspirin recommended is 1.2 mg/kg /day, aspirin is not found to be teratogenic. It can safely be given even during the phase of organogenesis. In fact for prevention of recurrent immunological losses this is the phase where aspirin administration is most desirable. Therefore, aspirin should be given and safely given all throughout pregnancy in this dose.

Q. Premature Closure of Ductus Arteriosus

A. It is well-known that prostaglandins keep the ductus arteriosus patent in the intrauterine life. On administration of NSAIDS was feared as these being antiprostoglandins they might cause a premature closure. It created an apprehension that ductus arteriosus would prematurely close with aspirin. But with the understanding of Cox-1 and Cox-2 pathways becoming apparent in the mechanisms of action of NSAIDS including aspirin this apprehension was summarily resolved. It was found that Cox-1 pathway is the one on which aspirin acts. On the other hand, it is the Cox-2 pathway that keeps ductus arteriosus patent. Therefore, aspirin does not cause premature closure of the ductus.

Q. How does One Handle Aspirin in Subjects of Recurrent Miscarriages who may Require a Cervical Cerclage? z

A. Cervical cerclage may be required in subjects of recurrent miscarriages who may develop an acquired cervical incompetence due to repeated dilation and evacuation for completing the process of miscarriage. However in subjects in whom aspirin is being given and a cervical cerclage is to be done, the current recommendation is to discontinue aspirin seven days before surgery. It can be restarted 24 hours after the surgery has been done. The rational for this is based on the effect of aspirin on the cyclooxygenase pathway of platelets has been extensively discussed in the section of use of antithrombotic agents in the prevention of obstetric vasculopathies.

HEPARIN

Another very vital weapon in the armamentarium of the obstetrician who deals with recurrent immunological miscarriages is heparin. This is started as soon as pregnancy is diagnosed or when the subject reports to the clinician whichever is earlier. Heparin is administered in a dose of 5000 IU subcutaneously. The duration for which heparin needs to be given and the wide spectrum administration has been discussed in great details in the section of prevention of obstetric vasculopathies. It is, therefore, not envisaged to discuss this again here. Nevertheless one or two points need to be quickly touched. One of this is the fact that as of now till the time that an effective antioxidant is found, aspirin plus heparin combination gives the best results in the treatment of recurrent immunological miscarriages. Also, there would be a large number of pregnant subjects in whom the clinician will have to decide so in favor of these agents solely on the basis of clinical features. In these subjects it is absolutely wise to start aspirin plus heparin in absence of any laboratory evidence. As of now there are no laboratory tests available that can diagnose alloimmune causes of recurrent pregnancy loss. Therefore, clinical features will be the sole basis for taking this decision.

PROGESTERONE IS TREATMENT OF IMMUNOLOGICAL MISCARRIAGES

No other treatment modality is as controversial in entire obstetrics as is progesterone use in obstetrics. The pendulum swings over a period of time from being of no use to most useful agent. It is also very strange but true that while the scientific world went on discussing this entire matter the clinicians never stopped or started using progesterone on the basis of trending scientific thinking. Clinicians continued their faith in them unwaveringly.

One reason for this scientific research to clinical practice disconnect could be the so-called TINA factor. TINA means *There is No Alternative*. In absence of any other alternative the clinicians continued to prescribe progesterone irrespective of the prevalent scientific recommendation at that moment in time. Progesterones have been examined for both their endocrinal action and the so called "immune-modulation" action. As regards the endocrinal action of progesterone, it comes from a very simple understanding of the physiology. In normal pregnancy, the corpus luteum secretes progesterones to support the pregnancy. This hormone precipitously falls in experimental animals in which corpus luteum was paralyzed or destroyed by luteolytic agents. Concurrently with falling levels of progesterones there consistently occurred miscarriages. By supplementing progesterone it was presumed that somehow the pregnancy gets supported in the same way as in normal pregnancy support. This accounted for their immense popularity in clinical practice.

With scientific research that followed it was found that this concept of support of pregnancy may not be valid. This swung the pendulum to the opposite end. The scientific world took a stand that progesterone's support may not be acting at all. Thus it was recommended that there is no need of progesterone use for pregnancy "support". This phase was followed by the phase of a different understanding about hormones. It was found that all hormones especially these involved in the process of reproduction had two personalities. One is the obvious endocrinal face and the other is the immunological face. The immunological face was believed to bring about such profound changes in the entire fetal allo graft to maternal host interaction that the fetus got immunologically tolerated by the maternal system.

This aspect has been covered in the light of HCG in the section of prevention of obstetric vasculopathies. When this concept was studied with progesterone, like HCG they were also found to have this immunological effect. The pendulum of recommendation swung back to supporting the use of progesterone in the treatment of recurrent pregnancy loss. However, the truth seems to be lying somewhere along the middle of the road. It seems that progesterones are neither a panacea nor useless agents. It also seems that progesterones act using both actions, endocrinal as well as the immunological action of this hormone.

As regards the evidence for the use of progesterone two RCTs are available which though had a small sample size, showed that progesterone supplementation helps in pregnancy sustenance in its early phase.

Difficulties in Interpreting Scientific Data

It is very challenging for the scientific world to interpret data obtained from studies for evaluating the efficacy of some agent or otherwise in pregnancy support. The simplistic way in which one may tend to draw conclusions is by comparing the outcome in subjects who had miscarriages in the past. In these subjects the agent under study is administered in subsequent pregnancies. If there was no miscarriage and the pregnancy continued unhindered it was concluded that the agent in question was effective in preventing a miscarriage.

However this way of drawing conclusions is not free from errors. Every pregnancy is unique. Every conceptus has its own intrinsic unique configuration which will cardinally decide if those pregnancies will fare uneventfully or will hit a road block. In such a situation giving credit to a particular extraneously administered agent for a favorable obstetric outcome may be misplaced credit.

Also, ethical principles limit the scientists in going too deep in the study of early pregnancy outcome. There is always a strong possibility of any conceptus being very normal and healthy. As a result, any intervention (including administration of any drug) cannot be studied beyond a limit of normalcy. There is a fear of affecting the course normally running pregnancy, adversely.

Another limitation comes from the fact that inspite of miscarriages in the past every pregnancy has a large possibility of spontaneous resolution. This means that intrinsically by its own mechanisms of protection any pregnancy will protect itself from getting miscarried. This holds true in subjects with spontaneous recurrent miscarriages also. Thus any pregnancy can have therefore a spontaneous resolution and not be miscarried. In such an eventuality trying to judge the efficacy of an extraneously administered agent is fraught with the danger of committing an error. If in a given subject who had miscarriages in the past, administration of a particular agent prevented a miscarriage or was there a spontaneous resolution is a question which is so tough to answer.

In the light of these challenges the swing of pendulum of efficacy of progesterone is preventing a miscarriage, from very effective to totally ineffective is quite understandable. We, therefore, keep this in mind while prescribing recurrent miscarriages including immunological miscarriages. Thus, while we do use progesterone's we do not give them undue and excessive credit if miscarriage did not occur in the pregnant subject this time.

TREATMENT OF A SUBJECT OF MISCARRIAGE ALWAYS FOR PREVENTION

It is interesting and true that a miscarriage once it occurs cannot be reversed. Therefore in strict sense of the word *treatment*, a miscarriage cannot be treated. A miscarriage can be prevented. Therefore all attempts in this direction are to prevent a subsequent miscarriage. A similar situation arises in the *treatment* of eclampsia. Once a subject has thrown a fit she is labeled as eclampsia. All measures are then after for prevention of subsequent fit. Therefore like miscarriages, eclampsia is to be prevented and not treated. Consequently in strictest sense of the term all that is required to do once fetal demise occurs in a given subject of miscarriage is to assist nature and complete the procedure. This is done by performing an evacuation procedure. Thenafter measures are introduced to prevent a subsequent miscarriage. Therefore not much is written here under the head treatment of miscarriages. Relevant aspects have been covered in prevention of obstetric vasculopathies.

REFERENCES

1. Desai P, Desai M, Modi D. Recurrent spontaneous abortions of immunological cause: a case of work-up after two losses. *Jr O & G India*. 1997;47:303-6.
2. Backos M, Rai R, Baxter N, Chilcott IT, Cohen H, Regan L. Pregnancy miscarriages associated with antiphospholipid antibodies: Treated with low dose aspirin and heparin. *Br J Obstet Gynaecol.* 1999;106(2):102-7.

CHAPTER

22

Treatment of Obstetric Vasculopathy—Preeclampsia

CHAPTER OUTLINE

- Limitations of Blood Pressures as an Indicator of Severity
- Early Diagnosis and Alert Surveillance
- Do Subjects of Preeclampsia Need Admission
- Management on Hospitalization
- Antihypertensives
- Induction of Labor in Pregnancy Induced Hypertension
- Methods of Induction of Labor
- Cesarean Section in Pregnancy Induced Hypertension
- Post Delivery Care

INTRODUCTION

The basic aspect of treatment of preeclampsia includes controlling hypertension and preventing complications. It needs to be clarified that in treating hypertension no attempts are made to bring the BP to prepregnant level. This is important because not only will the BP never come back to the prepregnant level till the pregnancy is on but it can downright harm the mother and the fetus if such energetic measures are taken to sink the BP to these levels. Consequently, it will be in the interests of ongoing pregnancy to continue BP at stages of mild hypertension till as long as possible. This is due to the fact that the ongoing processes of vasculopathies have produced a widely pervading vasospasm. The rise in BP is a reaction to that vasospasm. Now if through antihypertensives the BP is energetically pulled down the blood flow to the different systems of the gravida and the all important fetomaternal interface would get impoverished and hampered. As a result these systems and interfaces that are now working or tuned at the raised pressure of blood can react stormily including rendering them dysfunctional. One sees some similar effects in complications of accidental hemorrhage. (It will be dealt within the section of treatment of accidental hemorrhage separately).

LIMITATIONS OF BLOOD PRESSURES AS AN INDICATOR OF SEVERITY

In the entire clinical spectrum of preeclampsia, hypertension is the major and cardinal factor in its diagnosis. Across the board any pregnant subject with systolic blood pressures of 130 and/or diastolic BP of 90 or more and therefore a MAP of 103 or more is labeled as hypertensive. In clinical practice in most pregnant subjects this indeed hold true. However, there can be situations where BP may not reach their levels and still some manifestations of preeclampsia and milder changes and complications may appear.

Also, in some subjects the worsening of BP can be timely detected to label it as worsening of this obstetric vasculopathy. But in some subjects complications may occur without much changes or rise in BP A pregnant subject may show changes on fundoscopy which are characteristic of severe preeclampsia at levels of BP much below the recommended levels of hypertension for labeling in this class of preeclampsia. In such situations proteinuria can be of great help. It is therefore felt that presence of proteinuria greater than 300 mg/24 hours should be comprehensively considered with hypertension to label it as preeclampsia. The two together can be very important indicator for worsening of the condition. Therefore in subjects with preeclampsia a rise in BP and/or increasing proteinuria to singly or in combination are better measures to label a subject as having a worsening preeclampsia.

Leveno and Cunningham while authoring the chapter on *Management of Eclampsia* in Chesley's Hypertensive Disorders of Pregnancy have succinctly defined the basic management goals of a subject with preeclampsia. They have stated that the basic management objectives for any pregnancy complicated by preeclampsia are:

1. Termination of pregnancy with the least possible trauma to the mother or the fetus
2. Birth of an infant who subsequently thrives
3. Complete restoration of health to the mother.

They further add that in certain cases of preeclampsia, especially in women at or near term all three objectives are served cqually well by induction of labor. Therefore, the most important information that the obstetrician has for successful management of pregnancy and especially a pregnancy that becomes complicated by hypertension is *precise knowledge of the age of the fetus*[1].

These three principles of management of preeclampsia have been by and large achievable in nearly all subjects of preeclampsia in modern obstetrics. However, to reach this stage has never been an easy journey. Besides, very elaborate understanding of the etiopathology and pathophysiology involved new drugs and influx of modern technology in obstetric practice have made all this possible. The principles of management of preeclampsia focusing on the aforesaid three goals begin with the concept of early detection and vigilant surveillance.

EARLY DIAGNOSIS AND ALERT SURVEILLANCE

The cutout BP of 130/90 that has been described in the preceding pages may be just one factor (**P**···). However, in subjects with antenatal care of good quality more appropriate cutout are 30 mm of Hg systolic and/or 15 mm of Hg diastolic taken on two consecutive readings at least six hours apart after adequate bed rest. The importance of each of these subclasses to the registering of rise in BP has been discussed in details elsewhere.

However, this aspect of diagnosing hypertension without waiting for the absolute cutout of 130/90 is very important. This is more so for petite mothers especially in the Indian subcontinent and other parts of East Asia. These mothers have a very low set BP physiologically. Many of these subjects comfortably maintain their physiology of all organs and systems at BP as low as 90/70 mm of Hg. There will always be situations that can befool the clinician if he/she waits for the absolute figure of 130/90 mm of Hg.

The other point which comes in alert surveillance is the point related to the midtrimester fall in BP registered in normal pregnancy. In hospital-class patients in India whose quality antenatal care coverage is poor the failure of fall of this BP can be missed to get recorded. These subjects may register late for antenatal care, if at all they do. In such situations a clinician may not be able to provide them with the advantages of alert surveillance.

The two sets of pregnant subjects can help detect an impending preeclampsia much early: those that register a rise in 30 mm of Hg BP systolic and/or 15 mm of Hg BP > rise in diastolic BP and those subjects in whom there is no fall in midtrimester BP In both these subjects quality antenatal care providers can give an advantage to these pregnant subjects of early prenatal detection.

The other aspect where quality surveillance can help is at the late stage of impending eclampsia. Clinical and laboratory features like worsening proteinuria, rising BP, sudden severe weight gain, complaints like epigastric pain or dimness of vision and the entire list of features of an impending eclampsia. These can be used for early intervention before it is too late. In these subjects termination of pregnancy with least possible trauma to the mother and the fetus can be planned much before the situation goes out of hand.

DO SUBJECTS OF PREECLAMPSIA NEED ADMISSION

In clinical practice in India there are two distinct groups of pregnant subjects: One group of public hospital-class patients who do not have the awareness of the need for antenatal care. The other group is the well educated and adequately resourced subjects who register for antenatal care (usually in private hospitals and clinics) as early as possible. Expectedly the outcome in both these group of subjects is bound to be different. As a result some principles of approach would be a shade different.

Subjects in whom the importance of antenatal care is not known and their reliability of coming for a regular antenatal care cannot be guaranteed, in them admission for preeclampsia even if mild, becomes necessary. However, with the same BP subjects in whom adequate follow-up for antenatal care can be ensured, admission may not be necessary at the hospital and they may be treated at home.

MANAGEMENT ON HOSPITALIZATION

Needless to say, once admitted these subjects need a very systematic management plan. This includes:

- Twice a day measurement of BP

- Bed rest with restricted activity: By restricted activity it is meant that she can be allowed to go to the toilet for her daily and periodic clean up and wash needs as well as for passing urine and stool.
- Testing urine for albuminuria is also to be done every day. A worsening (increasing) proteinuria may be the first sign of a worsening preeclampsia. It may indicate a need for an early intervention.
- Biophysical profile: On admission and thereafter daily there will be need to perform a biophysical profile of the pregnant subject. It may sound a trifle too soon, but sudden precipitous deteriorations of these subjects are known. It is also wise in subjects of severe preeclampsia, to individualize performing a biophysical assessment. There can be situations where, if the patients preeclampsia is steadily worsening there might be a need to perform biophysical profile especially CTG tracings even six hourly.
- Steroids: Antenatal administration of steroids to improve the fetal systemic maturity especially lungs should be given to the mother. 24 mg of Betamethasone administered intramuscularly over an internal of 24 to 36 hours is the standard schedule.

We administer steroids upto 34 weeks in late II trimester and upto mid third trimester. The controversy related to repeat dosage of steroid administration and other aspects is not being touched here as it is beyond the scope of this discussion. However, one controversy that is discussed here is related to the organ and systemic maturity occurring faster in preeclamptic subjects. There had been reports and studies which suggested that babies born to mothers with severe preeclampsia and eclampsia have much better systemic maturity when matched for the new borns of non-preeclamptic subjects. They seem to develop RDS and complications like necrotizing enterocolitis at a much less frequency. Nevertheless this claim could not be fully substantiated. It was found that this advantage of early maturity of newborns in subjects with preeclampsia was not universal. It was only for subjects who had persistent proteinuria along with hypertension. Thus proteinuria seems to be the key deciding factor in enhanced systemic maturity.

This is not to suggest that in some mysterious way proteinuria enhances the fetal lung and other systemic maturity. Development and persistence of proteinuria indicates a severe form of preeclampsia. Due to this challenge the fetus in itself develops a faster systemic maturity. This may be a natural preparation for the possible early delivery that may occur due to a rapidly developing hostile intrauterine environment.

Besides administration of steroids to subjects of preeclampsia, admitted subjects may also be needed to be subjected periodically to colour Doppler studies. Although CTG may be able to give the status of the fetus over a period of a week or so, colour Doppler will give the fetal status at the precise moment. When the results of the two are reviewed in combination, one gets a more accurate idea for the need to terminate the pregnancy.

ANTIHYPERTENSIVES

Amongst many controversies that are associated with obstetric vasculopathies one that generates maximum controversy is related to the use of anti-hypertensive. This is due to the fact that one school of thought is very conservative on this aspect and the other quite contrastingly radical. In such a situation carefully conducted RCTs have guided us in taking decisions.

The trickiest question is related to the timing of starting antihypertensives. While many seem to emphatically state that mild preeclampsia does not need antihypertensives for treatment we do not completely agree to this in the situations where we have worked. The recommendation for not starting antihypertensives in mildly preeclamptic subjects came from results which showed that fetal outcome in particular and general obstetric outcomes do not alter by starting antihypertensives in such subjects. However those recommendations may not be applicable to setups where pregnant subjects may not come for follow-up regularly and are ill informed of the dangers of preeclampsia.

Even these RCTs and meta-analysis on the subject matter recommend a need for longer trials and more data to take a final stand. Therefore they rightly state and we too agree that as of now there is no need for practitioners of the subject to change the policy. If they are prescribing they may continue to do so and if not they may do so. We individualize the cases based on the follow-up and comprehensive view of the fury of preeclampsia. By this we mean that if a subject is rapidly developing clinical features of preeclampsia, than in these subjects even if the disease process at the material moment of time is labeled as mild, we still prefer to start antihypertensives. However, if the subject is already showing an insidious progression of the condition we do not start antihypertensives. Besides this if we feel that labor induction is imminent in any given subject, the need to start antihypertensives is much more liberal. This is because control of BP in these subjects once in labor tends to go haywire.

Which Antihypertensive

This seems to be a perpetual debate. Volume of research papers have been generated on this. The constant influx of antihypertensives in pharmacological science makes the obstetrician inquisitive if anyone could be better than the others. Thankfully in this matter the situation is now quite clear and shall be crystallized in the paragraphs to follow.

Challenges before any Antihypertensive in Pregnancy Induced Hypertension

Any antihypertensive when used in pregnancy faces some peculiar requirements to be fulfilled. The foremost is that it should not be teratogenic. Teratogenicity in antihypertensives confines not much to their effects in first trimester (albeit that is important) but in subsequent trimesters too. This is because the need for giving an antihypertensive in first trimester is not common. It is usually confined to those subjects in whom there is chronic hypertension.

In this regard most antihypertensives in current domain of physicians are by and large safe. However, ACE-inhibitors are teratogenic. They can cause renal effects if given in first trimester and can precipitate an IUGR or worsen an already existent IUGR later in pregnancy. Therefore, if a hypertensive subject is planning a pregnancy and she is on ACE-inhibitors, a transition to safer agents should be immediately undertaken before she conceives. In the eventuality of a subject already pregnant with early pregnancy and on ACE-inhibitors, immediate change over to safe agents needs to be done.

Besides, this challenge of teratogenicity, the other challenge before any antihypertensive when put to use in pregnancy is its need to be rapidly effective. In this regards it has been found that α-methyldopa may be a little "lazy" in generating it full pharmacological effects. However, this agent is very popular and has nothing much against it.

One more challenge before an antihypertensive to be employed for use in obstetrics is it should not reduce the BP. precipitously. By precipitous reduction it is meant that it should not be so powerful that BP falls within seconds of its administration and can even be pushed down very close to hypotensive levels. Classical example in this regard is sodium nitroprusside. This antihypertensive is very potent and very rapid in action. Its use was primarily confined to subjects in whom there was an eclamptic fit. In eclampsia there is a need for controlling BP fast. However, sodium nitroprusside was found to be very precipitous in pushing down the BP Such a rapid fall in BP and that too to suboptimal levels at times precipitated accidental hemorrhage in pregnant subjects. It also caused acute fetal distress and even fetal death.

Apprehensions were expressed regarding nifedipine, one of the most popular calcium-channel blocker, that it can precipitously cause a fall in BP. Over a period of time this has been disproved and fears allayed.

Another challenge before any antihypertensive was to be able to maintain good and effective control over BP during labor. It is well known that the entire control of BP can go completely awry during the stress of labor. Violent uterine activity can quickly shunt large amounts of blood from and into the maternal circulation. In such a situation, the BP control gets severely challenged and may be lost. A good antihypertensive must be able to control her BP even during this phase.

A challenge that has only recently been met with is the route of antihypertensive administration. Eclamptic subjects are unconscious and hypertensive. They can convulse again if the situation is not managed efficiently. Oral administration of antihypertensives in them is nearly impossible. Attempts made by some to administer antihypertensives through the nasogastric tubes were also futile and even dangerous. This is because a convulsive subject may not be able to tolerate the nasogastric tube for long. Also, eclamptic subjects have a reduced gastric emptying time. In such a situation administering anything orally can be vomited out. Vomiting in an unconscious subject is very dangerous as it can precipitate Mendelson's syndrome. This can be fatal.

For long, hardly any antihypertensive which can be safe for use in pregnancy parenterally was available. This problem was first solved by the availability of hydralazine. Nifedipine in the mean time was able to solve this problem even before parenteral labetalol became available. This was because nifedipine could be administered sublingually and so nonoral administration of antihypertensive became a reality even before injectable hydralazine became universally available.

One more problem that antihypertensive face is the problem of mechanism of action. One mechanism by which many antihypertensives act is by reducing the cardiac output. This could be unacceptable to the pregnant subject as it can seriously jeopardize the fetal circulation. In all of these therefore agents which reduced peripheral resistance by vasodilatation were found to be most useful. This explains the popularity of nifedipine and hydralazine in PIH as well as eclampsia.

Alpha methyldopa and labetalol have also been showing very good efficacy in management of hypertensive disorders of pregnancy. Beta blockers like propranolol did gain some popularity for some time. However the fear that it may be worsening neonatal jaundice if given just before delivery made them out of circuit.

Thus amongst all antihypertensives that are currently in use the safest, effective and popular are nifedipine (calcium channel blockers) alpha methyldopa, atenolol and labetalol. The question that was asked at the commencement of this chapter (P···) is which of these is the best? The answer to this is none and all. This means none of these agents are superior to one another and therefore all of them are effective and can be used safely in pregnancy. As has been mentioned there is no antihypertensive amongst those currently recommended for safe use in pregnancy that is superior or inferior to others. Therefore, the choice is left to the clinician. However in large meta-analysis and Cochrane review it is found that while no antihypertensive is superior or inferior to others, it seems that Labetalol may be a shade better than others for better control of BP in labor.

Monotherapy Versus Multidrug Therapy

By and large monodrug therapy in preeclampsia is a rule. However second drug can be added if BP is not adequately controlled by the highest permissible dose of the single drug started. It is therefore recommended that the dosage of the same drug is increased gradiently if the BP is not under control. Only if the maximum dose is unable to adequately control the blood pressure should the second line of defense be added.

For nonoral administration currently three drugs are available for use: (A) Sublingual nifedipine, (B) Intramuscular labetalol, and (C) Intramuscular (or intravenous to be verified) hydralazine.

Dosage Schedules

Nifedipine

Nifedipine is given in the dose of 10 mg 8 hourly orally. In subjects of eclampsia or those in whom oral administration is to be restricted, nifedipine is administered in a dose of 5 mg sublingually to be repeated every six to eight hourly. However, as soon as the pregnant subject is able to take orally one can switch over to the oral dosage schedule.

Atenolol

Atenolol is administered in a dose of 2.5 mg per day. Atenolol usually controls BP by once a day dose. However, if the BP is not controlled 2.5 mgm is given 12 hourly for that much time that BP comes under control.

Labetalol

Labetalol is given in a dose of 200 mg 12 hourly to commence with. But as soon as the BP comes under control, the dose is reduced to 100 mg 12 hourly.

Alpha Methyldopa

Alpha methyldopa is usually started in a dose of 250 mg 8 hourly. However, if this does not suffice to control BP dosage can be increased to 250 mg 6 hourly. This can be further increased upto 500 mg 6 hourly. Thus alpha methyldopa can be given upto 2 gm in 24 hours in 4 divided doses.

Hydralazine

Hydralazine is also recommended for use in pregnancy hypertension. In fact it was the only antihypertensive which could be used safely in pregnancy that was available for parenteral administration especially in the U.S. market. Its recommended dose is an IV bolus at a dose of 5 to 10 mg, depending on the severity of hypertension, and may be administered every 20 minutes up to a maximum dose of 30 mg.

When to Stop Antihypertensives

This seems to be an easy question to answer. As soon as the diastolic BP goes less than 90 and/or systolic goes less than 130 and the mean arterial pressure below 103, antihypertensives can be stopped safely. However, the problem arises in some subjects in whom BP suddenly goes to normal immediately after delivery. These are usually subjects who have severe form of the condition including eclampsia. In these subjects BP can and usually does rise after this "Lucid Interval". It is a tricky situation. This is because thc subject is reeling under a severe attack of worst manifestations of hypertension in pregnancy and is not registering any hypertension. Why does the BP behaves thus is not exactly known.

As regards antihypertensives in these subjects, it is wise to discontinue antihypertensives if BP goes to normal levels even if for transient duration of time. However, close and periodic monitoring of BP should be continued. As and when the BP returns to the levels of hypertension, antihypertensives should be restarted in a graded fashion. By graded fashion it is meant that a full dose of antihypertensives may not be required at the first instance. It is a matter of wisdom and common sense to administer the drug dose graded to the rise in BP.

In most other subjects no such precipitous fall in BP is seen. In these subjects antihypertensives should be continued till the subject registers hypertension. However some subjects show a gradual decline in BP. In these subjects the dosage of antihypertensives needs to be gradually reduced. It is felt that if subjects having P.I.H. registers hypertension even after three months postpartum this could be a case of chronic hypertension or superimposed preeclampsia. This is more so in subjects in whom prepregnancy BP is not known. It is also believed that pregnancy may unravel a hidden hypertension in some subjects. The crux of the matter is if any subject registers a hypertension that needs antihypertensives even after three months postpartum, it is wise to seek an opinion of a physician and start investigating and treating these subjects as a chronic hypertensive.

Having managed the hypertension of a subject with PIH the next critical decision making for the clinician is induction of labor.

INDUCTION OF LABOR IN PREGNANCY INDUCED HYPERTENSION (PIH)

While it is not envisaged here to discuss the mechanism of onset of labor, the currently available labor inducing agents used for softening of cervix and simultaneous stimulation of uterine activity. Thus induction of labor is essentially initiation of uterine contractile activity on a softened and dilatable cervix in a patient of PIH so as to achieve a delivery.

When to Induce Labor in Pregnancy Induced Hypertension (PIH)

This question can have one of the easiest answers on one side, and the most difficult answer on the other side of the spectrum. The easiest answer is at 37 completed weeks of pregnancy.

37 Weeks

This 37 weeks cutout has been accepted over a period of time following many studies on the basis that at this duration of pregnancy, the fetus actives its systemic maturity especially that of the critical systems. This mainly includes the lungs. Once the fetus achieves its systemic maturity all it gains in the uterus is in terms of weight gain at the rate of about 23 grams/day. Maternal systems confer both the maturity as well as weight to the growing fetus. Most of the challenges that a prematurely born newborn encounters are essentially due to a deficient maturity. This precipitates life threatening problems like Respiratory Distress Syndrome (RDS), Necrotizing Enterocolitis (NEC) and generalized infections including septicemia.

In subjects of PIH in particular especially severe PIH if 37 weeks of pregnancy has already been achieved, labor should be induced. However, the bigger challenge lies in subjects who have not yet reached 37 weeks and labor for various reasons needs to be induced. It will be more challenging a decision-making.

Eclampsia

This is one easier decision-making situation. By and large in most of the pregnant subjects once a convulsion following PIH occurs it is wise to induce labor. The concept of inter current eclampsia waxes and wanes. There are times when some enthusiasts start advocating controlling the convulsions, preventing subsequent convulsions and allowing the pregnancy to continue. This is intercurrent eclampsia. It is argued that if the pregnancy has not yet reached a stage where neonatal survival chances are good, such pregnancies are continued beyond the convulsion. Most believe that allowing the maternal system to bear the fierce onslaught of the hypertension in its most severe form is unnecessary and unjustified. We do not believe in the concept of intercurrent eclampsia. We induce labor in any subject of eclampsia irrespective of the duration of pregnancy. We only wait for a few hours of a convulsion maximum two for the convulsing mother to settle and then initiate measures of inducing labor.

Severe Pregnancy Induced Hypertension (PIH)

Having had seen the two relatively easy indications for labor induction. Now some tougher areas need to be reviewed. Severe PIH is one such area. There are some groups of research workers who club severe PIH and imminent eclampsia together. Therefore in their subjects a severe hypertension characterized by BP at or above 110 diastolic and proteinuria of >1g/day or greater than 4 plus in a spot sample of urine are principle factors deciding in favour of induction of labor. These may be coupled by minor factors like sudden severe weight gain or oliguria or epigastric pain or persistent headache or visual alterations and the like. This bunch of features are clubbed as minor and therefore contribute to decision making though themselves do not clinch the issue on their own.

Induction of Labor in Pregnancy < 37 Weeks and no Severe Pregnancy Induced Hypertension (PIH)

This is the toughest decision making situation. In this the BP has still not crossed the limits to be labeled as severe PIH. Also, there are no life-threatening complications to the mother. To make matters worse the pregnancy has still not reached the comfort zone of 37 weeks and beyond. These are the pregnancies where decision-making is toughest.

In these subjects the need for induction arises purely because the unborn fetus is developing features of compromise including IUGR. The other feature which may or may not be accompanying IUGR is oligohydramnios. Thus IUGR and oligohydramnios singly or in combination are indication for labor induction in subjects of PIH. However the toughest part is to decide when to induce labor in such a pregnancy. It is therefore rightly said that when the intrauterine environment is more hostile for the fetus as compared to the extrauterine environment, the pregnancy needs to be terminated. Having had understood this principle, now the challenge lies in deciding and correctly diagnosing this hostility of the environment.

For this purpose clinical as well as technological inputs and their correlation becomes critical. Relying solely on any one of the two could invite a grave possibility of iatrogenic prematurity which is completely preventable and understandably unnecessary. As regards the clinical diagnosis it is based on parameters like a symphysio-fundal height (SFH). If the pregnancy has a difference of 6 cm or more of SFH at or after 30 weeks of pregnancy, IUGR and/or oligohydramnios should be suspected. This method has its own limitations of reliability but is often the first sign alerting the clinician.

Even a regular antenatal checkup can alert the clinician to a possibility of the baby not thriving within. This needs average experience and no extra ordinary expertise. Most clinicians have done away with the practice of measuring the symphysio-fundal height. In such a situation even a regular alert palpation of the fundus and assessing its height with context to the weeks of gestation as per the menstrual age is sufficient for the same.

The other vital help that is received is from colour Doppler and cardiotocograph tracings. These two have been extensively discussed elsewhere. On basis of ultrasonography oligohydramnios is diagnosed easily. Also, ultrasonography will help in diagnosing a head-sparing type of IUGR by automatically plotting the ratio of head circumference to abdominal circumference. If this is increasing (even if within the normal range) will give out the diagnosis of an IUGR and alert to a possible need of early intervention. Besides the HC:AC ratio and Amniotic fluid Index (AFI) serial ultrasound will also show a decline in expected birth weight (EBW). When plotted on the graph this decline is so obvious that it can't be missed.

Once the clinician is alerted to the possibility of the baby suffering from chronic hypoxia, the vital decision-making that is required relates to if and when to deliver this baby. In this situation colour Doppler and CTG together help significantly. If the colour Doppler reveals a compromised baby with the cerebro-placental ratio approaching 1, there is an urgent need to intervene and affect a delivery. Cerebro-placental ratio or CPR as it is popularly expressed as is the ratio of pulsatility index of the middle cerebral artery to the pulsatility of umbilical artery. This ratio holds a very impressive promise in deciding the need and haste at which induction of labor may be required. The advantage of this ratio is that it takes both the critical arterial flows into consideration. Thus it gives a comprehensive view of the situation improving the quality of decision making in the matter.

Another technological help that can be of great use in decision-making for the timing of intervention is CTG. This technology which analyzes the behavior of fetal heart rate and rhythm gives an idea of fetal oxygenation status over a small period of time. Any significant alteration in variability of the fetal heart rate and rhythm is ominous. Also if the fetal heart rate refuses to accelerate with fetal movement it is ominous. If during the course of evaluation if the fetal heart rate registers a deceleration on a Non Stress Test (NST) it is ominous. Any one or more of these features indicate that the fetus is in trouble and needs to be brought out.

These three technological inputs give the idea of the fact that the intrauterine environment is hostile for the fetus and therefore it would be wise to induce labor. So, the clinical situation of pregnancy being less than 37 weeks and if the decision-making about induction of labor is necessitated, it is the most difficult of all indications of induction labor in PIH.

The Need for Involving a Neonatologist

As a part of improved antenatal care and quality obstetrics it is now a rule in all good obstetric units to involve the neonatologist in decision-making about induction of labor in difficult situations. There are important inputs which are obtained from the neonatologist the main being how early or preterm child will the neonatal unit be able to handle. In this context most average units are now reasonably confident in handling average birth weight of 1200 g or more. However with betterment of technology, ventilatory support and the availability of surfactants, still younger and lighter babies can be salvaged. However this is absolutely within the preview of the neonatologist, his/her input only can decide on the basis of his experience with the neonatal intensive care unit that he/she handles.

The second reason to involve a neonatologist in this decision-making is based on the fact that the unit gets prepared for handling of such a baby. Gone are the days when obstetricians used to operate in isolation. It is no more only their concern when to induce labor. Working in isolation can open up scenarios where an unprepared and overloaded neonatal intensive care unit receives a sick baby it is unable to take in or adequately handle. It is therefore necessary to involve the neonatologist in decision making regarding the timing of induction in pregnancies less that 37 weeks in duration. As has been stated the obstetrician needs to evaluate if the intrauterine environment is more hostile for the fetus than the extra-uterine environment. The neonatal backup services therefore are most critical in making the extrauterine environment favorable and less hostile for the newborn. Understandably therefore the neonatologist needs to be involved in the entire decision-making process for inducing labor before 37 weeks of pregnancy.

METHODS OF INDUCTION OF LABOR

Discovery of prostaglandins has made induction of labor easier, more controlled and less arduous. In reality prostaglandins as so easily available for the purpose that now the onus is on the obstetrician to ensure that it is not misused or overused. Also the safety profile becomes a matter of concern with this relatively new pharmacological technology.

Trachleodynamics in Induction of Labor

While on methods of inducing labor it is necessary to understand the cervix, its dynamics and physiology for a successful and safe labor induction. The cervix needs to be evaluated for its favorability for labor induction. In this context Bishops score has been of great help in clinical practice for decades now. Bishop's score subsequently modified by Calder has been now well established. A god birthing unit will always mention the Bishop's score of the subjects before deciding for induction of labor.

Parameter/score	0	1	2	3
Position	Posterior	Intermediate	Anterior	–
Consistency	Firm	Intermediate	Soft	–
Effacement	0–30%	31–50%	51–80%	> 80%
Dilation	0 cm	1–2 cm	3–4 cm	> 5 cm
Fetal station	–3	–2	–1, 0	+1, +2

Universally accepted now, a score of more than 6 indicates a favorable cervix for induction of labor and will result in a successful outcome more after than not.

The concept to of trachleodynamics needs to be carefully understood in subjects with obstetric vasculopathies including PIH. This is so because on more occasions than not labor inducing interventions need to be employed. For success of any labor induction cervical compliance and subsequent synchronous dilatation has to happen. Cervical ripening agents are expected to bring about a series of changes in the ultrastructure and biochemical milieu in such a way that cervix becomes shortened, softened and dilated to let the passage of the fetus. This transforms the cervix from a sphincter organ which preserves the pregnancy to a dilated conduit letting the fetus pass through it. In this process prostaglandins have proved to be the "game changers".

Before the introduction of prostaglandins in induction of labor most pharmacological agents like oxytocin used to act on the uterus. Their uterine predominance activated the activity in the uterus secondary to it, the cervix dilated. However, in the physiology of labor, this is not the way labor progresses and initiates. In physiology of labor, cervix becomes compliant, softens and dilates proactively. The uterine activity is occurring in symphony with the cervical and in rhythm. None is secondary to the other.

Therefore, drugs and methods which envisaged inducing labor by bringing about uterine activity and letting the cervix respond secondarily to the uterus took a long time for labor to get induced. Very often these methods failed. They also had a tendency to need other ancillary measures to activate the process. These included methods like stripping of membranes or artificial rupture of membranes.

Prostaglandins

Both prostaglandins PGE2 and PGF2α are used to activate cervix and induce labor in PIH. However, PGE2 has been found to be predominantly active on cervix. Therefore, their action is more useful for cervical softening and ripening. PGF2α seems to be more selective for uterus in its action though it too has a weak direct action on the cervix. Therefore, PGE2 is used predominantly for labor induction by cervical ripening.

Intracervical and vaginal gets of PGE2 have less systemic side effects compared to oral and intramuscular routes of administration. As a result in modern obstetrics only these two methods are used for cervical ripening and inducing labor. Vaginal and cervical PGE2 complete the process by 24 hours. They lower the duration for which epidural analgesia needs to be administered and also decrease cesarean section rates. However, there is a small disadvantage of a possible hyperstimulation of the uterus. Over a period of time with obstetricians becoming more and more used to prostaglandin use, hyperstimulation is no more menacing and widespread. Carefully graded doses of administration of prostaglandins have nearly eliminated the fear of uterine rupture.

Dose

Intracervical PGF2α gels are available as 0.5 and 1 mg dispensation for cervical ripening. In subjects of PIH with an unripe cervix (Bishop's Score of less than 4) it is recommended to start with a dose of 1 mgm of intracervical or vaginal gel. This is to be repeated every six hourly for a maximum of a total dose of 4 mg in 24 hours. This dose may be reduced for multigravida proportionately. In multis the maximum dose recommended is 3 mg in 24 hours.

It is wise to monitor the uterine activity for initial half an hour to one hour of PGE2 gel administration. This is for diagnosing uterine hyperstimulation. There can also be fetal distress secondary to uterine hyperstimulation. Currently PGE2 is also administered in a dose of 0.5 mg initially as cervical or vaginal gel followed by 0.5 mg every six hourly. This has nearly eliminated the fear of uterine hyperstimulation and a consequent fetal distress.

Once the cervix becomes ripe and Bishop's score becomes more than 6, it is advised to give PGF2α in a dose of 25 micrograms per vaginum. This is given every four to six hours. PGF2α has its predominant uterine action. This action coupled with a compliant cervix creates a completely physiological situation for a proper and successful labor induction.

Most of the times labor with these doses of PGE2 gel supplemented by PGF2α induces labor within 24 hours, successfully. Not more than 10% subjects would warrant these labor inducing agents to be administered for more than 48 hours. This is more so in subjects of obstetric vasculopathies especially PIH and IUGR. Even in accidental hemorrhage labor induction occurs readily and swiftly.

System Readiness for Labor Induction in Pregnancy Induced Hypertension (PIH)

It is very interesting to note that the maternal system is always very ready to get labor induction going in situations of severe PIH and eclampsia. This is attributed to process of decidual activation that is the key harbinger of labor. With the understanding of the process of labor becoming more and more clear, it has become obvious that labor is induced not by the mother but by the fetal systems. It has now been known that if the intrauterine environment is non-conducive to pregnancy continuation labor gets induced much more easily. This does not need the fetus to be alive. The onus therefore is not on the live fetus. It is comprehensively on the fetal systems. As a result, even if the fetus has had a demise, labor gets readily induced to eliminate the product of conception.

The concept of the fetal unit having a key and decisive role in inducing labor came from the observation that fetuses with anencephaly in pre-ultrasound days could not be diagnosed so easily. As a result labor induction in anencephalic fetus would not happen readily. Anencephalic fetus was a known cause of postdatism in those days. It was found that induction of labor is principally the onus of the fetus. Therefore a challenged and endangered fetal system in obstetric vasculopathy supports attempts at labor induction readily.

Other Methods of Labor Induction

Before prostaglandins got established in this indication the principle pharmacological agent that was used was oxytocin. Oxytocin infusions in titrating doses were used for years with consistently poor results. As has been seen this was due to its primary effects on uterine musculature and only secondary effects on trachleodynamics.

Other than pharmacological agents, mechanical agents were also used in the process. These included hygroscopic cervical dilators, balloon catheters and the like. These were met with reasonably good success.

Another set of methods of labor induction included milieu-altering methods. These were methods that envisaged inducing labor by disturbing the stable environment of an ongoing pregnancy. In such a set of methods membrane stripping and artificial rupture of membranes was included. These met with inconsistent success. Besides their popularity was only because better methods were not available. There was always a grave risk of chorioamnionitis. If after an artificial rupture of membranes labor failed to get induced within a reasonable time (24 hours) there would be a real risk of chorioamnionitis. This could prove fatal both for the fetus as well as the mother. As soon as prostaglandins became available for labor induction these methods quickly fell by the wayside.

Once labor got induced, the progress monitoring in PIH is always more vigilant. This is because a compromised fetus would get distressed much earlier compared to low-risk pregnancy fetuses. Continuous CTG monitoring in labor is not out of place. Cesarean section incidence is therefore likely to be higher in subjects of severe PIH.

CESAREAN SECTION IN PREGNANCY INDUCED HYPERTENSION (PIH)

The when, why and how of cesarean section in PIH is a very interesting aspect of obstetric management of a subject with PIH. Though cesarean section rates may be little higher in subjects with severe PIH, this is not an absolute indication. Infact the only absolute indication for cesarean section in preeclampsia and eclampsia is status eclampticus. Needless to say, obstetric indications of cesarean section like cephalo-pelvic disproportion, mento-posterior and the like will warrant a cesarean section irrespective of preeclampsia. They need not be discussed in details as this will render the subject out of focus.

Cesarean section for PIH is a much more complicated and challenging issue which needs the fundamentals to be very clearly understood. If one revisits indication for doing PIH purely for PIH then the list is very small with either one or two entries. The most common amongst all is when PIH gets complicated with IUGR. In such cases if CTG and colour Doppler indicate a rapid intervention the obstetrician may need to carry out a cesarean section.

Rarer amongst the two is a situation where severe PIH continues to worsen inspite of antihypertensives and other concurrent treatments. BP not coming under control with or without systemic complications like renal compromise or coagulation failure is a reason which may need a quick intervention to end the pregnancy. This is debatable and thankfully rare. However, in an above average clinical practice load, obstetricians will have some subjects like these periodically wherein view of a rapidly developing situation, cesarean section may be carried out. However, it would always be wise to individualize the decision-making. Except for these two, there is hardly any situation where PIH may need a cesarean section.

POST DELIVERY CARE

In this section the entire discussion was around what all needs to be done for a subject of PIH on admission. Therefore aspects related to examination, investigations and treatment in hospital set up have been extensively discussed. The final management comes in related to post delivery management.

Pregnancy Induced Hypertension (PIH)

Once the subject has delivered there are a series of problems that need to be vigilantly dealt with by a clinician. The biggest dread is a possibility of PPH. For reasons still not amply clear, subjects with severe PIH have a tendency to develop atonic postpartum hemorrhage. This is a tricky situation to handle. Methyl ergometrine the known strong uterotonic is notorious for shooting up the blood pressure. In subjects of PIH, one can ill afford this situation. It would therefore be a challenge to the dexterity of a clinician to weigh between administration of methyl ergometrine for prevention and treatment of atonic PPH in subjects of PIH on one side and handling a sudden shooting up of blood pressure on the other.

Usually methyl ergometrine is avoided for preventing of atonic PPH in severe PIH. Instead milder agents like syntocinon are administered. However, when and if atonic PPH actually occurs the clinician does take a calculated risk and does administer methyl ergometrine. At that moment the critical decision is to weigh between allowing a potentially fatal blood loss and managing a fresh rise in BP The decision usually goes in favor of stopping blood loss. The rise in BP is usually handled by a sublingual nifedipine or parenteral labetalol.

BP

Irrespective of PPH, BP tends to behave erratically at times, postpartum. In most subjects the BP gradually falls in a graded pattern and returns to prepregnant levels by the time puerperium ends. Accordingly the clinician will be required to taper the dose of antihypertensives. However, there will be some subjects in whom BP can suddenly appear normotensive in early puerperium about 48 hours post delivery. But it then catapults to the pre-delivery levels quickly thenafter. The pathophysiology behind this has been extensively explained in the chapter relevant to the same. For a clinician, however, it would be necessary to be aware of adjust the dose of antihypertensives. It is possible that in the phase in which the BP suddenly falls down to "normal" levels immediately postpartum it may necessitate a complete withdrawal of antihypertensives. Then after they may be required to be reintroduced once BP has commenced to rise again.

There would be a small number of subjects, who had severe PIH just before delivery, whose BP strikes the base immediately postpartum. Thereafter the B.P may just not rise again. They will not require any antihypertensive support then after.

Coagulation Failure

Severe PIH can be complicated by a relatively rare complication of coagulation failure in postpartum phase. This process starts just when the process is at its peak before delivery but may get menacingly manifested as postpartum hemorrhage post-delivery. Replacement of coagulation factors in the form of whole fresh blood or blood components is the established form of treatment. However, it can severely challenge an already precariously balanced system.

Renal Failure

This complication of PIH also becomes manifested most of the times postpartum. A precariously balanced renal function gets ticked off with the added load of blood loss in subjects of PIH. Consequently there can be a renal failure getting clinically manifested in such conditions. Thankfully these are most of the times glomerular failure. However, if cortical failure occurs, it can be difficult to reverse. The subject may need dialysis and renal transplantation.

It is noteworthy that effect of PPH and precipitation of renal failure occurs much more readily in subjects with preeclampsia/eclampsia. This vulnerability arises from reversal of a physiology in hypertensive disorders of pregnancy. The increase in blood volume that occurs in pregnancy as a part of physiological adaptation to pregnancy can be as high as 1.5 liter by term. In PIH, this increase in blood volume is either completely or partially stemmed. As a result the maternal systems work on low circulating blood volume. As a result of this renal failure can occur with relative ease in subjects of preeclampsia. An impoverished renal system of blood volume and sick kidneys innate to PIH precipitates renal shut down readily. Postpartum hemorrhage in preeclampsia also occurs readily with relatively less blood loss as compared to blood loss in non-hypertensive subjects. Consequently, subjects with preeclampsia are more vulnerable to these complications than subjects who are non-preeclamptic, in postpartum period.

Pulmonary Edema

One more complication that a clinician needs to be watchful about while managing the puerperium of a preeclamptic subject is pulmonary edema. The reasons of preeclamptic subjects being vulnerable to this complication have been discussed in the chapter related to cardiovascular changes. Fluid imbalance can also readily occur in postpartum period of preeclamptic subjects. This is because of two reasons:

1. The extracellular fluid which had increased (manifesting clinically as edema) now starts reversing in postpartum period.
2. The process of hypertension itself makes the subject vulnerable to this imbalance.

In such a delicately balanced scenario if the clinician is not careful in administering fluids the cardiovascular system can get readily off-balance producing a pulmonary edema. It would therefore be a challenge for the clinician to have a sound understanding of the pathophysiology of hypertensive disorders of pregnancy to dexterously manage her puerperium.

REFERENCES

1. Leveno K, Cunningham G. In: Lindheimer M, Roberts J, Cunningham F, (Eds) Chesley's Hypertensive disorders of pregnancy. Stamford, Appleton and Lange. 2nd edn. 1998; Page 547.

CHAPTER

23

Treatment of Obstetric Vasculopathy: Accidental Hemorrhage

CHAPTER OUTLINE

- The Etiopathology of Accidental Hemorrhage
- The Clinical Effects of Accidental Hemorrhage
- Cardiotocography Changes in Accidental Hemorrhage
- Ultrasonography in Accidental Hemorrhage
- Obstetric Management of Accidental Hemorrhage
- Cesarean Section in Accidental Hemorrhage
- Medical Management

INTRODUCTION

All obstetric vasculopathies occur over a relatively long period of time. The entire pathophysiology involved in their occurrence itself is insidious and gradual. However as an exception to this is accidental hemorrhage. In an ongoing process of vasculopathy usually preeclampsia, there comes a time when the placenta suddenly separates from its base. This leads to bleeding from the base and a series of events which can endanger the life of both the mother as well as the fetus. The etiopathology and pathophysiology involved has been discussed in the respective sections (See Chapters 3–6). However when the management of accidental hemorrhage is being reviewed, it becomes necessary to touch them briefly.

THE ETIOPATHOLOGY OF ACCIDENTAL HEMORRHAGE

Being one of the vasculopathies, the pathophysiology involved in the process of accidental hemorrhage has to be at the fetomaternal interface. The anchoring cytotrophoblasts are responsible to affix the placenta within the uterus. The entire process occurs following implantation at that point in the uterus where the implantation window opens at the time of arrival of the zygote in the uterine cavity. Following a complex process where intricate immunology and apoptosis get involved, the placenta affixes itself and remains so till that time as the delivery of the newborn occurs. Following some strange and hitherto unknown signals once the baby is born, the placenta senses that its role is over and it readily separates from the uterus and is expelled from the uterine cavity. In accidental hemorrhage however this process of separation and expulsion of the placenta occurs much earlier even before the baby is born. Like any premature process in nature this can lead to devastating complications.

As is by now so clear that the basic pathology of any obstetric vasculopathy is vasospasm. This vasospasm in subjects of accidental hemorrhage leads to denuding of small segments of the anchoring mechanism to be of its vitality. Such devitalized segments of the anchorage of the placenta get challenged when reperfusion occurs. Needless to say, the process of vasospasm is never continuous. Intermittent waves of vasospasm alternate with reperfusion. It is during reperfusion that the walls of the anchorage mechanisms snap. This leads to bleeding at the uteroplacental surface. This is accidental hemorrhage.

THE CLINICAL EFFECTS OF ACCIDENTAL HEMORRHAGE

Consumptive Coagulopathy

Once this premature separation of the placenta occurs, there is collection of blood in the retroplacental space that is now created. Attempts are made by the body to stop this bleeding by initiating the coagulation process. Yet this bleeding usually never stops but consumes the coagulation factors massively in the bargain. It leads to rapid deletion of coagulation factors from the maternal system. The situation becomes all the more grave if accidental hemorrhage is occurring concurrently with preeclampsia. In the process of preeclampsia, blood coagulation system is already challenged. An added massive load on the coagulation system can therefore have disastrous and even fatal consequences.

The entire pool of coagulation factors can get consumed in the retroplacental clot leading to what is accurately named as consumptive coagulopathy. Before this pathophysiology became clear, the coagulation failure witnessed in accidental hemorrhage was termed as disseminated intravascular coagulation. In reality this coagulation alteration is not due to consumption of coagulation factors in the maternal vascular bed. It is only confined to the retroplacental clot therefore the word consumptive coagulopathy is more accurate.

As a result of consumptive coagulopathy the mother develops an acute and scary bleeding tendency. It is very prominently seen in the uterine musculature producing the state of Couvelaire uterus. If not arrested consumptive coagulopathy can prove to be fatal.

Renal Failure

Another dreadful effect of accidental hemorrhage is renal failure. It has been extensively discussed in the chapter related to renal changes in obstetric vasculopathies that one of the most affected and critically hurt systems in obstetric vasculopathies especially preeclampsia is the renal system (See Chapter 9). Already challenged, the kidneys get severely affected in accidental hemorrhage. This is because the blood is getting pooled in the retroplacental bleed. The kidneys which are already running low on their reserves are unable to handle this drying up of its blood supply. As a result the kidneys end up with a failure.

This failure could be both, reversible or permanent depending upon the type of renal damage. If it is a medullary failure it is by and large reversible. However, the cortical renal failure is permanent. It may not be reversible and the kidneys may not be able to get back their function to a large extent.

There were some papers which hinted at the possibility of coagulopathy and renal failure in accidental hemorrhage. However, it seems that this association is a result of severity of the condition that causes both rather than the two being internally linked. More severe the accidental hemorrhage, more the chances of both consumptive coagulopathy and renal failure. In subjects of accidental hemorrhage blood transfusion is very critical. Rapid and proportional replacement of blood loss can prevent renal failure in most if not all subjects. Wasting time in estimating the blood loss can be extremely damaging. It is better to overestimate blood loss in accidental hemorrhage than underestimate it. One fact that always goes against the pregnant subject with accidental hemorrhage is the fact that a large portion of this bleeding remains concealed. Therefore, the crude attempts of the clinician in estimating the blood loss on clinical assessment is bound to be erroneous.

Most subjects thankfully end up in medullary renal failure which may need dialysis by the time the kidneys regain their full function. However, in those few who may land up in cortical renal failure there may be need to perform renal transplants at a later date as the kidneys may not be able to resume their optimal functioning.

Fetal Demise

The worst combination for the fetus in obstetric vasculopathy is preeclampsia IUGR topped up by accidental hemorrhage. The vasospasm of obstetric vasculopathy at the fetomaternal interface leads to impoverished oxygenation and vascular flow. If accidental hemorrhage now supervenes it is like adding insult to injury for the fetus. Consequently, a chronically hypoxic fetus is unable to bear this acute add-on hypoxia leading to severe fetal compromise and demise. In closely monitored pregnancies this feature of an impending disaster can be foreseen. On CTG monitoring and color Doppler ultrasound feature of acute sudden compromise appears and is enough for the clinician to become alert and intervene before the fetus is irretrievably lost.

Consumptive coagulopathy and renal failure, the two of the three major complications of accidental hemorrhage are by and large linked to the severity of the disease. However fetal demise may not be so linked. Minimal accidental hemorrhage may be enough to tip the scales against the fetus inviting fetal demise. Besides there three major complications of accidental hemorrhage other complication are either due to obstetric vasculopathy process itself or due to these complications.

CARDIOTOCOGRAPHY CHANGES IN ACCIDENTAL HEMORRHAGE

Sudden unexplained deceleration in a subject with preeclampsia on non-stress monitoring or even during intrapartum monitoring should alert the clinician of an accidental hemorrhage. These subjects may or may not show a reduced variability or any other feature of fetal compromise. But sudden unexpected decelerations should warrant alertness and accidental hemorrhage can be picked up on CTG. Most of the subjects who have accidental hemorrhage usually develop it during labor induced or spontaneous. However this is not a rule. It can develop even without labor. Therefore, a close monitoring team of preeclampsia or IUGR will be able to diagnose this condition through CTG irrespective of labor.

ULTRASONOGRAPHY IN ACCIDENTAL HEMORRHAGE

The diagnosis of accidental hemorrhage before the days of USG was essentially clinical. As no good methods were available to "see" what is happening within, all grading and types of accidental hemorrhage were based on clinical features and manifestations of the condition. With USG now profusely available it is possible to image the happening within. It is most of the times unnecessary to use USG for diagnosis of accidental hemorrhage. However, in some subjects of preeclampsia, when on close monitoring the CTG shows a sudden unexplained deceleration USG can be used to image what is happening inside.

In such a situation accidental hemorrhage can be seen in the form of a retroplacental clot. The actual process of bleeding in the retroplacental space can be seen as well as a distinct space between the placenta and the uterine wall whose it was attached. In subjects with oligohydramnios there can be a sudden deceleration on monitoring with CTG. This as has been described in the chapter on CTG, will present as atypical deceleration. This can confuse the picture of deceleration due to retroplacental bleeding and USG can help differentiating the two.

OBSTETRIC MANAGEMENT OF ACCIDENTAL HEMORRHAGE

The standard management for accidental hemorrhage is intervention. This is usually in the form of labor induction. Most of the subjects of accidental hemorrhage develop this process of abruption in labor. Thus the obstetrician is required to augment this labor process. The standard treatment protocol warrants doing an artificial rupture of membranes (ARM) and starting of syntocinon (pittocin) drip.

Interestingly, the labor in subjects with accidental hemorrhage does not follow the partogram. By this it is meant that it moves faster than normal. By processes of ARM plus pittocin the labor gets paced up readily and moves quickly.

Why Labor in Accidental Hemorrhage does not Follow the Partogram

This is a very interesting phenomenon. It s a well-known fact that the entire process of labor is generated and maintained by a series of processes and substances at the level of the cells of the smooth muscles of the uterine musculature. Amongst these is intracellular or in-vivo oxytocin released by the body itself. This oxytocin is short acting and is immediately replaced at the smooth muscles by an enzyme called oxytocinase. This oxytocinase has a graded activity and eliminate the oxytocin to enable a fresh supply of oxytocin to get released, act at the synapses, bring about the uterine contraction and get quickly eliminated.

Interestingly in accidental hemorrhage this oxytocinase gets blunted. The reasons for this are not clear. However its effect is clear. Blunting or partial dysfunction in the activity of oxytocinase leads to oxytocin being in action for a longer time without getting eliminated. As a result the process of labor occurs faster and without being any method line. This means that one can expect labor to get over much faster in accidental hemorrhage. Therefore, ARM plus pittocin is the treatment of choice in these subjects. Vaginal delivery is therefore to be expected.

CESAREAN SECTION IN ACCIDENTAL HEMORRHAGE

In mid 1990s cesarean section rate in accidental hemorrhage was not expected to be more than 5%. However this scenario has undergone some change over a period of time. With the salvage of the fetus being more and the diagnosis of accidental hemorrhage being quicker and earlier, cesarean sections are done a little more readily in subjects with accidental hemorrhage. Previously, many a times the fetus in accidental hemorrhage used to be dead even before the subject used to present at the obstetric unit. This scenario has changed now. Subjects present early and diagnosis is easier, earlier and quicker. In such a situation, the bias is towards cesarean section in the interest of the fetus.

Another situation where cesarean section is required is very scary and may warrant a very dexterous handling. In some subjects of accidental hemorrhage in presence of coagulation failure, if the labor augmentation fails, cesarean section may be required to quickly eliminate the prematurely separated placenta from the uterus. Cesarean section and removal of the baby and the placenta is the most definitive way of stopping further process of retroplacental bleed. Till this occurs consumptive coagulopathy does not stop and the maternal condition gets severely challenged. In this dreadful scenario, with fresh blood replete with coagulation factors (< 6 hours of tapping) or blood fractions including platelets being administered simultaneously, a cesarean section quickly performed and readily completed can be life-saving for the mother. Needless to say, in such acute situations, fetus has more often than not undergone demise.

These subjects can have a grave risk of renal failure. Adequate and quick replacement of blood with blood can save the patient from this complication. Technically this cesarean section can be difficult as there would be more than expected bleeding in the operative field. Also, ignoring this bleed the obstetrician will be required to go in quickly and complete the process. Thus, dexterous and experienced obstetrician may be requested to help if not already present.

MEDICAL MANAGEMENT

This includes management of all medical accompaniments of accidental hemorrhage. Blood loss should be replaced by blood whole or fractionated. Renal failure if could not be prevented may need dialysis or even renal transplant at a later date. Sepsis can be occur due to life-threatening morbidity and should be prevented by asepsis and antibiotics. Consumptive coagulopathy should be diagnosed early and treated efficiently by blood components and fractions.

Index

Page numbers followed by *f* for figure and *t* for table, respectively.

A

Abdominal
- route 149
- uterine artery Doppler 168

Absent end-diastolic flow in umbilical artery 193*f*
Accelerations in heart rate 205
Accidental hemorrhage 235
Ace-inhibitors 223
Act through procoagulant mechanism 34
Activated partial thromboplastin time 117, 180
Acute hypoxia 207
Adverse drug reactions 175
AFLP-triad 122
Age of fetus 219
Agents of oxidative stress 45
Albumin 140
Alpha methyldopa 225
Alteration
- in coagulation factors 114
- other cellular components of blood 115

Amniotic fluid index 228
Amorphous characterizations of pathogenesis 149
Angiogenic factors 40
Angiotensin-converting enzyme 86, 87
Animal
- experiments 128
- studies 5

Anticardiolipin antibodies 20
Antihypertensives 171, 221, 222
Antiphospholipid antibodies 19
Antithrombotic agents 177, 184
APL antibodies 22
Application of
- genetic models 89
- predicting systems 149

Arngrimsson 88
Artificial rupture of membranes 238
Aspirin 173, 177
Atenolol 224
Autoimmunity in recurrent pregnancy loss 19

B

Balanced atom 43*f*
Barr cell 115
Basal heart rate and variability 204
Basic process of normal placenta and placentation 80
Basis for reviewing role of genetics in obstetric vasculopathies 86
Bearings
- in abnormal pregnancy 47
- of low dose aspirin 178

Beauty of lysophosphotidyl choline 76
Benefit out of preventive measures 167
Biological false seropositive for syphilis 20
Blood pressure 5
Blunted vascular response 127
BP 233
- hypertension 137
- in labor 224

Brain 112
- undergoing ischemic changes 58*f*

C

Calcium
- channel blockers 224
- supplementation 171

Canulated vessel and anatomy involved 58*f*
Cardiac Doppler in obstetric vasculopathies 200
Cardiotocographies
- changes in accidental hemorrhage 237
- in obstetric vasculopathies 204
- in subjects with APA syndrome 208

Cardiovascular changes in normal pregnancy 4
Cellular fibronectin 36
Central and peripheral cause of visual alterations 125
Cervical
- branch, descending 161
- intraepithelial neoplasia 166

Cesarean section in
- accidental hemorrhage 239
- pregnancy induced hypertension 232

Challenges
before antihypertensive in pregnancy induced hypertension 222
to genetic studies in obstetric vasculopathies 87
Changes in
intercellular matrix during vasospasm 47*f*
venous system 9
Chesley's hypertensive disorders of pregnancy 166, 219
Chronic hypertension 144
Chronic hypoxia 208
Circulating markers of endothelial activation 33
Clinical
bearing 37
effects of accidental hemorrhage 236
profile of obstetric vasculopathies 136
Closer to cell wall 46*f*
Coagulation
alterations in obstetric vasculopathies 116
failure 233
Color Doppler
and cardiotocography correlation 208
for discontinuation of antithrombotic agents 199
fundoscopy 126
in early pregnancy 187
in obstetric vasculopathies 159, 187
indices in early pregnancy 190
Components of fibronectin 36
Concept of competence
alteration of platelets 117
of reducing systems 139
Consumptive coagulopathy 236
Corticosteroids 212
CTG assessments 196
Cyclic adenosine mono phosphate 119
Cytokines 39

D

Decelerations in heart rate 205
Defective generation of syncitiotrophoblasts 24
Development of
preeclampsia 171
thrombocytopenia 114
Diastolic
BP 137
flow 201
notch 159, 160, 188
disappeared in first trimester itself 191*f*
Dietary
calcium 171
deficiency and animal experiments 130
Difference between disease and derangement 165
Different APL antibodies 22
Differential diagnosis of obstetric vasculopathies 144
Difficulties in interpreting scientific data 216
Disappeared diastolic notch in II trimester 189*f*
Disposition of fat globules normal late pregnancy 46*f*
Disruption of thromboxane prostacyclin mechanism 21
Diuretics 170
Diurnal variations in BP 6
Doppler assessments 196
Dosage schedules 224
Dose of heparin 181
progesterone 175
Doubts on veracity of pathognomonic lesions 101
Ductus venosus 193

E

Early
decelerations 206
diagnosis and alert surveillance 219
Eclampsia 226
Edema 141
in preeclampsia 170
Effect of preeclampsia on offspring 97
Effective renal plasma flow 107
Embryo
decidua crosstalk in immunology of obstetrics vasculopathy 22
donation 159
Endothelial
activation and prostaglandins 33
cell adhesion molecule disturbances 35
cell dysfunction and obstetric vasculopathy 31
cells 67
Endothelin 37
Epigastric pain 122
Epigenetic features in preeclampsia 92
Etiopathology of accidental hemorrhage 235
Exclusivity of human pregnancy 133
Exercise and prevention of obstetric vasculopathies 74
Expression of genes of prolactin 23

Extracellular reducing systems 70
Extremes of maternal age 159

F

Family of free radicals 61
FAQs on aspirin 214
Fasting blood sugar 196
Faults in fetomaternal linkage placenta and obstetric vasculopathy 84
Fetal
- aortic Doppler studies 201
- contributions 89
- demise 237
- heart rate 207

Fetus 235
- allograft 11
- unique allograft 13

Fibronectin 157
Focal segmental glomerular sclerosis 105
Folic acid 213
Formed elements in blood 39
Forming lipid radical 56*f*
Free radical 43

G

Gene variation 133
General aspects of obstetric vasculopathies 1
Generated images of brains 59*f*
Genetics of obstetrics vasculopathies 86
Gilson capsule 120
Glomerular
- endotheliosis 129
- filtration rate 98, 107

Gradual hypoxia 207
Graft versus host 14
Gross changes in kidneys 102

H

Hand-grip test 153
Handling of urinary excretion of proteins in preeclampsia 108
Hard facts emerging from animal experiments 134
hCG in prevention of obstetric vasculopathies 175
Heart rate 6
HELLP syndrome 121, 123, 144
Hematological cellular and non-cellular indices 154
Hemodynamics in normal pregnancy 95
Heparin 173, 177, 215
High density lipoproteins 48
Hormonal basis of hCG administration 176
Human
- chorionic gonadotropin 175
- females 129
- leukocyte antigen 91

Humphries 88
Hydralazine 225
Hydrogen peroxide 61
Hydropic degeneration of placenta 159
Hypertension 136
Hypertriglyceridemia 51
Hypochlorus acid 61
Hypoimmunogenic embryo 13
Hypoxia and fetal heart rate 207
Hypoxia-inducible factor 63

I

Ideal reducing system 74
Immunoglobulins 172
Immunological
- antibodies 38
- basis of hCG 176

Immunology
- and genetics 91
- of obstetric vasculopathy 11

Impending eclampsia 120
Implantation not right of embryo 23
Incompetent GnRH activity 25
Inconsistency of reducing systems 73
Inconsistent
- notch 189
- presence of diastolic notch 168

Indications of heparin 183
Induction of labor in pregnancy 227
Inefficient second wave of trophoblastic invasion 63
Innate maternal reducing systems 59
Inputs from animal models 92
Insulin
- growth factor binding protein 23
- resistance 159

Intramuscular
- hydralazine 224
- labetalol 224

Intrauterine
- growth retardation 100
- insemination 23

Intriguing observations from animal experiments 132

J

Jaundice 122

K

Kallikrein 154
Kidney lesions 101

L

Labetalol 225
Labor in
  accidental hemorrhage 238
  pregnancy induced hypertension 226
Late decelerations 206
Leads recurrent spontaneous abortion 11
Left ventricle 6
Limitations of
  blood pressures indicator of severity 218
  reducing systems 72
  venous Doppler 197
Limited sperm exposure 159
Lipid
  hydroperoxides 56*f*
  metabolism in normal pregnancy 47
  peroxides 45
Liver
  enzymes 121
  in hemolysis elevated liver enzymes low platelets syndrome 122
Longitudinal changes in cardiac functions 6
Low
  concentrations of lipid hydroperoxides 56
  density lipoproteins 48
  dose aspirin 180, 214

M

Major histocompatability complex 13
Mammalian studies 88
Management
  of eclampsia 219
  on hospitalization 220
Manifestation of endothelial cell activation 34
Marinobufagenin 40
Maternal
  environment preventing trophoblastic invasion 84
  infections 159
  low birth weight 159
  susceptibility genes 159
Matrix metalloproteinases 32
Mean arterial pressure 137, 152
Measures prevent occurrence or prevent worsening 169
Mechanisms of action antithrombotic agents 177
Medical management 239
Methods of
  induction of labor 229
  labor induction 231
Microalbuminuria 153
Middle cerebral artery 191, 193, 194
  flow 194
Midtrimester BP 151
Mild preeclampsia 143
Mischief of free radicals in vascular walls 45
Modulate matrix metalloproteinase 81
Molecules contributing to endothelial cell activation 38
Monitoring subjects on heparin 181
Monotherapy versus multidrug therapy 224
Mother's body 12

N

Nausea 122
Negative to positive predictive value 151
Neonatal intensive care unit 2
Neonatologist 228
Nifedipine 224
Nitric oxide 65, 67, 68
  in obstetric vasculopathy 65
  synthase 68
Non stress test 228
Normal
  flow through ductus venous 196*f*
  middle cerebral artery flow 194*f*
  pregnancy 21
  uterine artery flow 192*f*
Notch
  depth index 189, 190*f*
  index 189
Nuchal translucency 187
Nullipara 167

O

Obesity 159
Obstetric
  management of accidental hemorrhage 238
  vasculopathies 2, 51, 80, 95, 164
  vasculopathies and effects
    on central nervous system 111
    on heart 95
    on hematological system 114
    on liver 120
    on renal system 98
Obstetrician's nightmare 136
Oocytes donation 159
Ophthalmic features in obstetric vasculopathy 124
Oscillatory
  and propulsive pressures 8*f*
  pressure 8

Overview of available predicting measures 148
Oxidative stress 42
- and health 44
- and obstetric vasculopathies 42

Oxygenation 83

P

Paralysis of maternal protector systems pregnancy 13
Partner specificity in miscarriages 18
Pathological
- changes in liver 121
- lesions in preeclampsia 112

Peripheral vascular resistance 9
Peroxidized LDLs 69
Peroxynitrite anion 61
Phenomenon of endothelial cell activation 32
Physiology and cardiotocography 204
Pittocin drip 238
Placenta 80
Placental
- atherosis in obstetric vasculopathy 69
- ischemia 128
- lipid peroxidation 54

Plasma urea 143
Plasminogen and allied procoagulant activity 34
Platelets 21, 155
- activation 155
- activation and thromboxane A2 production 118
- count 155
- in normal 116

Policemen model to understand uric acid 71
Polyunsaturated fatty acids 55
Postdelivery care 232
Postglucose blood sugar 196
Power house reductant 71
Practical clinical challenges with heparin use 183
Predict obstetric vasculopathies 159*t*
Predicting obstetric vasculopathies 148
Preeclampsia 6, 86, 132, 133, 144
- need admission 220

Preeclamptic pregnancies 116
Preexisting thrombophilia 159
Pregnancy
- after donor insemination 159
- induced hypertension 1, 232

Premature closure of ductus arteriosus 214
Prenatal brain lesions 113
Presence of
- nasal bone 188
- protein 140

Prevalence of APL 20
Preventing obstetric vasculopathy challenge 167
Prevention of
- eclampsia 184
- obstetric vasculopathies 177
- preeclampsia 164

Preventive measures of obstetric vasculopathies 173
Primary aborters and non-immunological basis 19
Primi paternity 159
Privileged status of
- central nervous system 111
- syncitiotrophoblasts 25

Procoagulants 114
Procopciuc LM 88
Progesterone 8, 174
- in prevention of obstetric vasculopathies 174

Propulsive pressure 8
Prostaglandins 230
Protective mechanisms
- in placenta 17
- shared placenta and uterus 18

Protects fetus 12
Protein C activation 22
Proteinuria 140
Prothrombin time 117
Psychiatric complications obstetric vasculopathies 113
Pulmonary edema 234
Pulsatility index 160, 190, 191, 202

Q

Quantification of fetomaternal interface vascular activity 131

R

Rational medical practitioner 213
Reactive oxygen species 32, 61, 64, 71
Reason for edema in preeclampsia 142
Recurrent miscarriages 212
Reducing radical extra proton balances 44*f*
Reduction of obstetric vasculopathy 187
Renal
- diseases 146
- failure 233, 236
- function alterations in preeclampsia 107
- handling of proteins in preeclampsia 108
- pathogenic model for other forms of hypertension 106
- system 93

Renin-angiotensin system 86
  in preeclampsia 109
Reperfusion 57
  damage of obstetric vasculopathies 112
Respiratory distress syndrome 226
Results of crosstalk 23
Retinal edema 125
Rheumatic disease 159
Riots 71
Role of
  cofactor 20
  oxygen tension in trophoblastic invasion 81
  uric acid in obstetric vasculopathies 157
Roll-over test 152

S

Salient results emerging from animal experiments 131
Salt restriction 170
Severe
  preeclampsia 143
  pregnancy induced hypertension 227
Shouldering 207
Side effects of progesterone 175
Small
  dense LDL phenotype in obstetric vasculopathy 52
  for gestational age 189, 191
Special features of renal failure in obstetric vasculopathies 99
Spontaneous resolution 27
Starting of syntocinon drip 238
Stop
  antihypertensives 225
  heparin 182
String of beads 105
Stroke volume 6
Studies from aberdeen 88
Subatomic structure of
  bound 43*f*
  free radical 44*f*
Subjects with obstetric challenges 169
Superoxide
  anion radical 61
  dismutase 54
Suppressor mechanisms in protection 16
Symphysio-fundal height 227
System readiness for labor induction in pregnancy induced hypertension 231
Systolic to diastolic ratio 160, 190

T

Teratogenicity of aspirin 214
Terms of prothrombin time 142
Third trimester color Doppler in obstetric vasculopathies 192
Thrombotic microangiopathies 103, 106
Tina factor 215
Toxins 39
Trace elements like
  magnesium 172
  zinc 172
Trachleodynamics in induction of labor 229
Transforming growth factor-β 17
Transient hypertension 146
Transition metals in lipid peroxidation 55
Treatment
  bearings 76
  of accidental hemorrhage 218
  of immunological miscarriages 215
  of obstetric vasculopathy 212, 235
    preeclampsia 218
  of subject of miscarriage always for prevention 217
Trophoblastic differentiation 83
Trophoblasts 80
Tumor necrosis factor-α 39
Two together in
  intrauterine growth retardation 210
  preeclampsia 208

U

Ultrasonography in accidental hemorrhage 238
Umbilical
  artery 193, 199
    flow 193
  venous flow 198
Unpaired electron of free radical 44*f*
Uric acid 71, 156
Urinary
  calcium 154
    creatinine ratio 153
  kallikrein 153
  tests 153
Uterine artery diastolic notch 188*f*
Uteroplacental blood flow 131

V

Vaginal route 149
Variable decelerations 206

Vascular
  endothelial growth factor 37, 64
  endothelium and oxidative stress 62
  response to increase cardiac output 7
  responses in obstetric
    vasculopathy 127
Vasospasm and reperfusion damages 178
VEGF type specific functions 65*t*
Venous Doppler 195
  for deciding route of delivery 198
Visual alterations of special mention
  recurrent 125
  unilateral 125
VLDL and LDL molecules sink
  between cells in intercellular
  matrix and undergo denaturation 47*f*
Vomiting 122
Vulnerability of renal system 98

W

Weight gain 153

Z

Zona pellucida 13